# FIT
## FOREVER

30 DAYS to Healthy Habits
You Can Handle—for Life!

# FIT FOREVER

## BY JEANNE ERNST

### WITH INSPIRATIONAL ADVICE FROM
### CARMEN RENEE BERRY

### FOREWORD BY JANE FONDA

CONSULTING EDITORS:
Mary Hise, *Registered Dietician*
Patrick Williams, *Chef*

A BYRON PREISS BOOK

QVC PUBLISHING, INC.

# DEDICATION

This book is dedicated to my love, life partner, and manager, Jim Neuman, without whom this book would not have been possible. His tenacity and belief in this project made *Fit Forever* a reality.
To Jim's darling little girl Aubrey Neuman who lights up my life every day.

Published by QVC Publishing, Inc., 50 Main Street, Suite 201, Mt. Kisco, NY 10549.

QVC Publishing, Inc.

Jill Cohen, Vice President and Publisher

Ellen Bruzelius, General Manager

Karen Murgolo, Director of Rights and Acquisitions

Cassandra Reynolds, Publishing Assistant

**Q** Publishing and colophon are trademarks of
QVC Publishing, Inc.

Printed in the United States of America
First Edition: March 2002
10 9 8 7 6 5 4 3 2 1
ISBN:  1-928998-42-9
Cover and book design by Andy Omel

# Table of Contents

Foreword . . . . . . . . . . . . . . . . . . . . . . vii

Introduction . . . . . . . . . . . . . . . . . . . 1

The Key to Fitness: A Body
in Motion Stays in Motion . . . . . . . . . . 7

The Philosophy Behind
Energy Balance Nutrition . . . . . . . . . . 15

Energy Balance Basics . . . . . . . . . . . . . 21

Getting Started . . . . . . . . . . . . . . . . . 31

Day 1 . . . . . . . . . . . . . . . . . . . . . . . . 32

Day 2 . . . . . . . . . . . . . . . . . . . . . . . . 38

Day 3 . . . . . . . . . . . . . . . . . . . . . . . . 44

Day 4 . . . . . . . . . . . . . . . . . . . . . . . . 50

Day 5 . . . . . . . . . . . . . . . . . . . . . . . . 56

More from Chores . . . . . . . . . . . . . . . 62

Day 6 . . . . . . . . . . . . . . . . . . . . . . . . 66

Day 7 . . . . . . . . . . . . . . . . . . . . . . . . 72

Core Four Cardio . . . . . . . . . . . . . . . . 78

Day 8 . . . . . . . . . . . . . . . . . . . . . . . . 80

Day 9 . . . . . . . . . . . . . . . . . . . . . . . . 86

Day 10 . . . . . . . . . . . . . . . . . . . . . . . 92

Taking a Break . . . . . . . . . . . . . . . . . 98

Day 11 . . . . . . . . . . . . . . . . . . . . . . . 100

Day 12 . . . . . . . . . . . . . . . . . . . . . . . 106

Day 13 . . . . . . . . . . . . . . . . . . . . . . . 112

Day 14 . . . . . . . . . . . . . . . . . . . . . . . 118

Core Four Upper Body . . . . . . . . . . . 124

Day 15 . . . . . . . . . . . . . . . . . . . . . . . 126

Balance Ball Workout . . . . . . . . . . . . 132

Day 16 . . . . . . . . . . . . . . . . . . . . . . . 136

Day 17 . . . . . . . . . . . . . . . . . . . . . . . 142

Day 18 . . . . . . . . . . . . . . . . . . . . . . . 148

Day 19 . . . . . . . . . . . . . . . . . . . . . . . 154

Day 20 . . . . . . . . . . . . . . . . . . . . . . . 160

Internal Workout . . . . . . . . . . . . . . . 166

Day 21 . . . . . . . . . . . . . . . . . . . . . . . 168

Core Four Lower Body . . . . . . . . . . . 175

Day 22 . . . . . . . . . . . . . . . . . . . . . . . 180

Day 23 . . . . . . . . . . . . . . . . . . . . . . . 186

Day 24 . . . . . . . . . . . . . . . . . . . . . . . 192

Day 25 . . . . . . . . . . . . . . . . . . . . . . . 198

Shopping and Travel . . . . . . . . . . . . . 204

Day 26 . . . . . . . . . . . . . . . . . . . . . . . 206

Day 27 . . . . . . . . . . . . . . . . . . . . . . . 213

Day 28 . . . . . . . . . . . . . . . . . . . . . . . 220

Core Four Abdominals . . . . . . . . . . . 227

Day 29 . . . . . . . . . . . . . . . . . . . . . . . 230

Day 30 . . . . . . . . . . . . . . . . . . . . . . . 236

Your Day . . . . . . . . . . . . . . . . . . . . . 244

Conclusion . . . . . . . . . . . . . . . . . . . . 246

Index . . . . . . . . . . . . . . . . . . . . . . . . 247

# Foreword

WHEN I MET JEANNE she was doing a very successful TV exercise show, *Body Buddies*. She was one of the first people I picked to help me open the Jane Fonda Workout and was still there at the closing. I remember the gifts of joy and enthusiasm that she brought to teaching. I relied on her sound judgement, intuition, and professional knowledge to help us with the many management and employee responsibilities that are part of a successful business.

Jeanne's greatest gift to me and her students was her easygoing way of encouraging everyone to do only what they could handle at the time, to take it slow and be kind to yourself in order to reach your goals.

I, like her, found that a commitment to personal health and fitness was a constant source of strength and energy.

I hope the Fit Forever program will encourage you to discover your core strength to commit to a healthier way of living and emerge a happier, healthier woman.

—Jane Fonda

# Acknowledgements

My life has been blessed with an extraordinary support system, filled with colleagues, friends, clients, and family.

A very special thanks to Byron Preiss of Byron Preiss Visual Publications, who never gave up and continued to push until *Fit Forever* found the right home with QVC.

To my gifted editor Dinah Dunn, whose insight and knack for editing is truly remarkable. Without your hard work and that of your staff, including Kelly Smith, J. Vita, and Jeanine Campbell, this book would never have been the same.

To Jill Cohen, Vice President/Publisher of QVC, who saw the value to the QVC audience and made *Fit Forever* a reality: A very special thank you. To Ellen Bruzelius and the staff of QVC Publishing, thank you for your excellent and encouraging comments.

To Daniel Kosich, Ph.D., a mentor, professor, and friend. I wouldn't be the fitness professional I am today without your excellent tutelage.

To Dr. Bernie Ernst, my former husband, for introducing me to the wonderful world of fitness.

To Harry Langdon, a magician with a camera. Your patience and extended friendship is most appreciated.

I will be forever grateful to Mark Brunetz, MS, my former Inventing Fitness partner. Thank you for making a difference in my life as I've hopefully made in yours.

And to my dear friends who have through the years enhanced the many changing seasons of my life, including:

A special thanks to Julie La Fond, Jane Fonda's partner and my very special friend who constantly inspired me to be more than I could have ever imagined. She pushed me to move beyond all limitations. I bless the day I met you.

And to my friend Joni Cowdin who read every page of this book and gave me valuable feedback.

I am profoundly grateful to Irene Mink, my stylist, who kept me sane with her wealth of information on how to dress for a successful mid-life transition.

A million thanks to my wonderful father and my twin brother who kept me laughing when I needed it the most.

A special mention to my friends of 30 years, Jan Sheridan and Mary Ellen Mayer. We have shared love, loss, and joy, and supported each other through the ups and downs of life. I love you very much.

To my Jane Fonda video workout buddies Laurel Turell, Susie Casey, and Kurt Gombatz. Thanks for the memories.

Finally, a special thanks and mention to Jane Fonda, who gave me not only her friendship but also the chance to work with her for ten wonderful years. The times spent teaching, training, and performing with you were some of the best years of my life.

# Introduction

I HAVE STRUGGLED WITH my weight all my life—as a child I remember being described as "pleasantly plump." The women in my family naturally veer toward lush, more like Marilyn Monroe than Twiggy. But as a teenager I became surprisingly slim—I swam and dove competitively and was named best dancer in my senior year of high school. With nonstop energy and an athlete's body, I ate like a truck driver but didn't seem to gain an ounce. What fun! But it wasn't destined to last.

When I got married right out of high school, I was one of the few in my circle of friends who didn't want children right away. My doctor prescribed birth control pills (the first high potency pill on the market) which caused me to blow up like a balloon. I gained 20 pounds in two weeks—and that was just the beginning. I continued to gain weight until I tipped the scales at 150 pounds. I'm only five feet two, so it really showed. And I couldn't seem to lose the weight, which made me even more miserable. This unhappiness combined with a lot of other problems in my too young marriage gave me the incentive to file for divorce.

Overweight, unhappy, and alone, I went looking for a way to rekindle the joy I remembered from my happy teen years. I joined a gym, where I met Bernie, who later became my second husband. He was a bodybuilder, which increased my awareness of the body beautiful. The message was strong and clear: An average healthy body was not enough; you had to be perfect. I worked out like mad, dieted like crazy, and gradually inched closer to that ideal.

As the years passed, I lived in a state of uneasiness: a life of constantly battling my natural genetic makeup and the impossible criteria set by the fitness world. Heck, I probably helped pioneer it, with one of the first television shows about fitness, *Body Buddies*, which I cohosted with Bernie. Every day I was in front of a camera showing America not only how to stay fit but how fit I was—talk about pressure!

## NO MORE "NO PAIN, NO GAIN"

In the wake of my success with *Body Buddies,* Jane Fonda asked me to help her start an aerobics studio in Beverly Hills, which later became the world-famous Jane Fonda Workout Studio. I soon became the manager and was responsible for the One-on-One Personal Training department, handling all nutritional and weight-loss counseling and overseeing the instructors. Unlike producing *Body Buddies,* where I was isolated in a television studio, I was now working closely with people from all over the world who wanted to stay young-looking and in good health. I had the thrill of watching women who were shy and unsure become outgoing and confident after losing twenty, ten, or even five pounds.

Although my job enabled me to look good on the outside, on the inside I was a mess. In 1990 I went through a very painful divorce that ended my 23-year marriage to Bernie. In an effort to block out what was happening to me emotionally, I put every waking hour into my job and training for one of Jane Fonda's upcoming videos. During this time, constant exercise was the one thing that helped me feel as if I had some sort of control over my life. Exercise became my comfort zone.

Before I knew it, I was overdoing it. I had adopted a "no pain, no gain" philosophy in order to get in video shape, cycling 125 miles a week through mountainous terrain along the California coastline. I dropped from 135 to 110 pounds. At age 46, this was a difficult task, since I was battling not only genetics and my age but also my lifelong self-perception of always being ten pounds too heavy. I was on a low-fat, low-calorie diet, which left me constantly starving. I went to bed hungry and woke up hungry, but I didn't care. I just ignored the pangs in my stomach and went on another bike ride.

The week we taped the video, I worked out on camera 10 to 12 hours a day for five consecutive days. The strenuous workouts, coupled with the emotional strain of my recent separation, drained me. As the stress mounted, I became numb to the physical pain. It wasn't until the day after we had finished taping the video that I discovered I had suffered a debilitating knee injury.

My orthopedic surgeon diagnosed me with chondramalasia of the patella, an injury that meant I'd basically have to remain inactive for a minimum of two months. Many people would have welcomed the opportunity to take a break from the rigorous work-outs and exhausting schedule. I, on the other hand, equated my self-esteem with my ability to exercise. And without that capability, I saw myself as worthless. I spent week after depressing week doing paperwork at the gym or staring at the television, feeling like I was getting flabbier by the day.

After two months of convalescence and inactivity, I was finally allowed to take a leisurely walk. I remember that day like it was yesterday. I was in good spirits, my mind was clear, and I walked along with the music walking tape I had made while laid up. The sky was slightly overcast, with a crispness in the air that I appreciated for the first time. I was so eager to be out and moving that I paid no attention to how far or even how hard I walked. This was unusual because mentally noting mileage and intensity was a habit I had formed over the years. That day, it was as if someone were guiding me and telling me to slow down, to take it easy and let go of the "no pain, no gain" philosophy. This walk marked the beginning of a whole new chapter in my life.

I began to listen to my body more, ate a balanced diet, and finally returned to my healthy weight. For the first time in my life, gaining a few pounds didn't bother me. Hand in hand with my new diet, I designed a series of basic exercises to accompany my walking routine that I called my core program. I soon discovered that I could feel as healthy with this moderate program as I did when I was working out like mad. For the first time, diet and exercise were fun, easy, and doable.

Around this time, a physical therapist recommended a new client to me. Ellen had a frozen shoulder that needed a gentle stretching and strength-training program. During my evaluation of her health history, Ellen described her hard-core workouts with a trainer many years ago. She had been in fabulous shape; she'd loved how she looked then. However, as her job and family responsibilities changed, she found she didn't have the time or energy to maintain such a rigorous training schedule. So she quit working with a trainer and decided to work out on her own. Without knowledge of exercise or a plan, she maintained her resolve about two weeks before she gradually stopped exercising. Her belief was "If I can't do that kind of hard-core workout, what good is it? I'm wasting my time." She gradually began to pack on pounds. When I told her we could get her into good shape without an intensive program, she looked at me like I was crazy.

Who could blame her? Like many of us who emerged from the compulsive fitness culture of the late 1980s, she still believed that "harder is better" and that you couldn't be fit without "going for the burn." I could see how difficult it was going to be for her to break through that old way of thinking—after all, I had denied my struggle for years. She was just one of the many women I met who were afraid that by slowing down and making more sensible choices, they would become flabby and gain weight. They felt that their bodies had to be perfect. No matter how much it compromised their health, perfect was more important than future consequences. I knew then that there was a great need to reeducate the public. I began my mission with Ellen.

The first hurdle was helping Ellen accept that she could not work out or look like she did when she was 20 years old. She was older, and her body couldn't take the beating she had put it through in previous years. Her life had more stress and time constraints, which also put her in a different fitness category. On top of those considerations, she also had an injured shoulder. If we tried to do the kind of hard-core workout she did when she was younger, Ellen would either hurt herself and/or burn out within a few sessions. I was not going to let that happen.

Since she had not exercised in years, I began her program sitting down, with a routine I call Sit and Be Fit. With this kind of easy and gentle workout, I was able to increase Ellen's energy, strength, and endurance. I assigned her homework to do between our sessions. In only a few weeks, her shoulder became more flexible, the strength in her entire upper body increased, and she lost a few pounds of fat.

We also discussed her nutritional habits, which were fairly typical for a woman so busy: little or no breakfast, a sandwich for lunch, a few quick snacks during the day, and dinner with her family a few times a week. Oh yes, and she loved chocolate. By tweaking some of the ingredients in the meals she tended to eat and making a few changes in her habits, she gradually began to lose more weight. But more importantly, my balanced program gave her the nutrients to feed her brain, muscles, and bones and maintain a high energy level. Research has supported my belief that sensible workouts not only provide the same benefits as more rigorous exercise but also significantly reduce the risk of sustaining lifelong injuries.

Now Ellen is fit and healthy. All her friends comment about how they wish they could learn her secret. She has plenty of energy to play 18 holes of golf, and she enjoys her career and family.

Shortly after my encounter with Ellen and my personal epiphany about the need for moderation, I made the decision to retire as a full-time employee of the Jane Fonda Workout. I started a personal training business, one that targeted the baby-boom generation that needed a more down-to-earth approach to diet and fitness. That approach evolved into *Fit Forever*.

## TRUST ME: YOU CAN DO THIS

What do you think about when you hear the words exercise and fitness? Maybe you feel guilty—many do. You know you should lose weight and work out more, your doctor tells you it would increase your energy, and the media is constantly reminding you that being healthy and strong will prolong your life. So what is stopping you?

Did you exercise and find it to be too much of a time commitment? Maybe your muscles hurt so much afterward that you never wanted to repeat that experience. I've heard hundreds of reasons over my years in the fitness business, the most common being a version of "Exercise is boring and painful, and I can't find the time to go to the gym." These misconceptions are the obstacles I knew I'd have to overcome in order to have any success with *Fit Forever*.

The fitness and nutrition recommendations outlined in this book have been developed through years of working with thousands of my personal training clients and seminar participants. The result is a well-rounded program that builds bone mass; burns fat; protects your joints, tendons, and ligaments; and leaves you feeling good and full of energy. And most importantly, the program doesn't take over your life, but works around it.

This program fits exercise and balanced food choices into your preexisting schedule. You don't have to wear special clothes, go to a gym, or weigh your food. With small changes, you will slowly integrate movements and nutritional tips that will allow you to build health into your life a little bit at a time and with as little effort as possible. No matter what your fitness level, lifestyle, or schedule, in 30 days or fewer this program will improve your energy and health.

You can also create your own personal program by picking and choosing menu suggestions and fitness movements. The nutritional suggestions will be based on foods you already like that will balance your blood sugar level all day long. Through a combination of recipe suggestions and menus that fit with your lifestyle and food preferences, we will create an eating regime that is an energy balancing, fat-burning program. This program will be combined with a series of small movements throughout your day that will improve every major muscle group. The daily routine contains a variety of exercises that will condition the muscles that women often overlook: the upper body, the lower back, the abdominal region, and the often neglected muscles involved in posture.

To address the emotional side of body image, I've teamed up with Carmen Renee Berry, a warm and wonderful psychotherapist and body worker. She's also a best-selling author, whose book *Coming Home to Your Body* deals with many of the issues women face with their bodies. Her insights are sprinkled throughout the book, under the heading "Carmen's Advice."

Before you begin, keep the following guidelines in mind.

## BASIC GUIDELINES

➤ Good health is created by the choices you make moment to moment, day to day. Health can be found in the simple choice between taking a ten-minute walk or sitting through a long commercial break on TV. Or the choice between food that is energy enhancing or food that will make you feel good for 30 minutes and then put you to sleep. Every choice affects how you feel all day long.

➤ Do only the exercises you want to in the program, as long as you do something every day. There is no overarching goal to the program beyond incorporating new movement into your life. The variety of the routines I've outlined allows you to pick and choose the movements you enjoy, creating a Can-Do fitness program.

➤ Take your time and make all the muscle-conditioning movements slow and controlled. Think "Take it slow" at all times, no matter what exercise you choose to do. Remember that most injuries occur when movement is rushed or when you try to do too much too soon.

➤ Read the instructions completely before attempting any movements. I have detailed the correct form and safety cues to protect you from doing something that could possibly hurt or injure you.

➤ If you have not exercised in a while, be aware that your body needs time to adjust. Listen to its limitations, and your body will reward you with painless progress. Also, check with your doctor before you begin any exercise or fitness program.

➤ If you currently exercise on a regular basis, pick the routines that will complement your program.

➤ Moderation is the key to consistency, and consistency is the only way to achieve long-lasting healthful fitness. With a movement program you enjoy enough to continue, you will reach a level of health that is energy charged and makes life a lot more enjoyable.

➤ Do not allow yourself to become hungry. The Energy Balance eating program is not a diet but a way of eating that promotes long-term health and energy. Starvation and depravation are not part of the program.

➤ Follow the plan of eating six small meals a day. By eating smaller portions throughout the day, you will stay in the Energy Balance, where your blood sugar level stays steady for longer periods of time.

➤ Choose foods that satisfy. Many times you have finished a meal and you are full, but something is missing—it's called satisfaction. When you choose foods you enjoy, you will be less likely to reach for energy-depleting foods that will raise and lower blood glucose (sugar) levels rapidly.

➤ Choose foods that give you as much variety as possible. I have found that if you eat at least three different items at each meal, you are more satisfied than if you eat only one or two. This abundant variety will also help keep you in the Energy Balance. (See meal plans and recipes in the following chapters.)

➤ Jump-start your day with breakfast. People who skip breakfast usually see an energy drop midmorning and feel as if they are on an energy roller coaster all day long, until they drop into bed exhausted and burned out.

➤ Changing a habit can change your life. It takes anywhere from 30 to 90 days to make or break a habit, so don't beat yourself up if you occasionally return to former unhealthy eating habits.

➤ Plan for a snack attack. If you have a backup list of favorite snacks that satisfy, you will be better equipped to handle any and all situations.

➤ Drink at least 4 to 8 glasses of water a day. Water helps curb cravings, and one side effect of dehydration is fatigue. Your body may seem tired or hungry, but you really may just need a big glass of water. You will be amazed at the difference in how you feel and think when you drink enough water.

With these basic guidelines in mind, let's get started!

# The Key to Fitness:
## A Body in Motion Stays in Motion

**M**UCH OF YOUR WEEK is made up of routines, whether getting ready for work, sending the kids off to school, or putting your home in order. With your daily responsibilities, you probably don't have a large block of time to dedicate solely to exercise.

With this in mind, I've created the following exercises to work within your routine. While going through your day, whether combing your hair, brushing your teeth, or drinking your morning coffee, you'll find you can consistently incorporate these quick and easy movements, which will condition your muscles while relieving stress and tension. If you follow this program for 30 days, these movements will become part of your routine, a habit that will lead to a stronger and leaner you.

And remember: Exercise should be easy. Any pain or strain means you have overextended yourself and you should return to an easier level of exercise. But consistency is key. A recent study of nearly 40,000 women 45 and older showed that routinely walking at least an hour a week cuts the rate of heart disease in half! That's quite a benefit from only 60 minutes a week.

## FITNESS ESSENTIALS

In the day-by-day plan, the following elements serve as the backbone of the program.

### Wake-up Affirmation

Initially, one of the hardest parts about fitness is keeping your motivation strong. Therefore, each day in this 30-day program begins with a fact or a quotation to keep you moving toward your goal.

But you can also create a morning ritual with your own goals and affirmations. Before you begin, write on index cards the reasons you want to be more healthy and fit, from wanting to be more comfortable in your clothes, to ridding yourself of back pain, to having more energy at the end of the day. Place these cards close at hand, maybe under your pillow or on your nightstand, and read them before you go to sleep and when you wake up. Remember: Once the mind is in line, the body will follow.

### Wake-up Workout

Before you roll out of bed in the morning, take a few minutes to let your body slowly wake up and prepare for the day. Jumping out of bed too quickly can cause injury, especially if you suffer from back problems. These miniexercises will strengthen injury-prone areas, including your lower back. If you don't have time to do all the movements, do at least one a day.
1. While still lying down, take several deep, refreshing breaths.
2. To increase circulation, tighten and release all the larger muscles in your body. Point your toes and release. Tighten your thighs and buttocks and release. Squeeze your shoulder blades together then raise your arms straight up toward the ceiling and stretch. Exhale deeply as you release.

3. To stretch out your lower back in bed, place your hands and forearms behind your knees and draw them as comfortably close to your chest as possible. Hold them there for 30 seconds, release, and repeat two more times.

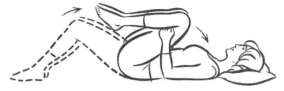

4. Lower your legs to the bed and do a pelvic tilt by squeezing your buttocks together. Don't arch your back; press your lower back into the mattress as you lift your buttocks. This movement will strengthen your buttocks and thighs, as well as release tension in your lower back. Over time, work up to 20 repetitions.

5. This itsy-bitsy sit-up uses the mattress and your pillow to support your neck and back. Lie on your back, push your lower back into the mattress, and place a small pillow behind your neck. Interlacing your fingers behind the pillow, slowly lift your head toward your knees until you feel a slight tightening of your abdominal muscles. Release and lower your head to the bed. Over time, work up to 20 repetitions.

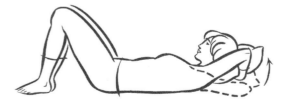

6. For a hamstring stretch, lie on your back and bend both knees. Keep your feet flat on the mattress at hip distance apart. Take your right leg and slowly bring it toward your chest. Straighten your left leg as much as your range of motion will allow and hold for 30 seconds Always keep a slight bend in your knee to prevent

stretching your hamstrings too far and placing undo strain on your knee tendons and ligaments. Repeat the exercise with your left leg.

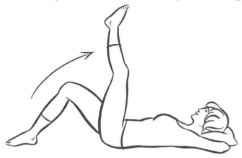

7. Finally, roll onto your stomach and push yourself up onto your hands and knees. Sit back on your heels and stretch your arms out in front of you, palms down on the mattress. This is a yoga stretch of the back, shoulders, and sides of the waist that I have found relaxes as well as wakes you up.

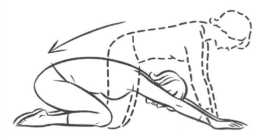

## Core Four

The Core Four ten-minute routine is designed to strengthen the major muscle groups of your entire body. By doing these four simple exercises each day, you will see a difference in both your energy level and the ease with which you do everyday chores.

When you do the routine is your choice. The movements are designed for every fitness level, increasing in difficulty. A regimen of progressive resistance is helpful because muscles will grow stronger when they are challenged by harder levels of exercise. Advance to the next level when the exercise you are currently performing feels too easy. If you are happy doing a level one exercise, then stay with it. If at any time you advance to the next level and it is uncomfortable, return to the previous level that felt good to you. Sore muscles are not an indication of good exercise. Sore muscles mean you did too much too soon.

## The Core Four Routine

### 1. PUSH-UP

This exercise will condition and strengthen your chest, the fronts of your shoulders, and the backs of your arms.

**BEGINNING, LEVEL ONE** Kneeling on a pillow about 12 inches from your bed, place your hands on the edge of the mattress with your arms straight, shoulder width apart. Slightly tighten your buttocks and your abdominals to protect your lower back. Make sure your lower back is not arched but flat like a tabletop. Bending your arms, slowly lower your chest to the bed and push back up. Breathing: Inhale on the down movement and exhale as you push up. Work up to 20 repetitions.

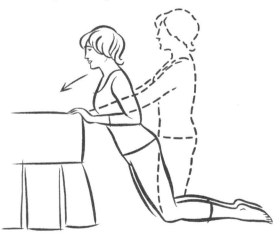

**MODERATE, LEVEL TWO** On your hands and knees on the floor, slightly tighten your buttocks and your abdominals to protect your lower back. Make sure your lower back is not arched but flat like a tabletop. Slowly lower your chest to the floor until you almost touch your nose, then push back up. Do not lock your arms at the top of the movement, but keep your elbows slightly bent. Breathing: inhale on the down movement and exhale as you push up. Over time, work up to 20 repetitions.

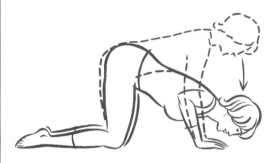

**CHALLENGE, LEVEL THREE** On your hands and knees, walk your hands forward until you are no longer bent at the waist and your back, thighs, and head are in a straight line. Slightly tighten your buttocks and your abdominals to protect your lower back. Make sure your lower back is not arched but flat like a tabletop. Bending your arms, slowly lower your chest and touch your nose on the floor and slowly push back up to the starting position, keeping your elbows slightly bent. Breathing: Inhale on the down movement and exhale as you push up. Over time, work up to 20 repetitions.

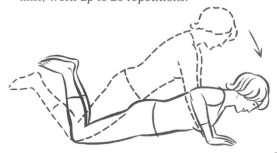

## 2. SIT-UP

This movement will strengthen your abdominal region, facilitate movement, and enhance your posture. A strong abdominal region also provides support for your lower back.

**BEGINNING, LEVEL ONE** Sit up straight on the floor with your legs bent in front of you and your hands on your knees. Inhale and slowly lean back as far as your comfort level will allow while tightening your stomach muscles. Round your back and pull in your abdominals. Hold for a few seconds, exhale, and return to the starting position. Work up to 10 repetitions. When 10 repetitions is easy, move on to level two.

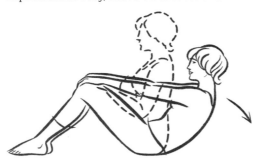

**MODERATE, LEVEL TWO** Lie on the floor on your back with your knees bent and your feet flat on the floor. Place a small pillow beneath your head and your hands behind the pillow, elbows pointing to the sides. (This will support your neck.) Inhale as you press your lower back into the floor. Using your abdominals, exhale as you slowly lift your head and, if comfortable, your shoulders and hold for a count of 2 before returning to the starting position. Look at a spot on the wall slightly above your knees and keep your gaze fixed on that spot. This will help you keep your head and neck in a straight line as you gently lift to a contracted position. (Note: If you only curl your head up off the pillow and hold, you are still toning almost 75 percent of your abdominal wall.) Work up to 20 repetitions.

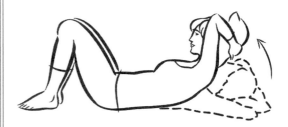

**CHALLENGE, LEVEL THREE** Lie on your back on the floor with your knees bent and your heels on the seat of a chair, making sure your knees are directly over your hips. Place a small pillow beneath your head and place your hands behind the pillow. Look at a spot on the wall slightly above your knees and keep your gaze fixed on that spot. This will help you keep your head and neck in a straight line as you gently lift the pillow and your head and shoulders to a contracted position. Hold for a second and return to the starting position. Do as many as comfortable, gradually working up to 20. When 20 repetitions are easy, do another set. When two sets of 20 repetitions are easy add one more set of 20.

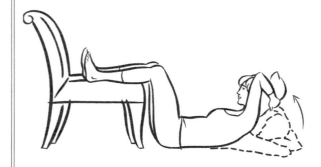

### 3. SIT AND STAND

This exercise will firm and tone your buttocks and thighs, while burning fat and increasing your heart's strength. Strong thighs will enable you to move throughout your day with ease. **BEGINNING, LEVEL ONE** Stand with your back to a chair as if you are about to sit down. Exhale as you slowly lower yourself into a seated position, and then inhale as you stand back up. If you feel off balance, hold on to another chair or a table with one hand. Once you feel comfortable with the sit and stand routine, don't hold on to anything. When you are strong enough to do 15 repetitions, move on to the next exercise level. **MODERATE, LEVEL TWO** Stand with your back to a chair. Exhale as you slowly lower yourself into a seated position, and inhale as you stand up while squeezing your buttocks. Start with 10, working up to 20 repetitions. **CHALLENGE, LEVEL THREE** Stand with your back to a chair. Exhale as you slowly lower yourself to touch the edge of the chair with your buttocks and then inhale as you stand back up and squeeze your buttocks. Keep your knees slightly bent in the upright position. Do 15, working up to 20 repetitions. When one set is no longer difficult, add two more sets of 20 for a total of 60 repetitions.

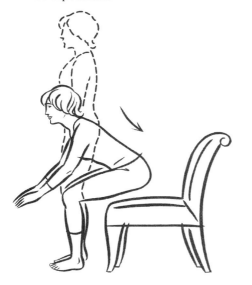

### 4. POSTURE SQUEEZE

This combo will strengthen the fronts of your arms and your back muscles. **BEGINNING, LEVEL ONE** In a seated position, straighten your back and lift your rib cage, keeping your shoulders down and relaxed. Take a deep breath and squeeze your shoulder blades together. Exhale and collapse your rib cage. Repeat this rib cage lift and squeeze 10 times. **MODERATE, LEVEL TWO** Sit with your arms at your sides, elbows glued to your waist, palms facing forward. Slowly curl your hands toward your chest until they are level with your waist, holding this position. Lift your rib cage, inhale, and squeeze your shoulder blades together for two seconds. Lower your arms, relax your rib cage, and repeat 10 times. For more resistance, hold on to 3- to 5-pound weights. **CHALLENGE, LEVEL THREE** You will need 5- to 8-pound weights for this exercise. Sit in a chair, hold a weight in each hand, with your fists facing each other and your thumbs facing in front of you. Bend over slightly with your arms straight, tighten your stomach muscles to support your lower back. Bend your elbows, exhale and pull your hands toward your waist, and squeeze your shoulder blades together. Hold for a second and inhale as you return to the starting position. Do 15 repetitions, working up to 20. When a single set becomes easy, add two more sets.

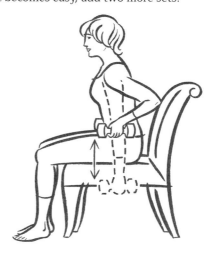

## Homemade Weights

You do not need to buy any equipment to get the benefits of free weights. Common household items will work just as well, especially products that come in plastic containers with handles. Just make sure to have the same weight in each hand. If the plastic is too rough on your hands, wrap a small towel around the handle to cushion any sharp edges.

### APPROXIMATE WEIGHTS OF HOUSEHOLD OBJECTS

➤ 16-ounce bottle of syrup or shampoo: 1 pound
➤ 33.8-ounce bottle of water: 2 pounds
➤ Small bottle of concentrated detergent: 3 pounds
➤ 64-ounce bottle of detergent: 4 pounds
➤ 1 liter of soda: 6 pounds
➤ 6- pack of soda: 6 pounds
➤ Cat litter in handled container: 7, 14, or 20 pounds, depending on size
➤ 3.5-quart detergent: 8 pounds
➤ Gallon of milk or water: 9 pounds
➤ 12-pack of beer: 12 pounds

You can also use plastic handled bags to combine products to increase weight one pound at a time. Be sure to load them evenly and lift without allowing your wrist to bend backward.

## Stretch, Relax, and Sleep

The stress hormones that course through our bodies all day cause a flight or fight syndrome that is extremely hard on our hearts and nervous systems. Mild movement at the end of the day can release the day's buildup of these hormones, rendering them harmless to our bodies and allowing us to fall asleep more easily.

The goal of the following stretches is to relax, not raise your heart rate, because rigorous exercise in the evening often makes it harder to fall asleep. Doing these movements just before going to bed will help you wind down from the day.

With that in mind, the following stretches should be done sitting on the edge of the bed.

1. **CHEST/POSTURE STRETCH** As we sit and walk during the day, our shoulders tend to slump forward, creating a closed-off feeling in our chest areas. By reversing the process with this stretch, you will open up the breathing pathways.
Place both hands behind you in the lower back region, palms facing out. Take a deep breath and squeeze your shoulder blades together, lifting your rib cage. Hold this stretch for a second or two, then exhale and return to the starting position.

2. **NECK AND UPPER SPINE STRETCH** Do this stretch any time you feel tension in your upper neck and back, especially if you are desk-bound and need a tension-releasing break.
Sit up straight and place both hands behind your head on the round part of the skull. Drop both elbows forward and let gravity and the weight of your arms gently pull your head down so your chin gently rests on your upper chest just above your collarbone. You should feel the stretch in your upper neck and radiating down your spine.

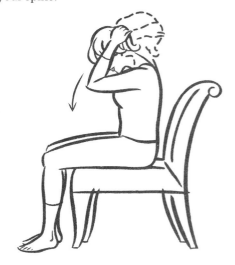

**3. LOWER SPINE STRETCH** This stretch will increase circulation and oxygen in your head and release accumulated stress in your lower back. Place a small pillow on your lap and bend over from the waist, so your chest rests on the pillow. Hang your head and arms down toward your feet. Feel the stretch all the way down your spine and into your lower back. Hold for just a few seconds. Slowly lift back up to the starting position.

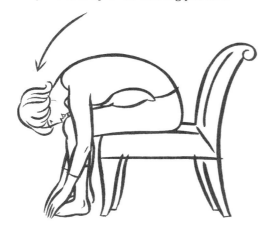

## Daily Routine

The Wake-up Workout, Core Four, and Stretch, Relax and Sleep will serve as the backbone for your daily routine. Over the next 30 days, I will show you a variety of additional exercises that condition all areas of your body, including Take Ten, Sit and Be Fit, and Energy Lift exercises. When the following movement breaks are woven into your day, you will be adding exercises that will take you to a higher level of strength and fitness easily and effortlessly.

**TAKE TEN** These small toning and conditioning movements spring from the research that exercise does not have to last for an extended time to increase fitness. In ten minutes or less, these fitness breaks will make a difference in how you look and how you feel.

**SIT AND BE FIT** Just because you are desk or house bound does not mean that you can not work out. These seated exercise breaks will work with resistance in order to improve your posture, balance, muscle strength, flexibility, and fitness level.

**ENERGY LIFT** These movements increase your energy by increasing your circulation, which also allows for greater blood flow to the brain and muscles, enabling you to think more clearly and move more efficiently. Movement also accesses the mood-elevating chemical endorphins and burns up stress hormones, so you will feel better, too.

Before you know it, you will be doing your fitness routine anywhere and everywhere!

# The Philosophy Behind Energy Balance Nutrition

I F YOU'RE LIKE MILLIONS OF WOMEN, you are tired of hunting for the next trendy diet or miracle pill that promises to take you to the seemingly wonderful world of size 6. To me, the word diet means deprivation, and pills often make your body work in unnatural ways, good reasons to avoid both of them. My clients often dieted for years before they came to me, and they usually stopped for one of the following reasons:

**1.** They regained weight as soon as they stopped.
**2.** They didn't like the food.
**3.** They didn't feel satisfied.
**4.** They couldn't stay on the diet forever.
**5.** They felt tired and hungry.
**6.** They couldn't eat with family and friends.

Sound familiar? Being unsatisfied by a meal creates a mental craving that translates to "What and when am I going to eat next?" How can you possibly lose weight if you are constantly thinking about food and what you can and cannot eat?

## HOW LOW-CALORIE DIETS CAUSE YOU TO GAIN WEIGHT

Besides giving you a near obsession with eating, low-calorie dieting or weight cycling (losing and gaining more than ten pounds over a period of many years) actually undermines your health. By breaking down muscle mass, which lowers your metabolism, these diets slow your weight loss down. When, discouraged, you start eating the way you want, the weight you are putting back on isn't the muscle you lost—it's FAT. Consequently, you end up heavier and fatter than you were before you initially lost the weight.

Being malnourished from dieting also causes an imbalance in your biochemistry, including your insulin levels, the hormone that regulates blood sugar levels. Insulin is up to 30 times more effective at turning extra calories into fat than it is at turning them into muscle. One way to stay lean is to control your insulin with effective eating and to activate your fat-burning hormone, glucagon. Let's take a closer look at how food and exercise affect these hormones and how they impact your fat gain and fat loss cycles.

## THE SCIENCE OF WEIGHT LOSS

### Carbohydrate

Carbohydrate, one of the three principal constituents of food, along with protein and fat, forms the bulk of the average human diet. The end product of the digestion and assimilation of all forms of carbohydrate is a simple sugar, glucose, commonly called blood sugar when found in the human body. The metabolism of some components of fats and certain protein substances can also lead to the production of glucose. Glucose is the principal fuel that muscles and other portions of the body consume to produce energy.

### Insulin

Regulating the flow of nutrients—including glucose, amino acids (proteins derived from dietary protein or muscle breakdown), and fatty acids (fats)— into the body's cells is insulin's primary job. This hormone is also responsible for shuttling glucose out of the blood stream and into your body's fat cells for use later as energy. When you eat too much carbohydrate and especially

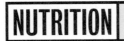 

carbohydrate that is in high-sugar, low-fiber foods, your pancreas will respond by secreting high levels of insulin. This will bring down your the blood sugar, store the sugar as fat, and keep it stored as long as insulin is present.

Insulin also inhibits the activity of lipase, the enzyme that breaks down fats in the digestive system. So the trick is to find the right balance of nutrients to keep insulin from being put on alert.

## Glucagon

Glucagon, also produced by the pancreas, is insulin's biological opposite. As your body's sugar- and fat-burning hormone, glucagon primarily releases stored carbohydrate in the form of glucose to feed your tissues. When your body has more insulin than glucagon, it begins storing sugar as fat, in the blood.

When insulin and glucagon are in balance, your body is able to burn stored fat as energy. In addition, the combination of dietary protein and exercise stimulates the release of glucagon. The Energy Balance program uses these scientific facts to enable your body to lose weight.

## THE ENERGY BALANCE AND THE MIDLIFE FAT CELL

Somewhere between the ages of 35 and 55, our bodies begin to change. We start a shift of fat weight from our hips and thighs to our waistline, which our mothers might have called middle-age spread. It is unclear whether the blame for this gain lies with aging or menopause.

Whatever the cause, the weight gain is a natural phenomenon that is actually good for your health. When your body senses a drop in estrogen, it will begin to increase the storage of fat, because fat stores estrogen. Settling around the waistline, near the liver and upper body, this added fat aids in the midlife transition. The estrogen within it helps you get through menopause by lessening hot flashes, mood swings, sleep disturbances, dry skin, and

other signs of the end of your child bearing years.

Can you avoid this midlife fat gain?

The answer is yes and no. Every woman will experience some kind of shift in her fat weight, even if she starts out on the thinner side. However, an excessive increase in waistline fat can endanger your health by causing a greater risk of heart disease, hypertension, and breast cancer.

Combating middle-years fat is an art. If you exercise too much and eat too little to compensate for midlife fat, you are putting your body through additional stress, which can cause megamenopause. You are compromising your muscle mass, bone strength, metabolism, and health.

With my kinder, gentler way of treating your body, you will be able to outsmart the middle-years fat cell without sacrificing your figure or your health.

## THE ENERGY BALANCE IS NOT A DIET

My program is not a diet because it does not begin or end but is designed for the challenges of today's woman in a permanent way. A woman who is too busy to weigh and measure food or count calories. A woman who wants to eat with her friends and family. A woman who refuses to go on yet another diet that requires odd food choices, deprivation, and willpower. And this new approach to eating, with its balance of nutrients that boosts energy by leveling out your blood glucose will make you feel so good you'll stick with it. Instead of a diet that you go on and off, this program is so healthy and nutritious that you can make it part of your life.

Although the science behind it is not new, my time-tested approach stresses easy meals and snacks, works with your daily routine, and is based around foods you like (unless that happens to be plates of fudge, morning, noon, and night).

If you want to lose weight, you will, but it will be more fat than water weight or muscle. When I have run fitness seminars for corporate clients, participants achieve an average fat loss of 10 to 30 pounds in 12 to 15 weeks. This program is based on changing your habits, so don't jump on the scale daily. Use your clothes as an indication of what is happening to the fat stores in your body. When you burn your stored fat for energy, there will be a significant change in how you look over time. But in 30 days, you will be well on your way to losing the weight you want. And if your goal is not weight loss, this program will enable you to feel stronger, healthier, and more vital.

How many times has three o'clock rolled around to find you tired, cranky, and hungry, even though you had lunch at noon? In all likelihood, the reason you feel so tired that is you ate too many high-sugar carbohydrates or you didn't eat enough protein. With Energy Balance nutrition, you will avoid this slump and hunger will happen gradually, allowing you to avoid impulse eating. You will crave sugar less and think more clearly without the roller coaster of your blood sugar dictating your moods. Once you realize how your food choices make you feel two to three hours after eating, you will want to eat foods that promote longer-lasting energy and endurance.

The Energy Balance nutrition program helps you eat healthier because it teaches you how to look at food in a different way. The food choices enable you not to demonize food—it is neither good nor bad—but to think of what you eat purely as a source of energy. Before you fix a meal or a snack, you'll ask yourself this question: How do I want to feel in three hours? You will begin to choose your food with this criteria in mind:

➤ Does this meal or snack have the Nutritional Core Four? Think about protein first, then add high-fiber, low-sugar carbohydrate, and a little fat. A good example is a turkey sandwich: Turkey is your protein source, whole-grain bread is the high-fiber carbohydrate, and one slice of low-fat cheese with mustard, tomato, pickles, and any other condiments would round out this balance.

➤ Don't deny yourself anything. If you want to use mayonnaise, use just enough to make the sandwich taste good, and use one that is low-fat or fat-free.

➤ Eat six small Energy Balance meals or snacks a day. A 1998 Tufts study showed that eating six small meals a day (called grazing) can increase a woman's ability to burn fat faster. If those meals are a combination of protein, fat, and high-fiber carbohydrate, your energy levels will stay higher longer because those meals take longer to digest. This eating regimen will also slow down the impact of carbohydrate and sugar entering your blood stream, thereby keeping your energy balanced. By keeping your sugar-induced mood swings in check, you will lessen the impact of eating out of boredom, reward, fear, and anger.

If you can consistently choose food with these criteria in mind, you will begin to feel more energetic and have fewer cravings. The most dramatic results are felt at the midday energy slump, where most of my clients report an incredible increase in productivity. As one of my clients said, "Now I don't feel like crawling under my desk at 3 P.M. and taking a nap."

## NUTRITION ESSENTIALS

### How Hungry Are You?

Do you sometimes find yourself eating simply because it's lunchtime or because you're bored or maybe because there's a bag of chips sitting right in front of you. Before you make a food choice, pick a number between 1 and 10 that signifies your level of hunger, with 1 being not very hungry and 10 being starving.

➤ If you are at level 1-3, wait a few minutes and drink a large glass of water. It could be false hunger, based on habit, boredom, or dehydration.

➤ If you are at 4-6, eat an Energy Balance meal or snack.

➤ Try to eat before your hunger level gets to 7-10.

When you are this hungry, your Energy Balance is thrown off and you start to lose control of your food choices. You will eat without thinking about your fat-burning progress. If you eat when you are slightly hungry and before your blood glucose starts to descend, you will be using the science of the Energy Balance program, not impulse, to make the right choices.

## Drink All the Time

Drink 4 to 8 glasses of water a day, no matter what. Your kidneys work hard to keep salts and minerals in your body in proper balance, but they work slowly. By the time your brain says, "You are thirsty," your body's water supply is already seriously depleted.

Besides preventing sagging skin, building new tissue, metabolizing stored fat, and relieving ailments such as constipation, drinking lots of water is one way to prevent or relieve kidney problems, such as kidney stones and urinary tract infections.

Not drinking enough water actually stops you from losing weight. In a pilot study at the University of Utah in Salt Lake City, scientists found that when participants were just slightly dehydrated, they had a 2 to 3 percent decrease in their resting metabolic rate, which in turn slows the burning of calories. Also, when your water stores are too low, your body responds to the drought by increasing fat stores in your liver.

Drinking water also helps you lose weight by
➤ filling you up so you eat less
➤ ridding your body of the toxic by-products of metabolism, products such as ketone bodies, which can harm blood and tissues
➤ helping with digestion and assimilation of nutrients so you aren't chronically hungry.

If you're tired during the day, try drinking a big glass of water. One of the side effects of dehydration is fatigue, in addition to:
➤ memory loss
➤ dizziness
➤ poor cognitive function

➤ headaches
➤ light headedness
➤ dark urine with a strong odor
➤ muscle fatigue

## Plan for a Snack Attack

If you have favorite snacks that satisfy on hand, you will be better equipped to handle any and all situations. Throughout the book I'll list some of my favorite soul-satisfying snacks and show you how to use your favorite foods to make your own.

## Eat Slowly

There is a fair amount of research to suggest that it takes about 20 minutes for your stomach to signal your brain that you are full. If you are going out for a late dinner, eat a small Energy Balance snack before you go. This will help keep you from devouring the bread when you sit down at the restaurant.

## Eat Acidic Foods

Foods such as oranges, grapefruit, lemon juice, and lime juice are digested slowly and help keep your blood sugar level. If you are drinking juice instead of eating the fruit, which has fiber, put a small amount in a large glass of water or seltzer. This dilution will soften the impact of the high-sugar of juice on your bloodstream.

## Eat Most of Your Food Before 7 P.M.

Proper timing will enable you to burn more calories during the day and help you wind down at the end. If you are hungry around 9 or 10 P.M., eat a small Energy Balance snack and you will sleep better and wake up more refreshed.

## Monitor Your Caffeine Intake

Caffeine will stimulate the production of insulin, causing your body to store more fat. More than two cups of coffee, cola, or tea a day will also leech calcium from your bones.

### Eat High-Fiber Foods

Foods such as whole grains, legumes, and some fruits and vegetables will fill you up while aiding digestion.

### Sleep at Least Eight Hours a Night

If you're sleep-deprived, you are setting yourself up for a host of ailments, one of which is a greater propensity to eat more and store fat.

### Learn to Manage Your Stress

When you are confronted with stress, the hormone cortisol will shunt more fat to your abdomen. Stress will also increase the fat-storing hormone insulin. At the end of each day in the program, I've added a movement or another way to decrease stress in your life.

### Take It Slow

A gradual day-to-day shift in balancing your eating and exercise habits will increase your body's appetite-controlling mechanisms. This shift will enable you to stabilize your blood glucose levels for longer periods of time.

If you overeat, binge, or give in to emotional eating, don't worry—you are just one meal away from being back in balance. I recommend taking a day off once in a while to eat whatever strikes your taste buds. Besides satisfying any cravings, you will feel the difference eating too much carbohydrate or sugar can make—it's almost as bad as having a hangover! This experience may make you think twice before going off the Energy Balance program.

## GETTING THE VITAMINS AND MINERALS YOU NEED

You need 13 different vitamins and 10 minerals to stay alive, to enhance your immune system, to build and repair muscle and bone, to enable you to relax, to help turn food into energy, and to do the thousands of chemical transactions that keep you healthy and strong.

Although a balanced diet is the key to good health, unless you are continually eating the most nutritious foods you can find, you will not be getting all the vitamins and minerals you need. Try as we might, most of us just can't eat this well every meal, every day. Our stressful, fast-paced lifestyle and health busters such as smoking, stress, alcohol, and sugar further erode our good intentions, undermining health.

The first line of defense against vitamin and mineral deficiency is to eat a nutritious, balanced diet such as the Energy Balance nutrition program. Then add a supplement. A multivitamin will ensure you are getting all 13 vitamins and 10 minerals that help turn food into energy. Make sure your multivitamin has the recommended daily allowance of all vitamins and minerals, especially the following.

➤ The American Medical Association states that 400 international units (IU) of natural vitamin E helps prevent heart disease, diabetes, and cancer and boosts your immune system. This antioxidant will protect your cell membranes against free radicals, which can ravage them and cause health problems. Vitamin E also helps the healing process and keeps arteries more flexible.

➤ Take at least 500 to 1,000 milligrams of vitamin C a day. I recommend a time-release C in a base of bioflavonoids that originates from a natural source. Among the 300 different uses of vitamin C in your body, it is needed to make collagen, the strong connective tissue that holds your skeleton together and attaches your muscles to your bones; to assimilate folic acid and iron; and to enhance your immune system.

➤ Take at least 1,000 to 1,600 milligrams of calcium a day. Women over 50 need at least 1,500 milligrams a day. If you don't get enough calcium, the 206 bones in your body will be susceptible to osteoporosis, which means they will break easily because they are thin, porous, and brittle. Osteoporosis has several related causes beyond lack of calcium, including not getting enough weight-bearing exercise and having lower estrogen levels.

Adding vitamin supplements while eating Energy Balance foods will ensure all the fat-burning, energy-converting vitamins are available to improve your health now and in the future.

## MORE ON CALCIUM

Without the proper amount of calcium each day, your body will not burn fat as effectively. Calcium blocks the formation of fat and helps break it down for energy. Your muscles, brain, and nervous system can't function without it. When your calcium levels fall, your body thinks it's in starvation mode. This mode causes an increase in strong hormones from the parathyroid that stops your body from burning stored fat for energy.

The supplement many doctors recommend, calcium citrate, dissolves easily even if you don't have much stomach acid. As we age we produce less stomach acid, so calcium citrate is the better choice for older women. Make sure your calcium supplement also has magnesium, vitamin D, and vitamin K. You need the vitamin D to keep your blood level of calcium normal and to help your bones hold on to the calcium. Vitamins D and K are essential to the complex process of remodeling bones. Magnesium helps your body absorb calcium and use vitamin D properly. To avoid getting too much vitamin D, don't take any other supplement that also contains D.

Calcium supplements that are not bone and body friendly:

➤ **BONE MEAL** The Food and Drug Administration warns that bone meal, a powder made from the bones of cattle, may contain high amounts of lead.
➤ **DOLOMITE** This compound, also known as calcium magnesium carbonate, also contains high amounts of lead.
➤ **OYSTER SHELL** These supplements, made from ground-up oyster shells, may also contain high amounts of lead and occasionally other contaminants such as mercury and cadmium. And don't use them if you are allergic to shellfish.

Now that you understand the basics behind Energy Balance nutrition, in the upcoming chapters you will learn how to use the Core Four (protein, high-fiber, low-sugar carbohydrates, and fat) to create the following:

➤ Recipes for Energy Balancing your life
➤ The right food portions to satisfy your appetite and food needs
➤ How to Energy Balance your whole family without their knowing it
➤ Guides for staying in the Energy Balance while eating in restaurants
➤ How to eat when you can't find Energy Balance food

# Energy Balance Basics

DO CALORIES CAUSE YOU to gain weight? Nutrition wisdom states that if you consume calories and don't burn them for energy, you will store them as fat, which is true. However, an abundance of insulin is also a factor in fat storage, no matter how many calories you are eating. The trick is to keep calories and insulin in a healthy range that will allow your body to burn fat as energy.

With Energy Balance foods, you won't need to count calories to stay within that range; instead, the blood-sugar-leveling choices and suggested portion sizes of the Energy Balance program will do that for you. When you are nutritionally fed and satisfied, you will not crave foods that contribute to weight gain. And with no type of food off-limits, you will never feel deprived.

The goal of the Energy Balance program is to help change your eating habits toward high-nutrition, high-energy foods. When you understand the reasoning behind Energy Balance, you can create your own meals, snacks, and menus. It may take time to get used to this way of eating, but once the habit is set and you have figured out how to balance your favorite foods, the Energy Balance will become part of your life. For every meal and snack, just think about low-fat protein first, low-sugar carbohydrates second, high-fiber carbohydrates third, and small amounts of healthy fat to round it out—it's that easy!

## THE ENERGY BALANCE CORE FOUR FOOD GROUPS

To stay in the Energy Balance, at every meal and snack include a favorite food from each of the Core Four food groups: protein, carbohydrate, fat, and fiber. In the following pages, foods are listed by type which will help you to understand why foods fall into certain groups. Although on this plan you can eat any food you like, try to keep in mind the suggested serving sizes.

## Protein

Protein is the basis of all life. Aside from of water, protein is the most plentiful substance in our bodies. As much as half your dry body weight—including most of your muscle mass, skin, hair, eyes, and nails—is made up of protein. Protein is the main structural ingredient of your cells, as well as the enzymes that keep them running. Even your immune system is essentially composed of protein! So you can see why it is an integral part of your diet.

Protein can commonly be found in foods such as dairy products, fish, legumes, poultry, and lean meats. Eating protein-rich foods does not cause your blood sugar level to rise significantly, which helps you feel satisfied longer. The longer you feel satisfied, the less likely you are to grab a snack to tide you over to the next meal.

### Suggested Serving Sizes for Protein

➤ **MEAT:** 6 ounces per meal and 2 to 3 ounces per snack, which for a meal is about the size of your hand. If you are eating in a restaurant that serves oversize portions, eat only half.
➤ **DELI MEAT:** 2 to 4 slices
➤ **POULTRY:** 1 chicken breast or 1 chicken leg with thigh
➤ **FISH:** 6 ounces or the average portion in a restaurant.
➤ If you find you are still hungry after you have finished your meal, you may want to eat a slightly larger serving of protein next time.

## Sources Include

➤ Beef from the round, chuck sirloin, or loin. Buy "choice" or "select" grades of beef rather than prime. Choose ground beef that is 85 percent lean or higher.
➤ Buffalo, which is low in fat
➤ Cheese, including low-fat cottage cheese and string cheese
➤ Chicken, Cornish hen, turkey, ground turkey, and turkey sausage and bacon
➤ Dairy products such as skim milk and low-fat yogurt
➤ Deli meat, such as low-fat turkey, chicken, turkey ham, turkey pastrami, and lean boiled ham. Try to find deli meat that contains no nitrites, which are preservatives that tend to raise insulin levels.
➤ Eggs, including egg substitutes and egg whites
➤ Fish and shellfish, such as tuna, lake trout, herring, mackerel, sardines, and salmon, including lox
➤ Game, including rabbit, venison, and pheasant
➤ Lamb, especially the leg, arm, and loin.
➤ Legumes, including white, kidney, and pinto beans and lentils (1 cup cooked)
➤ Pork, such as tenderloin, chop, and lean ham
➤ Tofu (soybean curd)
➤ Vegetarian soy-based "meats" that contain less than 4 grams of carbohydrate

## Protein Tips

➤ Avoid meats that have a large amount of visible fat. If you buy these cuts, trim the visible fat before cooking.
➤ Remove skin from poultry before cooking, unless it is a whole chicken or turkey. In that case remove the skin after cooking.
➤ Avoid goose, duck, and processed poultry products, which are high in saturated fatty acids.
➤ Liver, brains, kidney, and sweetbreads are high in cholesterol and should be limited or avoided.
➤ Use cooking methods that require little or no fat, such as broiling, baking, roasting, poaching, steaming, sautéing, stir-frying, and microwaving.

## Carbohydrate

You need a certain amount of carbohydrate in your diet to feed your brain and muscles, both of which use the glucose in carbs as a primary energy source. The liver's capacity to store carbohydrate in the form of glycogen is very limited and can easily be depleted within 10 to 12 hours. Therefore the liver's glycogen reserves must be maintained on a continual basis, which is one reason why our body craves carbohydrates.

Once the glycogen levels are high enough in both your liver and your muscles, excess carbohydrate has just one fate: to be converted into fat and stored in fatty tissue. Even though carbohydrates themselves can be fat-free, excess carbohydrates end up as fat.

Glucose is found in grains, pasta, bread, cereals, starches, and vegetables. Fructose is found in fruits. Galactose is found in dairy products. Although the liver rapidly absorbs all these simple sugars, only glucose can be released directly into the bloodstream. The sugar in glucose-rich carbohydrates, such as bread and pasta, virtually sprints from your liver into your bloodstream. Galactose and fructose enter your bloodstream at a slower rate because they must first be converted to glucose in your liver.

This conversion is a very slow process, especially for fructose. Carbohydrates that are fructose based (primarily fruits) have a low glycemic index (the rate at which sugar enters the bloodstream) compared to glucose- and galactose-containing carbohydrates. The Energy Balance program, therefore, limits the amount of glucose- and galactose-based foods, so your blood sugar does not rise and fall continually.

## Suggested Serving Sizes for Carbohydrates

➤ 3/4 cup grain or cereal
➤ 1 slice bread
➤ 1 small bagel or roll

➤ 1/2 cup pasta
➤ 2 cups leafy vegetables
➤ 1 cup solid vegetables
➤ 1 fruit

## Carbohydrate Sources Include

➤ Bread, such as rye, whole-grain, and whole wheat, which can take the form of bagels, English muffins, pita bread, crackers, and rolls. Each serving should contain more than 2 grams of fiber.
➤ Cereals, such as bran, shredded wheat, and **multigrain**. Limit your intake of granola, which can be filled with fat and sugar. Each serving should contain more than 3 grams of fiber.
➤ Grains, such as rice (preferably brown), bulgur, quinoa, barley, and couscous.
➤ High-fiber pasta. Look for pasta made of a combination of wheat and buckwheat flours, noodles made of alternative-wheat (spelt) flour, and noodles with no wheat at all, just brown rice, corn, or quinoa.

## Vegetables

Beans, such as green beans, peas, or snow peas
Bell Peppers (red, yellow, and green)
Broccoli
Cucumbers
Lettuce, such as romaine and red leaf (Avoid iceberg, which does not contain many nutrients.)
Mushrooms
Onions
Parsnips
Tomatoes

## Fruits

Apples
Apricots
Bananas (Make sure the banana is a small one. Bananas are higher in sugar than most fruit.)
Blackberries
Blueberries
Cherries

Cantaloupes
Grapefruits
Peaches
Pears
Pineapples
Plums
Strawberries
Tangerines

## Carbohydrate Tips

➤ Although most fruits and vegetables are good sources of low-fat carbohydrates, coconut meat, avocados, and olives are high in fat.
➤ Fruits that are fresh or canned in water are lower in calories than fruits canned in juice or syrup. Drain and rinse fruits canned in syrup to remove the extra sugar or use light canned fruit.

## High-, Medium-, Low-Sugar Foods

When you plan meals, note that carbohydrates will cause a high, medium, or slow release of insulin. When creating meals based on the carbohydrates listed, add low-sugar food to the meal to slow down high-sugar foods reaching your bloodstream. For example, when eating 1/2 cup white rice (high-sugar), add broccoli (low-sugar) or other low-sugar vegetables and a good-size portion of chicken, tofu, or fish to slow down the absorption of the sugar. With a small amount of low-fat cheese, you'll have a perfectly balanced meal that is in the Energy Balance range.

### HIGH SUGAR—RAPID INSULIN RELEASE
Bagels
Cakes and muffins
Cookies and crackers
Dates
English muffins
French fries
Graham crackers
Highly processed cereals
High-sugar sports drinks
Pineapple

Rice cakes
Russet potatoes
Tropical fruits such as bananas
Waffles and pancakes
Watermelon
White and whole wheat bread
White rice

### MEDIUM SUGAR — MODERATE INSULIN RELEASE

Apple juice
Applesauce
Barley
Beans: Butter beans, Lima beans, Navy beans, Pinto beans, White beans
Beets
Bran
Bulgur
Couscous
Custard
Grapes
Instant noodles
Multigrain Rices: Basmati rice, Brown rice, Long-grain rice
Oat bran
Oatmeal
Oranges
Orange juice
Pasta
Peas
Raisins
Rye bread
Sponge cake
Yams

### LOW SUGAR — SLOW INSULIN RELEASE

Apples
Baked beans
Broccoli
Cantaloupe
Cherries
Chocolate (in moderation)
Cucumbers

Grapefruits
Green beans
High-fiber bread (more than 2-3 grams of fiber per slice)
Hot chocolate
Ice cream
Kidney beans
Lentils
Lettuce
Milk
Peaches
Peanuts
Pears
Pita bread
Plums
Popcorn
Soybeans
Strawberries
Sweet potatoes
Tomatoes
Tomato soup
Yogurt

# Fat

Your body can't function without fat in your diet. The American Heart Association suggests you consume up to 30 percent of your total calories from fat. But what kind? Not all fat is good for you, especially those oxidized, hydrogenated, or heat-processed fats found in fried foods, margarine, and vegetable shortening, among other foods. You should also limit your consumption of foods high in saturated fat, such as full-fat milk products, fatty meats, tropical oils, partially hydrogenated vegetable oils, and egg yolks.

Not all fats are bad for you, either. Extra-virgin olive oil, canola oil, flaxseed oil, fish oils, nuts, seeds, and avocado are heart-healthy fats.

➤ Fats slow down the digestion and release of carbohydrates into the system, thereby helping keep insulin levels lower.

➤ Fats are a concentrated energy source (9 calories per gram) and help make food taste good.

➤ Fats cause the release of the hormone cholecys-tokinin (CCK) from your stomach, triggering the message of satiety to your brain. Without that message, you would continue to feel hungry even when your stomach is full.

➤ Fats assist in the absorption of the fat-soluble vitamins A, D, E, and K and calcium.

➤ Fats nourish the skin, nerves, and mucous membranes.

➤ The supply of essential fatty acids from omega-3s (flaxseed oil and fish oil) benefit the immune, cardiovascular, reproductive, and central nervous systems. Some of the more recent research suggests omega-3s prevent blood clotting, repair tissue damage caused by clogged arteries, lower the rate at which the liver makes triglycerides, and lower high blood pressure.

Less fat in the diet does not necessarily lead to less fat in the fat cells. One study found that dietary fat accounted for only 2 percent of weight gained—the balance was caused by underexercising, overeating, or overactive middle-life fat cells.

## Suggested Serving Sizes for Fat

➤ 1 teaspoon oil
➤ 1 tablespoon seeds
➤ 1/8 of avocado
➤ 1 tablespoon of mayonnaise or peanut butter
➤2 tablespoons nuts
➤5 large olives

## Fat Sources Include

Polyunsaturated and monounsaturated oils are the kinds of fats you'll want to include in your daily diet. Pay close attention to the kinds of fats and oils in packaged foods because many contain saturated fat, the kind you want to avoid.

**HEART-HEALTHY FATS**
Canola oil

Corn oil
Flaxseed oil
Oil-based salad dressing
Olive oil
Polyunsaturated margarine
Safflower oil
Sesame seed oil
Soybean oil
Sunflower oil

**LIMITED USE**
Bacon, salt pork
Butter
Chicken fat, meat fat
Coconut oil
Palm kernel oil
Palm oil
Shortening
Suet, lard

**OCCASIONAL USE ONLY**
Peanut oil
Vegetable shortening

**OTHER SOURCES**
Avocados
Nuts low in saturated fats are chestnuts (the lowest), walnuts, peanuts, filberts, almonds, pecans, and pistachios.
Olives (black or green)
Seeds, such as sunflower, sesame, and pumpkin

## Fat Tips

➤ Eggs have 213 milligrams of cholesterol per yolk, though egg whites don't have any. To keep cholesterol and fat to a minimum, eat no more than 3 egg yolks a week.

➤ To cut calories, use prune puree or applesauce in place of shortening or butter in brownies, muffins, and simple cakes.

➤ If you don't like the taste of low-fat or nonfat mayonnaise, mix equal parts regular mayonnaise and low-fat (or nonfat) yogurt.

➤ Use nonfat sour cream instead of milk or cream to enrich sauces and soups.

➤ Low-fat and heart-healthy products you can buy at the grocery include trans-fat-free margarine, low-fat or fat-free salad dressing and mayonnaise, low- or no-fat sour cream, and non-dairy creamer.

➤ Low-fat yogurt blended with 3 to 4 teaspoons cornstarch can substitute for heavy or sour cream.

➤ When cooking ground meat for sauces and stews, rinse the meat with warm or hot water after browning. This removes fat but does not affect the taste.

## Fiber

Dietary fiber is a general term for indigestible parts of plant foods. There are basically two kinds of fiber: soluble and insoluble.

Soluble fiber dissolves in water to form a soft gel in your intestines. As the gel moves through your intestines, it can pick up elements that could harm your health, such as cholesterol, while helping regulate insulin levels.

Insoluble fiber is cellulose, the main fiber in the cell walls of all plants. Insoluble fiber absorbs water, but it doesn't dissolve in it, so you need to drink more water when eating large amounts of fiber. Eating insoluble fiber helps alleviate colon and bowel problems. When your bowels and colon are clean, you may experience less bloating and less protrusion in the lower part of your abdominal area. The thin outer husks of whole grains such as rice, wheat, and oats (called bran) are insoluble fiber and rich sources of B vitamins and minerals.

According to a 1999 study in the *Journal of the American Heart Association,* people who eat a high-fiber diet weighed on average 8 pounds less than those whose fiber intake was in the lowest 20 percent of the study. One reason for this is that fiber slows the rate of absorption of carbohydrate into the bloodstream. Remove the fiber (like in juicing a vegetable or fruit) and the rate of entry accelerates.

## Suggested Serving Sizes for Fiber

It's not hard to get enough fiber in your daily diet. If you eat the fiber-rich foods listed in this chapter, you will easily reach the suggested daily amount of fiber of 25 to 30 grams. One way is with fiber-rich bread, which should contain at least 2 to 3 grams of fiber per slice. Three grams of fiber can also be found in a cup of oatmeal or oat bran or in an apple. But add fiber-rich foods to your diet slowly. If you are not used to large amounts of fiber, you may experience bloating and gas until your system gets used to it.

### SOLUBLE FIBER
Apples
Bananas
Carrots
Cauliflower
Citrus fruits
Cooked beans
Corn
Lentils
Oat bran
Oatmeal
Pears
Rice bran
Strawberries
Sweet potatoes (without skin)

### INSOLUBLE FIBER
Artichokes
Asparagus
Broccoli
Brussels sprouts
Carrots
Green beans
Nuts
Parsnips
Seeds
Sweet potatoes (with skin)
Wheat bran
Whole grains

Fiber Tips

➤ Oats may be a particularly beneficial source of soluble fiber. In one study, women who had 6 to 11 servings of whole grains a day reduced their risk of heart disease by a third.

➤ If you have trouble getting enough fiber in your diet, psyllium, a grain grown in India, is an excellent soluble-fiber supplement.

➤ Studies have singled out nuts, which contain omega-3 fatty acids and fiber, as being particularly beneficial for the heart by lowering LDL and total cholesterol without increasing triglycerides.

## EATING BY THE NUMBERS

To make shopping easier, here are the average grams of protein, carbohydrate, fats, and fiber in the Energy Balance meals and snacks.

### EATING BY THE NUMBERS

| | PROTEIN GRAMS | CARBOHYDRATE GRAMS | FAT GRAMS | FIBER GRAMS |
|---|---|---|---|---|
| Breakfast | 15 to 20 | 25 to 30 | 10 to 15 | 5 to 10 |
| Lunch | 15 to 20 | 25 to 30 | 10 to 15 | 5 to 10 |
| Dinner | 15 to 20 | 25 to 30 | 10 to 15 | 5 to 10 |
| Each snack | 10 to 15 | 15 to 20 | 5 to 10 | 3 to 5 |

## ENERGY BARS

Some people try to replace meals with energy bars, which are often mostly sugar and will give you an insulin surge, thus encouraging fat storing. Also, the thinking that a bar supplemented by a few vitamins and minerals covers your nutritional allotment for the day is WRONG! Eating a healthy well-balanced diet is the best way to get the vitamins and minerals you need, rounded out with a good all-around vitamin supplement.

However, these bars are a good alternative when faced with a quick need for an easy snack. Here is what to look for when choosing a bar that will fit into the Energy Balance Program:

**PROTEIN:** 10 grams or more
**CARBOHYDRATE:** no more than 25 grams
**FAT:** no more than 6 grams

## HAVE YOUR CAKE AND EAT IT TOO

Do you crave sweets? Do you reach for the cookies when you are sad and lonely? Maybe you just like the sweet taste of a dessert after dinner. There is so much behind your sweet cravings. The number one reason for sugar cravings is physical, not psychological—it is low blood sugar. When a sugar craving hits, ask yourself what you ate two to three hours ago. You can usually figure out why your blood sugar is low and fix it with an Energy Balance snack.

If, however, you just want a cookie, go ahead and have one. Yes, I said one. Make it part of your day, maybe a three o'clock decaf coffee break when you have your cookie. By allowing yourself to eat a small treat every day, you will not build a ravenous craving for cookies and eventually eat the whole box.

A trick I use to balance the sugar in the cookie is to put low-fat cottage cheese on it. I can hear you moaning, yuck! Stop that—it's very tasty. Cottage cheese is bland, and it will take on the taste of the cookie. It will also stop the sugar in the cookie from hitting your bloodstream so hard that you wake up insulin and the fat storing mechanism.

Another way to have your cake, cheesecake, pie, cookie, or ice cream (pick one) is to have it after an Energy Balance dinner. Why? Because the dinner slows down the dessert's sugar so you won't have an insulin rush. A small dish of ice cream would be your best bet, as it is slow to be digested and slow to enter your bloodstream. Ice cream is made from milk and has protein, carbohydrate, and fat, which is a pretty good balance.

When eating dessert at a restaurant, try sharing the dessert with your companion. That way you'll automatically limit your portion and still signal your brain that the meal is finished.

## VEGETARIAN TIPS

Vegetarians need to focus on including more quality complete proteins in their diets. Many vegetarian's diets are very high in carbohydrate and low in protein, causing their blood sugars to rise quickly and then drop just as fast.

There are a variety of ways to Energy Balance a vegetarian diet.

➤ Eat carbohydrates from the low-sugar, slow-insulin-release food group.
➤ Limit rice, pasta, and bread products.
➤ Get protein from eggs, beans, nuts, and low-fat dairy products.
➤ Tofu and soy products such as soy milk are excellent sources of protein and phytoestrogens, plant estrogens that aid in the midlife transition.
➤ Try soy "meat" products that contain less than 3 to 4 grams of carbohydrate.
➤ Keep your carbohydrate intake below 30 grams per meal and 20 grams per snack.

## FAST FOOD

Fast food is a health disaster waiting to happen, but you can eat anywhere and still stay in the Energy Balance. The biggest challenge today is the size of fast-food offerings, so keep in mind your serving size when ordering.

Rather than site specific foods, instead keep in mind the type of foods that traditionally contain the Core Four of nutrition:

➤ Order your sandwiches without the mayonnaise, tartar sauce, or special sauce to cut calories and fat.
➤ Order food that is grilled or broiled. Avoid food that is breaded or fried.
➤ Hold the cheese and opt for vegetables, such as lettuce, tomato, and onion.
➤ Use light or fat free dressing on salads and order it on the side.
➤ Don't drink your calories—avoid sugary sodas and milkshakes.

➤ At the salad bar, avoid premade dishes that contain mayonnaise or oil and instead fill up on fresh fruits and vegetables.
➤ Order pizza topped with vegetables instead of meat.

## IT'S PARTY TIME

These are helpful tips for staying in the Energy Balance and partying down at the same time.

➤ Eat an Energy Balance snack before you go to the event.
➤ At a buffet, eat shrimp, crab, or any other protein source you enjoy. Then add a little cheese and a few crackers.
➤ If you are going to drink, have a white wine spritzer (white wine and sparkling water in a tall glass with a twist of lemon). This drink takes longer to drink, and you are hydrating yourself at the same time.
➤ Try to stay sober. Once you've had too much to drink, you will eat everything in sight. If you do, dust yourself off and get back in the Energy Balance with your next meal.
➤ Drink a glass of water with a slice of lemon every hour.

## FINE DINING

When enjoying a meal in a restaurant, ask that the breadbasket be brought with the meal. Order a shrimp cocktail right away if you are starving. Now, for dinner:

➤ Small Caesar or dinner salad
➤ Fish, meat, or poultry (If they bring a huge piece, eat 1/2 and take the rest home.)
➤ Vegetables and 1/2 potato with a little butter or sour cream
➤ 1/2 dinner roll or 1 slice sourdough bread
➤ 1/2 a dessert
➤ Small decaf latte or coffee

## CHECK YOUR ENERGY BALANCE ALL DAY LONG

This test enables you to see what foods work best in your daily meal planning. In a chart like the one below, write down the food you eat, what time you eat it, and how you feel two to three hours later. If you were at a 1-3 hunger level, repeat that meal. It was in the Energy Balance and you will want to keep it. If you were in the 4-6 category, you didn't have enough protein in relationship to your carbohydrate or you didn't have enough fat. If you were in the "I'm starving" 7-10 category, you didn't eat in the Energy Balance at all. Rethink that choice.

After doing this exercise for a week or two, you will have a good idea of the foods that give you energy and the foods that take it away. This is how you will build your own arsenal of foods and meals that keep you in the Energy Balance.

|           | FOOD | TIME | HUNGER LEVEL 1-10 |
|-----------|------|------|-------------------|
| Breakfast |      |      |                   |
| Snack     |      |      |                   |
| Lunch     |      |      |                   |
| Snack     |      |      |                   |
| Dinner    |      |      |                   |
| Snack     |      |      |                   |

## HOW TO FOOL YOUR KIDS INTO EATING IN THE ENERGY BALANCE

Fooling kids into eating better is not an easy job. Take a look at any kids' menu in a restaurant. What are the food choices? Mostly fat and carbohydrate with macaroni and cheese, spaghetti and meatballs, grilled cheese sandwiches, hot dogs, hamburgers, French fries, malts, Cokes, hot chocolate, and other unhealthy food combinations. How, then, do you make this food healthier and still enable your children to eat with the rest of the world? I know parents who've tried to restrict these foods and failed miserably. When you restrict a child's food choices, you might be making the restricted foods more tempting. Remember that we don't want to make food the enemy.

Start with a smaller portion. When your child is finished, if he wants more give him an even smaller portion. This will enable you to control the size and amount without making him feel like you are denying him anything. This will also enable children to tap into their own unique hunger limits.

### Macaroni and cheese

**HOME** Use 1 ounce low-fat cheese with 1 ounce of regular cheddar cheese, and 1/2 cup cooked macaroni. Mix in a lot of the child's favorite vegetables and a breast of chicken chopped into fine pieces. This combo will make all the food taste better and the child will feel like she is eating her favorite food.

**RESTAURANT** Order macaroni and cheese and a side of chicken. Chop up the chicken and mix it into the macaroni and cheese. With this balance, your child won't eat as much, and the combination of fat and protein will slow down the macaroni as it hits the bloodstream.

## Spaghetti and Meatballs

**HOME** The goal here is to make the meal more protein heavy than carbohydrate heavy. Make a small amount of pasta with low-sugar tomato sauce and low-fat turkey meatballs. If your child doesn't like the turkey and wants beef, combine 1/2 lean ground beef and 1/2 ground turkey. Make small meatballs that kids can eat in one bite.

**RESTAURANT** When eating spaghetti and meatballs in a restaurant, it is more difficult to control the amount of fat and carbohydrate. The only thing you can do is limit how much he eats. So insist on a salad first. When the order arrives, your child may be more satisfied and not eat as much. If you can get him to eat more meat and less spaghetti, it will at least help lessen the insulin hit.

## Grilled Cheese Sandwich

**HOME** This is a tough one; however, it is possible to make it a little healthier. Use a butter-flavor vegetable cooking spray and spray the pan generously. Then, take a small amount of butter and coat the pan. Place 2 pieces of whole wheat bread in the pan and place 1 slice regular cheese and 1 slice low-fat or fat-free cheese on top of the bread. Cook until melted, place one piece on top of the other, and make a sandwich. Serve with a small fruit salad and 1/2 cup cottage cheese.

**RESTAURANT** When ordering this sandwich, ask them to use only 1/2 the cheese they would normally use. See if they could put a small chicken breast in the sandwich when grilling it. If this is not possible, you might get your child to split the sandwich with you and then split a salad with low-fat dressing.

## Hot Dogs

**HOME** Choose chicken or turkey and use a whole wheat bun. Let your child put his own condiments on the hot dog, including relish, onion, mustard, etc. Serve with a piece of low-sugar fruit such as a sliced apple.

**RESTAURANT** As the saying goes, "Just do it." The saving grace of a hot dog is that it has protein, fat, and carbohydrate in the same meal. Don't add any other high-fat, high-carbohydrate food to this meal because it's a deadly combination for insulin production and fat storage.

## Hamburgers

**HOME** For this staple of the American kid diet, use low-fat meat or make turkey burgers. Definitely cook French fries, but limit the portion.

**RESTAURANT** Order the hamburger well-done and ask for the mayonnaise on the side. Cut the burger in half and serve half to your child with a portion of French fries. If possible, add a small dinner salad before the hamburger, with the dressing on the side.

## Pizza

**HOME** When making pizza at home, cook a thin crust with lots of chicken and vegetables and a combo of regular and low-fat cheeses.

**RESTAURANT** Order a pizza with a thin crust, chicken, vegetables, and a small amount of cheese. Let your child have two pieces with a small salad.

With all this in mind, let's get started!

# Getting Started

**M**INUTES OF MOVEMENT A DAY—with this small investment, you'll be able to do more on a daily basis, like take longer walks or play more actively with your kids. The Fit Forever concept is designed to be easy, with fitness and food that work with your life, not against it.

But good health is sneaky—the more you do, the more you'll want and be able to do. With that in mind, the program begins with fundamental movements and dietary guidelines to get you started on the path to better health. As the days and weeks progress, the meals will vary and movements will be added to target key muscle groups. But there is no need to follow the program exactly. If you like a movement or a meal from one day, substitute it for something you don't enjoy on another day. To aid in creating a program that works for you, the end of the book includes a blank chart that will enable you to make up your own routine.

When exercising, flexibility or range of motion is determined by a number of factors, including the genetic make up of each joint, tendon, ligaments, bones and bony structures, as well as your age and daily activity. However, you can improve the range of motion of any joint by consistently stretching every day. I recommend static stretching, or holding a stretch for at least 20 to 30 seconds and release. Don't bounce or pulse because, in the untrained athlete, it could tear a muscle.

While most of the movements in the following days don't need equipment, I have suggested a few exercises that employ a resistance band or a Balance Ball, both of which can be found in sporting goods stores.

I recommend a resistance band because, when employed in place of weights, it provides resistance both on the first part and on the recovery phase of the exercise.

A Balance Ball workout is a highly effective and safe way to exercise. Although it looks like a toy, the Balance Ball is based on sound scientific principles that maximize muscle coordination, strength, and flexibility. A large ball for exercise was used in the 1950s in Switzerland to restore patients', motor skills after serious injuries. Today the exercises are recommended by personal trainers and physical therapists to strengthen the torso muscles in the back, abdomen, legs, and buttocks. I recommend the 65-cm ball for all of the exercises in this book, which is also often the best size when used as a desk chair.

Also included in the program are recipes that integrate the Core Four of nutrition: protein, carbohydrate, fat, and fiber. Most of the recipes are for a single serving. If your family is joining you in changing your eating habits, just multiply the ingredients by the number of people being served.

If you don't have access to a kitchen during the day, some of the meals and snacks need to be made in advance.

After each recipe, the average grams of the protein, carbohydrate, fat, and fiber per recipe is detailed based on the highest nutrient number in the food. For example, 1/2 cup cottage cheese has 14 grams of protein, 4 grams of carbohydrate, and 3 to 5 grams of fat. Because its largest nutrient number is protein, cottage cheese would be counted as a protein source. Don't worry about the other numbers—just use common sense. If you combine protein, complex carbohydrate, fat, and fiber into a meal, you will not be hungry. In 30 days, this way of eating will give you so much energy it will become part of your life.

# DAY 1

## WAKE-UP AFFIRMATION

**"Do not let what you cannot do interfere with what you can do."**

—*John Wooden, NCAA basketball coach*

## WAKE-UP WORKOUT

(See "A Body in Motion" chapter)

1. Let body slowly wake up
2. Take several deep breaths
3. Full-body tighten and release
4. Pelvic tilts
5. Pillow sit-ups
6. Hamstring stretch
7. Hands and knees yoga stretch

## CORE FOUR

(See "A Body in Motion" chapter)

1. Push-up
2. Sit-up
3. Sit and stand
4. Posture squeeze/biceps curl

## PORTION CONTROL TIP

Buy 4 or 5 tablespoons and keep them handy to familiarize yourself with that serving size and ensure that your portions are truly a tablespoon.

## ENERGY BALANCE BREAKFAST

Eggs, Toast, and Lox

1 egg and 1 egg white
Light vegetable cream cheese or trans-fat-free margarine
1 slice whole-grain bread (2 to 5 grams of fiber per slice)
2 ounces smoked salmon

1. Scramble the eggs.
2. Spread the cream cheese or margarine on toasted bread.
3. Place the smoked salmon on the toast and top with the eggs.

➤ If you want a larger meal: Increase to 3 egg whites and 1 whole egg.and have 2 slices whole-grain bread.

Drink water with lemon or 4 ounces of juice and 6 ounces of water, plus decaffeinated tea or coffee, if desired. Add low-fat creamer to taste.

| CORE FOUR APPROXIMATE BREAKDOWN | PROTEIN<br>➤ whole egg: 6 grams<br>➤ egg white: 3 1/2 grams<br>➤ salmon: 10 grams<br>CARBOHYDRATE<br>➤ slice of bread: 13 to 15 grams (depending on the size of the slice) | FAT<br>➤ egg yolk: 5 grams<br>➤ salmon: 4 grams of heart-healthy omega-3 oil<br>➤ light cream cheese or trans-fat-free margarine: 2 to 4 grams<br>FIBER<br>➤ slice of bread: 2 to 5 grams |
| --- | --- | --- |

## TAKE 10
Sit and hold

This knee bend will firm and shape the fronts of the thighs and the buttocks. You will also feel increased breathing and heart rates, indicating that you are conditioning your heart muscle and burning a small amount of fat.

1. Hold on to a steady surface with both hands for balance and sit back into a squat position.
2. Standing with your knees and feet pointed forward, sit back far enough so that your knees are directly over your heels. (If your knees are over your toes, there is too much pressure on your knees.)
3. Hold for a second and stand up. Repeat 10 times.

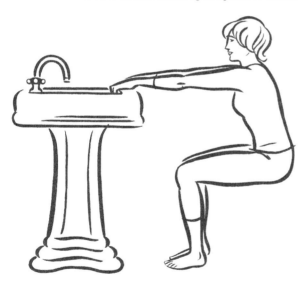

## SIT AND BE FIT
C is for crunch

Perfect for when you're seated in a chair or in your car stopped at a traffic light, this isometric hold and release will slowly condition your abdominals and help strengthen your lower back.

1. Lift your rib cage, straighten your back, and keep your shoulders back and down.
2. Contract your abdominals and push your back against the seat. It should feel as if you are making the letter C with your upper body.
3. Hold for about 5 seconds and release. Repeat 5 to 10 times, depending on your time constraints.

## WATER BREAK
Drinking water instead of soda or other sweetened beverages means you won't load up on excess calories and carbohydrates. Plus, the caffeine found in some sodas has a diuretic effect, which can upset the kidneys' ability to manage internal water balance.

## ENERGY BALANCE SNACK
Fruit and Cheese

1 small piece of your favorite fruit or half a small can of light fruit cocktail

1/2 cup low-fat cottage cheese or low-fat ricotta cheese

Sprinkle of sunflower seeds

CORE FOUR APPROXIMATE BREAKDOWN

**PROTEIN**
➤ cottage cheese: 14 grams
➤ ricotta cheese: 12 grams

**CARBOHYDRATE**
➤ fruit or light fruit cocktail: 12 to 15 grams

**FAT**
➤ cottage cheese: 2 1/2 grams
➤ ricotta cheese: 6 grams
➤ sunflower seeds: 3 grams

**FIBER**
➤ skin of the fruit: 2 to 5 grams
➤ sunflower seeds: 1 gram

# WATER BREAK

Water aids digestion, helps regulate body temperature, and serves as a natural appetite suppressant.

# ENERGY LIFT

## Fidgets

1. Squirm in your chair, moving your body in a haphazard motion for 20 seconds.
2. Circle each foot a few times, shrug your shoulders, release, and repeat.
3. Rock your body from side to side and bounce your heels on the floor (basically, do everything you were told as a child not to do) for 20 seconds.

# ENERGY BALANCE LUNCH

## DINING IN

### Chicken Caesar Salad

    3 cups lettuce
    1 cup chopped broiled chicken breast
    10 fat-free medium-size croutons
    1 tablespoon fat-free Caesar dressing
    1 tablespoon regular Caesar dressing
    1 small piece whole wheat pita bread

1. Cut up the lettuce.
2. Put the chicken and croutons in a bowl with the lettuce.
3. Toss with fat-free Caesar and regular Caesar dressing, which makes both taste better and cuts the fat in half.
4. Eat with the pita bread.

## DINING OUT

Order a Caesar salad with chicken, but ask for the dressing on the side. Dip your fork into the dressing, then take a bite of salad. If you like your salad tossed, ask for a light to medium amount of dressing. Take most of the croutons out of the salad.

➤If you want a larger meal: Add a decaf, nonfat latte.

| CORE FOUR APPROXIMATE BREAKDOWN | PROTEIN ➤ chicken: 15 to 20 grams CARBOHYDRATE ➤ lettuce: 4 to 6 grams ➤ croutons: 10 grams ➤ pita bread: 12 to 15 grams | FAT ➤ Caesar dressing: 10 to 18 grams FIBER ➤ lettuce: 2 grams ➤ pita bread: 2 to 3 grams |
| --- | --- | --- |

# SIT AND BE FIT

## Shoulder shrugs

This exercise will not only relieve tension, it will help strengthen your upper trapezius muscles. These muscles help support your head and neck, which can cramp or ache when you sit for long periods or are stressed and overly tired.

1. Sit in a chair, lift your chest, contract your abdominals, press your shoulders back and down, align your head and spine, and face forward.
2. Take a deep breath through your nose and allow your lungs to fill with air. Exhale through your mouth.
3. Lift your shoulders toward your ears as high as you can, hold for a second, and release.
4. Do as many as needed to increase circulation in the upper neck and release tension.

# WATER BREAK

In an average day, you can lose up to 3 liters of water through perspiration, your lungs, and urine. If you exercise or it's a very hot day, water loss can be significantly higher and may lead to dehydration. Replenish your stores right now with a large glass.

# ENERGY LIFT
## Up, down, and out

This little routine will help lift your energy for the rest of the day while also speeding up your circulation and raising your metabolism. It will also tone and strengthen your hips, buttocks, thighs, and lower legs.

1. **STAND AND SIT 10 TIMES** Place your feet at a comfortable and stable distance from your chair. Slowly stand up and squeeze your buttocks, release, and sit down. If you need help balancing, hold on to a table, a desk, or the back of another chair.
2. **LEG EXTENSIONS** Sit on the edge of your chair and hold on to the side of the chair with both hands. Slowly lift and extend your right leg in front of you and tighten the muscles on top of your thigh. Hold for a second and release. Do that side 10 times and then repeat with your left leg. This will help strengthen your thighs and your knees.
3. **HEEL LIFTS** Kick off your shoes, sit on the edge of your chair, and put your feet firmly on the floor. Keeping your toes on the floor, lift your heels as high as you can, hold for a second, and release. Do this 10 times. Now lift and lower your heels rapidly. This will help bring circulation to your lower extremities and firm and tone your calves. Take a deep, cleansing breath and move on to the next exercise.

4. **OVERHEAD ARM PUNCHES** Sit tall, lift your rib cage, and breathe deeply. Punch your arms overhead, left, right, left, right, continuously for 15 to 30 seconds. This will raise your heart rate and increase circulation to your upper neck area. If you suffer from any upper back or neck problems, punch straight in front of you. Any time you use your arms in an exercise, you raise your heart rate by approximately 10 beats per minute, which means extra calories burned.

# WATER BREAK

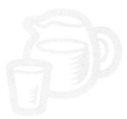

If you just can't stand to drink another drop of water, try decaffeinated tea or calorie- and sugar-free drink mixes or a mixture of both. But try to have less than two glasses of aspartame-sweetened drinks a day, since they can make you hungrier by imitating sugar. Your body doesn't recognize the difference between real sugar and artificial sugar and releases insulin, which clears the bloodstream of fat and sugar and stores them as fat. This process lowers your blood sugar, making you hungry faster.

# ENERGY BALANCE SNACK
## Crackers and Cheese

5 whole-grain crackers
2 ounces low-fat cheese or 2 tablespoons hummus

| CORE FOUR APPROXIMATE BREAKDOWN | PROTEIN<br>➤ low-fat cheese: 10 to 14 grams<br>➤ hummus: 5 grams<br><br>CARBOHYDRATE<br>➤ crackers: 10 to 15 grams | FAT<br>➤ low-fat cheese: 5 grams<br>➤ hummus: 5 grams<br><br>FIBER<br>➤ crackers: 1 to 3 grams |
|---|---|---|

## TAKE 10
### Just walk away

Take a ten-minute walk. Believe it or not, you always have the time. Just walk out the door, note the time, and walk for five little minutes, then return. This exercise is perfect before dinner because moderate exercise has an appetite-decreasing effect.

## WATER BREAK

If a full bladder wakes you up during the night, stop drinking water two hours before you go to bed.

## ENERGY BALANCE DINNER

### DINING IN
### Simply Stir-fry

> 6 to 8 ounces chicken breast, diced, or 6 shrimp or 6 to 8 ounces firm tofu, diced
>
> 2 1/2 cups chopped vegetables (try broccoli and red bell peppers)
>
> 1 tablespoon olive oil
>
> 2 tablespoons chicken broth
>
> 1 tablespoon soy sauce
>
> 1 tablespoon dry Sherry
>
> 1 teaspoon cornstarch
>
> 1/2 cup brown rice, cooked

1. Sauté the chicken, shrimp or tofu with the vegetables in a nonstick skillet in olive oil over high heat until tender.
2. Mix together the broth, soy sauce, sherry, and cornstarch until the cornstarch is dissolved.
3. Add to the chicken and stir at high heat until thickened (about 1 minute).
4. Serve over rice.

### DINING OUT

Order stir-fried chicken or lean beef with 1/2 cup brown rice.

➤If you want a larger meal increase the vegetables to 3 to 4 cups and the chicken, shrimp or tofu 2 more ounces.

| CORE FOUR APPROXIMATE BREAKDOWN | PROTEIN<br>➤ chicken or shrimp: 20 to 28 grams<br>➤ tofu: 14 to 20 grams<br>CARBOHYDRATE<br>➤ vegetables: 8 to 10 grams<br>➤ rice: 20 to 30 grams | FAT<br>➤ olive oil: 14 grams of heart-healthy fat<br>FIBER<br>➤ vegetables: 6 to 10 grams<br>➤ rice: 2 to 5 grams |
| --- | --- | --- |

## ENERGY BALANCE SNACK
### Yogurt Parfait

> 4 ounces nonfat, low-sugar yogurt (no more than 11 grams of carbohydrate per serving )
>
> 2 ounces low-fat cottage cheese
>
> 1/2 cup strawberries
>
> 2 tablespoons fat-free whipped topping
>
> Sprinkle of chopped walnuts

Layer first four ingredients in a parfait glass and top with walnuts.

| CORE FOUR APPROXIMATE BREAKDOWN | PROTEIN<br>➤ yogurt: 4 grams<br>➤ cottage cheese: 7 grams<br>CARBOHYDRATE<br>➤ yogurt: 11 grams<br>➤ strawberries: 6 grams | FAT<br>➤ walnuts: 6 to 8 grams<br>FIBER<br>➤ strawberries: 1 gram |
| --- | --- | --- |

## STRETCH, RELAX, AND SLEEP

1. Chest/posture stretch
2. Neck and upper spine stretch
3. Lower spine stretch

## HELPFUL HINT

Don't exercise too vigorously in the evening. It could raise your heart rate and blood pressure, giving you too much energy at the time when you need to calm down and relax.

# We Protect What We Love

I F YOUR HOUSE WERE ON FIRE, what would you try to save? Everyone answers this question a bit differently, depending on what we value. Certainly we'd all save our loved ones and our pets—but think of the "things" you'd rescue from the fire. Maybe you'd dash through the flames for the photo albums where you keep your children's baby pictures, or for the modern art piece you just hung in the living room. Would you endure the blaze for the 1852 edition of *Scottish Chiefs* entrusted to you by your uncle, or make a dive for that emerald ring left to you by your grandmother? What about those yellowed letters from the love of your life you keep tied with a ribbon? Or maybe you're a practical kind of woman and would head straight for the back-up discs on your computer table.

We protect what we love. Our behavior gives us away. As instinctively as we'd react in an emergency to salvage our most valued possessions, we demonstrate how highly (or lowly) we regard ourselves by how well we protect and care for our own bodies on a daily basis. Protest all you will. Words are cheap, but our actions tell the real story. If we value ourselves, we eat with intention, we move with regularity, make time for rejuvenating sleep, and take action to release and decrease the stress in our lives. If we don't value ourselves, we don't.

Starting this program is the perfect way to demonstrate that your self esteem has grown past your current behavior patterns. You love yourself enough to gather new information and commit to creating more affirming life patterns. That's terrific!

In the days ahead, at some moment you will groan, "Oh, this is tooooo hard!" (and you will groan, I'm certain of it). Remember today when you knew you loved yourself enough to change. In a very real sense, you are saving your own body from a burning building by taking the steps necessary to prolong your years of healthy, productive living. Congratulations and welcome to the program!

# DAY 2

## WAKE-UP AFFIRMATION

"Out of the strain of the doing, into the peace of done."

—*Julia Louise Woodruff, writer*

## WAKE-UP WORKOUT

**1.** Let body slowly wake up
**2.** Take several deep breaths
**3.** Full-body tighten and release
**4.** Pelvic tilts
**5.** Pillow sit-ups
**6.** Hamstring stretch
**7.** Hands and knees yoga stretch

## CORE FOUR

**1.** Push-up
**2.** Sit-up
**3.** Sit and stand
**4.** Posture squeeze/biceps curl

## PORTION CONTROL TIP

A four- to six-ounce portion of meat, fish, or chicken is about the size of an average adult's hand.

## ENERGY BALANCE BREAKFAST

### Bagel with Cream Cheese and Lox

1 small whole-grain bagel
1 to 2 tablespoons light flavored cream cheese
3 ounces lox, turkey, or cottage cheese
1 slice tomato

**1.** Spread the cream cheese on the bagel.
**2.** Top with the lox and tomato and enjoy.

➤ If you want a larger meal add 1 scrambled egg and 2 egg whites.

Drink water with lemon or 4 ounces of juice and 6 ounces of water, plus decaffeinated tea or coffee, if desired. Add low-fat creamer to taste.

### CORE FOUR APPROXIMATE BREAKDOWN

| PROTEIN | FAT |
|---|---|
| ➤ lox: 15 grams | ➤ lox: 6 grams |
| ➤ turkey: 15 grams | ➤ cream cheese: 2 to 4 grams |
| ➤ cottage cheese: 10 grams | ➤ egg yolk: 5 grams |
| ➤ 1 egg: 6 grams | **FIBER** |
| ➤ 1 egg white: 3 1/2 grams | ➤ bagel: 1 to 5 grams |
| **CARBOHYDRATE** | |
| ➤ small bagel: 30 grams, large bagel: 45 to 50 grams. If you choose a large bagel, eat only half. | |

## TAKE 10

### Ballet bend

This exercise will improve your balance and strengthen the muscles involved in everyday activities such as standing and walking. The stabilizing muscles being worked are the abdominals and lower back. The muscles being strengthened are the fronts of the thighs and the buttocks.

**1.** Stand with your feet hip distance apart, toes pointing out. Bend your knees slightly, lift your chest, contract your abdominals, press your shoulders back and down, align your head and spine, and face forward.
**2.** Look in a mirror to ensure proper alignment of your spine and torso.

3. Hold on to a countertop with one hand for balance.
4. Inhale while bending your knees over your heels (make sure your knees do not go past your toes!), as you lower your buttocks toward the floor.
5. Hold for two seconds while slightly squeezing your buttocks.
6. Exhale as you return to a standing position. Repeat 10 times.

## SIT AND BE FIT
### Posture pull and stretch

These contract-and-release movements will help stretch and strengthen your back and upper neck.

1. Sit on a chair with both feet on the floor and lift your chest, contract your abdominals, press your shoulders back and down, align your head and spine, and face forward.
2. Inhale and squeeze your shoulder blades together, hold for a second, exhale, and then release.
3. Clasp your hands in front of your chest, palms facing each other, as if you are praying.
4. Inhale as you push your arms straight out in front of your body as far as possible but no higher than shoulder level, palms up, and exhale, tightening your stomach muscles and feeling a slight stretch in your back. Allow your head to drop forward, breathe naturally, and hold as long as comfortable.
5. Repeat both movements 4 times.

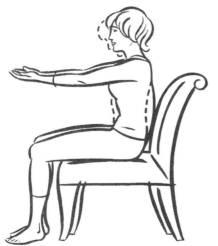

## WATER BREAK

Try herbal, green, or black tea, preferably decaffeinated. Research has found that both green and black teas have antioxidants that are heart healthy.

## ENERGY BALANCE SNACK
### Energy Bar

Half of an energy bar with at least 10 grams of protein and 1 gram of fiber and no more than 6 grams of fat, 22 grams of carbohydrate, and 220 calories.

## WATER BREAK

Research shows that inadequate water intake is a major factor in the development of kidney stones. Stop the stones with a drink right now!

## ENERGY LIFT
### Standing calf raise

This calf raise helps prevent poor circulation to your lower extremities; it will also improve your balance by strengthening your calf muscles and improving your ankle stability. The stronger your calves and lower legs the greater your balance.

1. Hold on to a chair for balance. Stand with your feet hip distance apart. Bend your knees slightly, lift your chest, contract your abdominals, press your shoulders back and down, align your head and spine, and face forward.
2. Take a deep breath and exhale as you rise up on your toes as high as you can without letting your ankles roll inward or outward. Feel the contraction in your calf muscles.
3. Inhale and lower your heels back to the floor. Make sure you don't bounce, and use controlled movements to isolate your calf muscles.
4. Do 2 sets of 12 times each.

As you become stronger, and if you have access to stairs, you can get a more challenging lift and stretch by standing on the balls of your feet at the edge of a step and then lowering your heels to just a little below parallel. Don't press down too far at first, as your Achilles tendon may not be ready for this much extension, and you could overstretch it.

# ENERGY BALANCE LUNCH

## DINING IN

### Salsa Pita

1 tablespoon low-fat mayonnaise
1 tablespoon prepared salsa
2 tablespoons diced red bell peppers
1 tablespoon fresh cilantro
1/2 cup diced cooked smoked turkey
1 small piece whole-grain pita bread
Shredded lettuce

1. Mix together the mayonnaise, salsa, red peppers, and cilantro.
2. Add the turkey, mix until coated.
3. Stuff the mixture into the pita and top with the shredded lettuce.

## DINING OUT

Ask for any turkey, tuna, or chicken stuffed pita with mayonnaise, lettuce, and tomato. If pita pocket bread is not available then place sandwich fillings on whole grain bread.

➤ If you want a larger meal: Add a 1 1-ounce stick of string cheese.

| CORE FOUR APPROXIMATE BREAKDOWN | PROTEIN ➤ chicken: 20 grams CARBOHYDRATE ➤ pita bread: 15 to 20 grams FAT ➤ low-fat mayonnaise: 2 to 4 grams ➤ string cheese: 6 grams | FIBER ➤ pita bread: 1 to 2 grams ➤ lettuce, tomato, bell peppers: 1 to 2 grams |
|---|---|---|

# SIT AND BE FIT
## Thumbs up

This exercise will increase the range of motion in the shoulder rotation, strengthen the rotator cuffs, and improve the stability of the shoulder joints.

1. Sit with your arms at your sides, thumbs pointing inward toward your hips. Lift your chest, contract your abdominals, press your shoulders back and down, align your head and spine, and face forward.
2. Inhale and slowly exhale as you raise your arms up and out to your sides. As you lift, keep your elbows slightly bent and your thumbs should be pointing down.
3. When your arms are at shoulder height, slowly rotate your thumbs to point toward the ceiling; the movement comes only from the rotation of your shoulders.
4. Hold for 5 seconds and release to initial position.
5. Repeat 12 to 15 times.

# WATER BREAK

Some people believe that drinking a lot of water will make them look bloated. The opposite is true: Drinking water helps to release salt and other waste, decreasing bloating.

# ENERGY LIFT
## Squat and lift

This exercise will improve your posture and balance and strengthen and stabilize your torso. You will use your abdominals and buttocks to stabilize your torso, which will help protect your lower back from injury.

1. Stand up straight, your legs hip distance apart. Bend your knees slightly, lift your chest, contract your abdominals, press your shoulders back and down, align your head and spine, and face forward. Place your hands on the back of a chair or on a table for balance.
2. In your squat, make sure your knees are over your heels, not over your toes.
3. Inhale as you straighten your legs and shift your weight onto your right foot. Exhale and tighten your buttocks, lifting your left leg out to the side, no higher than 45 degrees. Keep your supporting leg slightly bent and don't bend your torso to the side as you lift.
4. Inhale as you return to the starting position.
5. Repeat on the other side, then repeat 4 more times on each side. As this becomes easier, add more repetitions.

## WATER BREAK

A 2 percent loss of body fluid affects short-term memory, so don't forget to drink up.

## ENERGY BALANCE SNACK

An Apple a Day

> 1 small apple, sliced
> 1 tablespoon peanut butter or 1 ounce low-fat sharp cheddar cheese

Spread the peanut butter or put a slice of cheese on the sliced apple.

| CORE FOUR APPROXIMATE BREAKDOWN | PROTEIN<br>➤ peanut butter: 4 grams<br>➤ cheese: 6 grams<br>CARBOHYDRATE<br>➤ apple: 20 to 25 grams | FAT<br>➤ peanut butter: 7 grams<br>➤ cheese: 6 grams<br>FIBER<br>➤ apple: 2 grams |
| --- | --- | --- |

## TAKE 10

Knee lifts

This exercise will help raise your metabolism, burn fat, and increase the overall health and strength of your heart and lungs.

1. Stand up straight, with your feet shoulder width apart. Bend your knees slightly, lift your chest, contract your abdominals, press your shoulder back and down, align your head and spine, and face forward.
2. Hold on to a chair or table for balance if needed.
3. Lift your right knee toward your abdomen and exhale. Keep your hips level and still.
4. Return to initial position and inhale.
5. Lift the other leg and repeat. Continue for a count of 10 on each side or until your breathing rate has increased, allowing more oxygen into your lungs.
6. Rest for a moment and do 2 more sets.

## WATER BREAK

Water drinkers tend to eat less because the fluid fills the stomach, taking the edge off hunger.

## ENERGY BALANCE DINNER

### DINING IN

Beef Fajitas

4 to 6 ounces lean beef

1 cup mixed chopped bell peppers, zucchini, onions, and tomatoes

2 tablespoons olive or canola oil

1/4 teaspoon each cumin, paprika, garlic powder, coriander, and chili powder

2 small or 1 large whole wheat tortilla

2 tablespoons salsa

1. Sauté the beef and vegetables in oil in a non-stick skillet, over medium heat until tender.
2. Drain the fat and add the spices.
3. Roll the cooked beef and vegetables in the tortilla and top with the salsa.

### DINING OUT

Order lean-beef fajita. Eat the meat and vegetables and two small spoonfuls of the beans and rice.

➤ If you want a larger meal: Increase the meat to 8 ounces.

| CORE FOUR APPROXIMATE BREAKDOWN | PROTEIN ➤ beef: 15 to 20 grams CARBOHYDRATE ➤ tortillas: 30 grams ➤ salsa: 4 grams FAT ➤ olive or canola oil: 15 grams | FIBER ➤ vegetables: 5 to 10 grams ➤ tortillas: 3 to 5 grams |
| --- | --- | --- |

## ENERGY BALANCE SNACK

Crackers and Cheese

4 whole-grain crackers

1 1-ounce stick string cheese

| CORE FOUR APPROXIMATE BREAKDOWN | PROTEIN ➤ string cheese: 6 grams CARBOHYDRATE ➤ crackers: 12 grams | FAT ➤ string cheese: 7 grams FIBER ➤ crackers: 1 to 2 grams |
| --- | --- | --- |

## STRETCH, RELAX, AND SLEEP

1. Chest/posture stretch
2. Neck and upper spine stretch
3. Lower spine stretch

## STRESS RELIEF TIP

Get seven to eight hours of sleep a night. Chronic lack of sleep leads to the inability to handle stress. To ensure the deepest sleep, try some of the following tips:

➤ Go to bed at the same time each night.
➤ Make your bedroom dark and quiet.
➤ If noises wake you up at night, buy a white-noise machine that drowns out other sounds.
➤ Empty your head before going to bed: Write your concerns, goals, and dreams in a journal.
➤ Take a warm bath and use aromatherapy herbs that relax and calm the nerves.

# Drink to Serenity

STRESSED? NERVOUS? Maybe even have a panic attack now and then? Along with adding exercise to your daily routine, one of the best ways to manage stress is to drink yourself to serenity. You will assist your body in coping with anxiety if you:

➤ **DRINK WATER.** That sounds simple, but honestly… how much do you drink each day? Our bodies need between two and three liters of water every single day. That's a lot of liquid. Most of us wait until we're thirsty before we reach for a glass of water. However, when you feel thirsty, you are already dehydrated and dehydration makes it harder for your body to cope with stress. In fact, the lack of water can be a cause of anxiety. So keep a drink with you at all times and partake before that dry mouth lets you know you've waited too long.

➤ **CUT THE CAFFEINE.** I used to be a nervous wreck. I also used to drink two or three colas with every meal, and a few more during the day as snacks. My doctor strongly suggested I cut all caffeine from my diet. Amazing results! Without caffeine to overstimulate me on the inside, I discovered the stresses on the outside were much more manageable. You'll feel much calmer if you replace coffee, cola, or tea with iced or hot caffeine-free beverages that soothe rather than rev up your nervous system.

➤ **NIX THE ALCOHOL.** After a hard day at work or looking after the kids, is it tempting to pour yourself a glass of wine or something stronger to unwind? Since alcohol is a depressant, many people rely on it's dampening effect to cope with daily demands. Although alcohol may decrease your immediate sense of anxiety, it can also limit your body's ability to cope with stress on an ongoing basis. Even one glass can trigger insomnia, thirst and dehydration. Rather than becoming dependent upon alcohol, create a healthy body that can cope effectively with stress. Less is more when it comes to alcohol.

# DAY 3

## WAKE-UP AFFIRMATION

"There are two ways of meeting difficulties. You alter the difficulties or you alter yourself to meet them."

—*Anonymous*

## WAKE-UP WORKOUT

1. Let body slowly wake up
2. Take several deep breaths
3. Full-body tighten and release
4. Pelvic tilts
5. Pillow sit-ups
6. Hamstring stretch
7. Hands and knees yoga stretch

## CORE FOUR

1. Push-up
2. Sit-up
3. Sit and stand
4. Posture squeeze/biceps curl

## PORTION CONTROL TIP

A whole bag of prepared lettuce has only 5 to 8 grams of carbohydrate, so fill up on salad, vegetables, and low-fat dressing.

## ENERGY BALANCE BREAKFAST

*Cheddar Veggie Omelette*

   1 whole egg and 3 egg whites
   2 tablespoons grated cheddar cheese
   1/2 cup chopped vegetables, such as tomatoes, broccoli, bell peppers, or spinach
   Pinch of salt, pepper, parsley, and tarragon
   1 to 2 tablespoons salsa
   1 small whole-grain English muffin
   1 tablespoon light cream cheese

1. Beat egg and egg whites.
2. Put a pan coated with nonfat cooking spray over medium heat. Once the pan is warm, pour the eggs into it.
3. While the eggs are cooking, sprinkle them with the cheese, vegetables, and spices. Once the eggs are fully cooked, fold over the eggs to make and omelette.
4. Top with salsa to taste.
5. Spread the cream cheese on the English muffin and serve with the omelette.

➤If you want a larger meal: Add 2 more egg whites and 2 more tablespoons cheese.

Drink water with lemon or 4 ounces of juice and 6 ounces of water, plus decaffeinated tea or coffee, if desired. Add low-fat creamer to taste.

| CORE FOUR APPROXIMATE BREAKDOWN | PROTEIN ➤ whole egg: 6 grams ➤ 1 egg white: 3 1/2 grams CARBOHYDRATE ➤ English muffin: 30 grams ➤ vegetables: 10 grams | FAT ➤ egg yolk: 5 grams ➤ cheese: 5 grams ➤ cream cheese: 2 grams FIBER ➤ vegetables: 5 to 10 grams ➤ English muffin: 1 to 2 grams |
|---|---|---|

# TAKE 10

Doorway chest stretch

Many back problems occur when the front of the body is too tight and the back of the body is not strong enough to support proper posture. This exercise will stretch both your chest and the fronts of your shoulders while aligning the muscles in your upper back.

1. Standing with feet hip distance apart, place your hands on either side of a doorway at shoulder height.
2. Keeping your chest and head up and your knees slightly bent, move your upper body forward until you feel a comfortable stretch in your arms and chest.
3. Breathing easily, hold this position for 15 to 30 seconds.
4. Release and repeat 2 times.

# SIT AND BE FIT

Posture squeeze

This exercise will not only promote muscular balance by strengthening the backs of your shoulders but it will improve your posture by strengthening your upper back.

1. Sit in a chair leaning slightly forward from the hips, contract your abdominals, press your shoulders back and down.
2. Keep your head in alignment with your spine and place a pillow on your lap to support your upper body and decrease stress on the back.
3. Let your arms hang down from your shoulders, with your palms facing in and your elbows slightly bent.
4. Inhale as you raise your arms out to the side and up to shoulder height, leading with your elbows (which remain slightly bent). As your arms trace an arc, keep your palms facing down and keep your wrists straight.

5. Exhale as you squeeze your shoulder blades together, hold, inhale, and then slowly lower your arms to starting position. Repeat 12 to 15 times. As you become stronger with this exercise, you may want to hold 3- to 5-pound weights to add greater resistance and improve progress.
6. When you are finished, give yourself a big hug by wrapping your arms around yourself. This final stretch works your upper back while releasing the muscles you have just used.

# WATER BREAK

In the evening, fill half a 32-ounce plastic bottle with water. Place it in the freezer overnight. In the morning fill the rest of the way with water. Now you will have fresh, cool water with you all day.

# ENERGY BALANCE SNACK

Tall Decaf Latte

8 ounces 1 percent milk, heated
Decaf espresso or coffee
Sprinkle of cinnamon

| CORE FOUR APPROXIMATE BREAKDOWN | PROTEIN ➤ milk: 9 grams | FAT ➤ milk: 3 grams |
| --- | --- | --- |
| | CARBOHYDRATE ➤ milk: 12 grams | FIBER ➤ 0 grams |

# WATER BREAK

Drinking water dilutes urine, which helps prevent the formation of salt crystals that can lead to kidney stones.

## ENERGY LIFT
### Raise and squat

This combination of a calf raise and a half squat helps prevent poor circulation to the lower extremities, improves your balance by strengthening the muscles of your calves and increasing ankle stability, and strengthens and shapes your upper thighs and buttocks. By using the larger muscles of the body, you will also stimulate fat burning.

1. Stand, holding on to a chair for balance. Place your feet hip distance apart, bend your knees slightly, lift your chest, contract your abdominals, press your shoulders back and down, align your head and spine, and face forward.
2. Take a deep breath and exhale as you rise up on your toes as high as you can without letting your ankles roll inward or outward. Feel the contraction in your calf muscles.
3. Inhale and lower your heels back to the floor. Make sure you don't bounce and use controlled movements to isolate your calf muscles.
4. Bend your knees over your toes as if you were sitting down. Hold for one second and return to the starting position. Do this combination of heel raise and knee bend 8 to 10 times. Take it easy and work up to 2 sets of 12 times each.

## ENERGY BALANCE LUNCH

### DINING IN
### Tuna Pasta Salad

    1/2 head romaine lettuce, washed and chopped
    3 ounces water-packed tuna, drained
    1 ounce cooked pasta
    2 tablespoons low-fat Caesar dressing
    1 tablespoon croutons
    1 tablespoon Parmesan cheese

1. Combine the tuna and pasta with the lettuce.
2. Toss with the Caesar dressing and top with the croutons and cheese.

### DINING OUT

Order a Caesar salad with chicken, shrimp, or tuna and a small amount of dressing or ask for it on the side and use sparingly. Add one slice of bread.

➤ If you want a larger meal: Add more lettuce and 2 ounces of tuna.

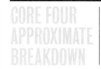

| CORE FOUR APPROXIMATE BREAKDOWN | PROTEIN<br>➤ Tuna: 20 to 25 grams<br>CARBOHYDRATE<br>➤ Pasta: 15 to 20 grams | FAT<br>➤ Dressing: 10 to 15 grams<br>FIBER<br>➤ Lettuce: 3 to 5 grams |
|---|---|---|

## SIT AND BE FIT
### Buttocks bounce and squeeze

This exercise will increase the range of motion in your waist and help release tension if you have been sitting for any length of time.

1. Begin seated with your arms at your sides. Lift your chest, contract your abdominals, press your shoulders back and down, align your head and spine, and face forward.
2. Inhale as you lift one arm up beside your head, with your elbow close to your ear and your palm facing the opposite wall.
3. Exhale as you reach over your head with a straight or bent arm and lean slightly to the arm's opposite side. Concentrate on reaching up and over. Make sure your buttocks and hips stay glued to the chair. Hold for 5 seconds and return to the starting position.
4. Repeat on the other side.
5. Continue, alternating sides, 8 to 10 times.
6. For the second part of this exercise, relax your upper body and squeeze and release your buttocks 30 times in rapid succession. This

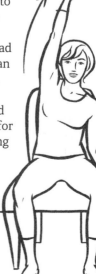

will help release tension in your lower back and bring circulation to and strengthen your buttocks.

## WATER BREAK

Drinking a large glass of water when taking aspirin, ibuprofen, or antibiotics such as tetracycline will hamper any stomach upset. The water disperses the medicine so it does not aggravate any one spot in your stomach.

## ENERGY LIFT

Side-to-side lunge

This exercise will not only strengthen both your inner and outer thighs but it will also help improve your balance.

1. Stand with your feet a little more than hip distance apart. Bend your knees slightly, lift your chest, contract your abdominals, press your shoulders back and down, align your head and spine, and face forward. Hold on to the back of a chair for balance.
2. Lunge to the right with your right leg and have your feet at about a 45-degree angle; make sure your knee does not pass your toes. This keeps the pressure off your knee and prevents injury.
3. Bring your leg back to the original position and lunge to the left with your left leg.
4. Keep the lunges small and make the movement somewhat fast paced.
5. Breathe evenly as you shift your weight from right to left.
6. Make sure you keep a lifted posture and don't lean forward.
7. This is an energy lift, so do as many as you can to raise your heart rate and improve your circulation.

## WATER BREAK

Hunger is often thirst in disguise, so drink before you eat.

## ENERGY BALANCE SNACK

Nuts

4 ounces natural almonds with no salt or oil

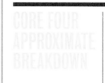

| CORE FOUR APPROXIMATE BREAKDOWN | PROTEIN<br>➤ 13 grams<br>CARBOHYDRATE<br>➤ 15 grams | FAT<br>➤ 35 grams. Yes, this is a lot of fat. However, it is unsaturated and is therefore heart healthy and won't raise insulin levels.<br>FIBER<br>➤ 4 grams |
| --- | --- | --- |

## TAKE 10

Standing stretch

This stretch allows for a greater range of motion in the fronts of your thighs, decreasing your chance of injury. Do this stretch after you have warmed up the fronts of your thighs with your daily activities.

1. Stand with your feet hip distance apart. Bend your knees slightly, lift your chest, contract your abdominals, press your shoulders back and down, align your head and spine, and face forward. Hold on to the back of a chair for balance.
2. From behind, place your right hand on the toe of your right foot and pull your heel to your buttocks, keeping your knees together. Don't arch your lower back. (If you are not flexible enough to reach your toe, wrap a towel around your foot and gently pull the towel toward your buttocks.)
3. Squeeze your buttocks while pressing your hips forward.
4. Bend your standing leg slightly to reduce the stress on the lower back. Hold for 15 to 20 seconds and repeat the stretch with your left leg.

# WATER BREAK

When your body processes water, it is a workout for your kidneys and internal organs, making them function better overall.

# ENERGY BALANCE DINNER

## DINING IN

Out-of-the-Ordinary Cheeseburger

4 to 6 ounces ground beef, turkey, or soy-based hamburger substitute

2 ounces goat cheese

Roasted red bell pepper

1 tablespoons low-fat mayonnaise

1 small hamburger bun or 2 pieces of whole-grain bread

Sliced tomato and onion

1. Form the meat into two thin hamburger patties.
2. Place goat cheese in between the two and press together until you have one patty with goat cheese in center.
3. Grill the burger to taste.
4. Rinse and dice the red bell pepper and mix it into the mayonnaise.
5. Dress the burger with the bun, mayonnaise, tomato, and onion.
6. Serve with a few low-fat chips and a big green salad with low-fat dressing.

## DINING OUT

Order a turkey burger or a lean hamburger made with top sirloin. Since you can't control the size of the bun, eat only the top half. Add a small green salad, and if you have the willpower, add a few French fries. If not, don't tempt yourself.

➤ If you want a larger meal: Add a small protein appetizer, such as a shrimp cocktail.

| CORE FOUR APPROXIMATE BREAKDOWN | PROTEIN ➤ ground beef or turkey: 20 to 25 grams CARBOHYDRATE ➤ hamburger bun, chips, salad: 30 to 40 grams | FAT ➤ ground beef or turkey: 15 grams ➤ goat cheese: 9 grams ➤ salad dressing: 1 to 2 grams ➤ chips: 2 to 5 grams FIBER ➤ salad: 5 grams |
|---|---|---|

# ENERGY BALANCE SNACK

Yogurt

4 ounces nonfat yogurt mixed with a small amount of sunflower seeds

| CORE FOUR APPROXIMATE BREAKDOWN | PROTEIN ➤ 4 to 8 grams CARBOHYDRATE ➤ 11 to 15 grams | FAT ➤ 5 to 10 grams FIBER ➤ 2 to 3 grams |
|---|---|---|

# STRETCH, RELAX, AND SLEEP

1. Chest/posture stretch
2. Neck and upper spine stretch
3. Lower spine stretch

# STRESS RELIEF TIP

Try to limit your caffeine intake. Too much caffeine damages your health by breaking down vitamins B and C and increases your susceptibility to stress by making you irritable and nervous.

# Let's Have a Heart-to-Heart

A FRANTIC MIND AND A STATIONARY BODY are two enemies of a healthy heart—much like the way gunning your car, without putting it in drive, will wear out your engine but not take you anywhere. Although public attention has recently been focused on breast, ovarian, and other cancers that can be deadly to women, we must not overlook the importance of a healthy heart. In fact, twice as many women die each year from heart disease than from all kinds of cancer combined.*

When we allow our minds to fret, our blood pressure increases and our muscles tense up. Powerful hormones pour into our bloodstreams, hormones designed to help us either fight for our lives or run for the hills. But if we don't put this increased physical energy to good use by fighting or fleeing, we put our hearts in danger. So don't fume over your problems while sitting behind a computer all day or flopped out on the couch all evening. Instead, focus on practical solutions to the challenges in your life and move your body every day. . . .if for no reason other than your heart's sake.

*"Boosting Heart Disease Awareness," Beth Israel Deaconess Medical Center, 2001

# DAY 4

## WAKE-UP AFFIRMATION

"I don't think being an athlete is unfeminine. I think of it as a kind of grace."

—*Jackie Joyner-Kersee, Olympic gold medalist*

## WAKE-UP WORKOUT

**1.** Let body slowly wake up
**2.** Take several deep breaths
**3.** Full-body tighten and release
**4.** Pelvic tilts
**5.** Pillow sit-ups
**6.** Hamstring stretch
**7.** Hands and knees yoga stretch

## CORE FOUR

**1.** Push-up
**2.** Sit-up
**3.** Sit and stand
**4.** Posture squeeze/biceps curl

## PORTION CONTROL TIP

Never eat standing up. There's a tendency to eat more, and a misconception that on-the-go snacks somehow don't count in your overall intake.

## ENERGY BALANCE BREAKFAST

### Waffle and Eggs

> 4 egg whites or 1/2 cup egg substitute
> 2 whole-grain waffles
> Light syrup
> 4 pieces turkey bacon

**1.** Cook the waffles and pour syrup on them.
**2.** Scramble the eggs.
**3.** Cook the bacon until well-done and crisp. Blot all grease with a paper towel.

➤If you want a larger meal: Add a whole egg and two more pieces of turkey bacon.

Drink water with lemon or 4 ounces of juice and 6 ounces of water, plus decaffeinated tea or coffee, if desired. Add low-fat flavored creamer to taste.

| CORE FOUR APPROXIMATE BREAKDOWN | PROTEIN | FAT |
|---|---|---|
| | ➤ egg whites: 14 grams | ➤ regular bacon: 7 grams |
| | ➤ turkey or regular bacon: 7 grams | **FIBER** |
| | **CARBOHYDRATE** | ➤ waffles: 1 to 2 grams |
| | ➤ waffles and syrup: 25 to 30 grams | |

# TAKE 10
## Twist and stretch

This exercise will stretch your entire torso and increase flexibility in your spine. If you play tennis or golf, this will help your swing and help prevent lower back injuries. Always remember to breathe freely during a stretch and elongate your muscles gently. Do not bounce, and be careful not to take a stretch too far.

1. Sit in a chair, lift your chest, contract your abdominals, press your shoulders back and down, align your head and spine, and face forward.
2. Inhale deeply as you slowly turn your upper body around and place both hands at waist height on the back of the chair, aiming your chin toward your shoulder. Exhale and hold for 10 to 15 seconds, breathing normally.
3. Release and slowly return to the original position.
4. Repeat the twist on the other side and hold for 10 to 15 seconds.
5. Release and repeat as many times as comfortable.

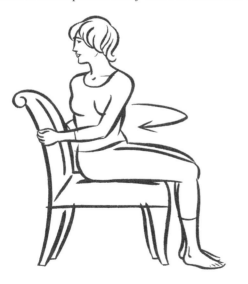

# SIT AND BE FIT
## Car care

Getting in and out of a car and driving can cause back pain. There are some ways to avoid injury:

1. Back into the seat, placing your buttocks on the seat first, keeping both feet on the ground. Swing both legs into the car at the same time.
2. When you are driving, your seat should give your back proper support. If your car seat does not, you can buy a lumbar support.
3. Do not rest your left arm on the car window for any length of time, because it makes your body lean too far to the left. This odd angle pulls your back out of alignment and can cause pain.
4. Keep your hands at the four and eight o'clock position on the wheel. This keeps your shoulders, neck, and back in a stable position, and if the air bag ever inflates, you will be in the proper position to prevent serious injuries.
5. When you get home from work or errands, take a minute to do the lower back bent-over spine stretch in Stretch, Relax, and Sleep (See "A Body in Motion").

# WATER BREAK

Planning a plane trip? The dry air on a plane can literally suck the water out of your body. Because of the lower levels of oxygen, you breathe harder, your lungs expel more moisture into the air, and your body loses water. Drink one 8-ounce glass of water before your flight and a glass every hour you're on the plane. This routine will also help to prevent fatigue caused by dehydration.

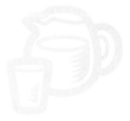

## ENERGY BALANCE SNACK

Grapes

1 cup grapes
1 1-ounce stick string cheese

| CORE FOUR APPROXIMATE BREAKDOWN | PROTEIN | FAT |
|---|---|---|
| | ➤ string cheese: 7 grams | ➤ string cheese: 6 grams |
| | **CARBOHYDRATE** | **FIBER** |
| | ➤ grapes: 15 grams | ➤ grapes: 1 gram |

## WATER BREAK

Beat a cold with more water! The mucus that protects your throat by trapping cold viruses dries out when you are dehydrated, so more water means fewer colds.

## ENERGY LIFT

Hand shake

This movement will not only help relieve finger fatigue, but it will also help strengthen your grip. Do this several times a day and you will eventually feel the difference a hand "break" can make.

1. Sit in a chair, lift your chest, contract your abdominals, press your shoulders back and down, align your head and spine, and face forward.
2. Shake both hands with loose wrists in front of you for 5 seconds.
3. Extend your fingers as far apart as they will go, hold for 5 seconds, and release.
4. Repeat 3 times.

## ENERGY BALANCE LUNCH

### DINING IN

Cranberry, Feta, and Walnut Salad

4 to 6 ounces cooked chicken, shrimp, or tuna
2 cups field greens or other lettuce

1 tablespoon dried cranberries
1 tablespoon feta cheese
1/2 teaspoon pepper
1 tablespoon chopped walnuts
2 tablespoons low-fat balsamic vinegar dressing

Combine ingredients in a bowl and toss.

### DINING OUT

Try a salad you have never tried before and have them add a chicken breast or 6 to 8 shrimp.

➤ If you want a larger meal: Add more chicken or a slice of cheese and a small dinner roll.

| CORE FOUR APPROXIMATE BREAKDOWN | PROTEIN | FAT |
|---|---|---|
| | ➤ chicken, shrimp, or tuna: 20 to 25 grams | ➤ feta cheese, walnuts, low-fat dressing: 10 to 15 grams |
| | **CARBOHYDRATE** | **FIBER** |
| | ➤ field greens, cranberries: 15 to 20 grams | ➤ field greens, cranberries, walnuts: 5 to 10 grams |
| | ➤ dinner roll: 15 grams | |

## SIT AND BE FIT

Forearm rotation

This exercise will strengthen your forearms and biceps, which will help improve your performance in tennis, golf, or any other game that requires forearm strength.

1. Sit and lift your chest, contract your abdominals, press your shoulders back and down, align your head and spine, and face forward.
2. Breathing gently and evenly, hold a fairly large book between your palms with your right hand on top of the book and left hand on the bottom.
3. Stretch your arms out straight in front of you at shoulder height.
4. Turn the book over so your left hand is on top and your right hand is on the bottom. Don't let go of the book and keep your hands glued to the top and bottom of the book.
5. Rotate your forearms left and then right until your arms are tired. Rest and repeat 2 more times.

# WATER BREAK

If you are tired of drinking plain water, for variety try some low-calorie designer waters that contain vitamins and herbs.

# ENERGY LIFT

Toe touch

This easy toe touch will not only give you an energy rush and raise your heart rate, it will help tone and firm your inner thighs. Do this when there is no one else around, because it is a little funny-looking.

1. Stand up straight, with your feet hip distance apart. Bend your knees slightly, lift your chest, contract your abdominals, press your shoulders back and down, align your head and spine, and face forward. Hold on to the back of a chair with your right hand for balance and lift your left arm straight out in front of you.
2. Lift your right foot toward your left hand, slightly rotating your knee out.
3. Bend your left knee slightly to keep stress off your lower back.
4. Lift your leg as high as possible, working up to tapping the inside of your right heel with your left hand.
5. Tap and lower 10 times.
6. Repeat on the left side.

# WATER BREAK

Constipation may be caused by not drinking enough water, especially if you are eating a lot of fiber. Water is needed to help fiber flush waste products through your system. So follow each high-fiber snack with some more $H_2O$.

# ENERGY BALANCE SNACK

Tuna Wrap

1 small piece whole wheat pita bread or 1 corn tortilla

Small amount of fat-free mayonnaise

2 to 3 ounces water-packed tuna, drained

1 slice low-fat cheese

1 slice tomato

1. Spread the pita bread or tortilla lightly with mayonnaise.
2. Place the tuna, cheese, and tomato on the pita bread.
3. Wrap it up!

CORE FOUR APPROXIMATE BREAKDOWN

| PROTEIN | FAT |
|---|---|
| ➤ tuna: 12 to 18 grams | ➤ cheese: 2 grams |
| **CARBOHYDRATE** | **FIBER** |
| ➤ pita bread or tortilla: 12 to 15 grams | ➤ pita bread or tortilla: 1 to 2 grams |

# TAKE 10

Foot massage

This massage relieves tension and helps make your feet and ankles more flexible. Do this whenever you have been on your feet for any length of time or you have been wearing a higher heel.

1. Kick off your shoes and place your right foot on your lap.
2. Hold your foot and massage the ball of your foot with your thumbs.
3. Massage your entire foot, paying attention to your toes. This should take only a few seconds.
4. Press your foot down into a pointed position and then back up into a flexed position as far as the flexibility of your foot will allow.
5. Release and repeat on the left foot.

## WATER BREAK

Drinking a lot of water inevitably makes restroom breaks necessary. But think of these breaks as positive—if you are confined to a desk for long periods of time, drinking water makes you get up every hour or so, which helps prevent desk-bound muscle tension.

## ENERGY BALANCE DINNER

### DINING IN

Lamb Chops with Couscous

4 to 6 ounces lamb chops
1 tablespoon Dijon-style mustard
1 tablespoon olive oil
1 tablespoon diced garlic
1 cup cleaned spinach
1/2 cup diced red bell peppers
1/2 cup prepared couscous, mixed with 1 teaspoon curry powder

1. Rub the lamb chops with the mustard and grill them until light pink in the middle.
2. Heat the oil and garlic in a nonstick skillet over medium heat.
3. Add the spinach and red bell peppers and sauté until the spinach is soft, 2 to 3 minutes.
4. Serve with lamb chops and couscous, a small dinner salad with low-fat dressing, and a small glass of wine.

### DINING OUT

Start with a salad and order the dressing on the side. Dip your fork into the dressing and then the salad. Order a small steak and a baked potato with vegetables. Cut the potato in half and top it with a small amount of sour cream and chives. Have one small glass of wine.

➤If you want a larger meal: Increase spinach to 2 cups and peppers to 1 cup.

| CORE FOUR APPROXIMATE BREAKDOWN | PROTEIN<br>➤ lamb chops:<br>20 to 25 grams<br><br>CARBOHYDRATE<br>➤ couscous, vegetables,<br>and wine:<br>25 to 30 grams | FAT<br>➤ dressing and oil:<br>10 to 15 grams<br><br>FIBER<br>➤ vegetables and<br>salad: 5 to 10 grams |
| --- | --- | --- |

## ENERGY BALANCE SNACK

Pretzel Trail Mix

1/2 cup mini pretzel twists
1/2 cup seedless raisins
2/3 cup almonds

This recipe makes about 5 servings, so save the balance for other snacks.

| CORE FOUR APPROXIMATE BREAKDOWN | PROTEIN<br>➤ almonds: 6 grams<br><br>CARBOHYDRATE<br>➤ pretzels: 15 grams | FAT<br>➤ almonds: 15 grams<br><br>FIBER<br>➤ raisins: 2 grams<br>➤ almonds: 1 gram |
| --- | --- | --- |

## STRETCH, RELAX, AND SLEEP

1. Chest/posture stretch
2. Neck and upper spine stretch
3. Lower spine stretch

## STRESS RELIEF TIP

If you have access to a steam room, sauna, or whirlpool, take advantage of the wonderful world of water, which will help relieve stress. Another option is a long, relaxing bath.

# Do's and Don'ts of Self-Love

L OVING OUR BODIES CAN BE DIFFICULT when we're bombarded from every direction by advertisers who desperately want us to dislike ourselves. Yes, they profit from our self-loathing. If we are dissatisfied with how we look, how we smell, how we're shaped, or how we feel, then we'll buy products that promise to make us lovable. But, hey, we're already lovable. Right now. And here are a few do's and don'ts that will increase the love you feel for yourself:

➤ Do focus your attention on your assets . . . and I don't mean your long legs or your naturally curly hair. I mean your inner assets, such as the way you pick up stray kittens and find good homes for them, or the flair you have for arranging flowers. Maybe you're a whiz at investing in the stock market or a wild woman behind the sewing machine. Are you the life of the party? Or a really good listener? We all have special qualities to offer, and these are to be valued far above our fat-to-lean-muscle ratio.

➤ Don't cut yourself into pieces… Hasn't every woman said something like "Well, I have pretty eyes, but my flabby thighs are horrid" or "My rump sticks out for miles, but at least my breasts are perky"? Why dissect yourself like a science experiment and announce which body parts are acceptable and which aren't? Your body is a whole entity — your body is you. And you are entirely acceptable.

➤ Do speak positively about yourself. . . Since you're no longer going to point out to yourself or anyone else which parts of your body are unacceptable, make a habit of speaking about yourself in kind, positive terms. If our friends spoke about themselves as negatively as most of us criticize ourselves inside our heads, we'd be horrified and plead with them to stop. Whenever you catch yourself saying something negative about your body, stick out your tongue. This will break the cycle of self-criticism and get you to smile if you're alone and probably trigger an interesting conversation if you happen to be standing in line at the bank.

# DAY 5

## WAKE-UP AFFIRMATION

**"Every day in every way, I'm getting better and better."**

—*Emile Coue (1857-1926), autosuggestion psychologist*

## WAKE-UP WORKOUT

1. Let body slowly wake up
2. Take several deep breaths
3. Full-body tighten and release
4. Pelvic tilts
5. Pillow sit-ups
6. Hamstring stretch
7. Hands and knees yoga stretch

## CORE FOUR

1. Push-up
2. Sit-up
3. Sit and stand
4. Posture squeeze/biceps curl

## PORTION CONTROL TIP

To limit your food intake at lunch and dinner, drink a cup of water or eat a cup of clear soup before you begin the meal.

## ENERGY BALANCE BREAKFAST

*Breakfast of Champions*

> 3/4 cup cereal that has less than 30 grams of carbohydrate
>
> 1/2 cup nonfat milk or vanilla soy milk
>
> Melon, strawberries, blueberries, or any fruit from the low-sugar fruit list (See "Energy Balance Basics" chapter.)
>
> 1/2 cup low-fat cottage cheese, farmer's cheese, or ricotta cheese

1. Combine the cereal and milk in a bowl.
2. You can serve the fruit on top of the cereal or with the cheese.

➤ If you want a larger meal: Add two scrambled eggs or 1/2 cup egg substitute.

Drink water with lemon or 4 ounces of juice and 6 ounces of water, plus decaffeinated tea or coffee, if desired. Add low-fat creamer to taste.

| CORE FOUR APPROXIMATE BREAKDOWN | PROTEIN | FAT |
|---|---|---|
| | ➤ cottage cheese: 14 grams | ➤ cottage cheese: 2 grams |
| | ➤ nonfat or soy milk: 4 grams | ➤ soy milk: 1 gram |
| | **CARBOHYDRATE** | **FIBER** |
| | ➤ cereal: 25 to 30 grams | ➤ cereal: 2 to 5 grams |
| | ➤ nonfat or soy milk: 6 grams | |

# TAKE 10
## Hip toner break

This exercise firms and tones the sides of the hips and strengthens a portion of the buttocks area that helps you maintain your balance. Do this whenever you encounter a counter.

1. Stand facing and holding on to a countertop, with your feet hip distance apart. Bend your knees slightly, lift your chest, contract your abdominals, press your shoulders back and down, align your head and spine, and face forward.
2. Inhale and exhale as you slowly lift your right leg 45 degrees to the side, keeping your upper body straight and your buttocks tucked under, with your supporting leg slightly bent. Don't let your lower back arch; maintain a neutral lower back.
3. Lower your leg and then repeat on the left side.
4. Repeat 10 times on each side, alternating back and forth.
5. If you feel any strain in your lower back, stop and check your lower back posture.

# SIT AND BE FIT
## Overhead extension

This exercise will not only firm and tone the backs of your arms, the lifted position will help open up your shoulder joints and increase flexibility in this area.

1. Sit in a chair and lift your chest, contract your abdominals, press your shoulders back and down, align your head and spine, and face forward.
2. Raise your right arm over your head with your elbow close to your ear and pointed toward the ceiling. Let your hand rest on your upper neck, behind your head.
3. Place your left hand on the back of your right arm beneath your elbow for support.
4. Exhale as you straighten your right forearm overhead. Do not lock your elbow at the completion of the movement. Inhale and bend your elbow back to the starting position.

5. Repeat 10 to 15 times.
6. As you become used to this movement, you can use 3- to-5 pound weights to add a little more of a challenge to the exercise. The more resistance, the better the toning results.

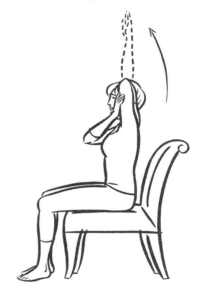

# WATER BREAK

Drinking water an hour before your workout can increase your endurance by up to 10 minutes, which will burn extra calories.

# ENERGY BALANCE SNACK
## Super Celery

   2 stalks celery
   2 tablespoons low-fat cottage cheese
   1 tablespoon peanut butter
   1 1-ounce stick string cheese
   8 ounces low-sodium tomato juice

1. Cut celery.
2. Stuff celery sticks with cottage cheese and peanut butter. Add string cheese on the side and serve with tomato juice.

57

| CORE FOUR APPROXIMATE BREAKDOWN | PROTEIN ➤ peanut butter: 7 grams ➤ string cheese: 7 to 8 grams ➤ cottage cheese: 7 grams CARBOHYDRATE ➤ tomato juice: 7 grams | FAT ➤ string cheese: 6 grams ➤ peanut butter: 7 grams ➤ cottage cheese: 2 grams FIBER ➤ celery: 1 to 2 grams |
| --- | --- | --- |

## WATER BREAK

If you have ever experienced a spaced-out feeling when you are running a fever, that's dehydration. The amount you perspire when breaking a fever severely dehydrates your brain as well as your body, so heed the doctor's advice and drink plenty of liquids.

## ENERGY LIFT
### Stationary lunge

This stationary lunge will not only firm and tone the fronts of your thighs and your buttocks, it will make walking a lot easier.

1. Stand with your knees slightly bent, lift your chest, contract your abdominals, press your shoulders down and back, and align your head and spine. Place your feet so that your right heel supports most of your weight. Hold on to the back of a chair for balance.
2. Extend your left leg straight behind you, toes on the floor and heel lifted.
3. Keep your right knee over your right heel— don't let it drift over your toes, which would place too much strain on your knee.
4. Bend both knees as you lower your body straight down toward the floor. Keep your left heel lifted and your right knee over your right heel.
5. Lift up to the starting position and repeat 5 times.
6. Change legs and repeat on the other side 5 times.

## ENERGY BALANCE LUNCH

### DINING IN
#### Smoked Salmon and Goat Cheese Sandwich

2 slices rye bread
4 to 6 ounces smoked salmon
1 ounce goat cheese
Arugula, watercress, or cucumber

1. Lightly toast both slices of the bread.
2. Place the salmon, goat cheese, and arugula on the toast.
3. Serve with cut-up fresh vegetables and low-fat dip.

### DINING OUT

Try any new and different sandwich with fish, meat, or chicken. Add a slice of your favorite cheese and go light on the mayonnaise. Have a small portion of potato salad or cole slaw.

➤If you want a larger meal: Add a small salad.

| CORE FOUR APPROXIMATE BREAKDOWN | PROTEIN ➤ salmon: 20 grams CARBOHYDRATE ➤ bread: 25 grams | FAT ➤ salmon: 10 grams ➤ goat cheese: 5 grams FIBER ➤ vegetables: 5 to 10 grams |
| --- | --- | --- |

## SIT AND BE FIT
### Biceps curl

This exercise strengthens the upper arms, making everyday activities like carrying groceries easier.

1. Sit in a chair, lift your chest, contract your abdominals, press your shoulders back and down, align your head and spine, and face forward.
2. Hold 3- to 5-pound weights or two books of the same weight in your hands with your palms facing upward. Keep your shoulder blades down and back throughout the movement.

3. Glue your elbows to your waist. Your arms are parallel to your thighs, with a slight bend in your elbows, and your wrists are rigid and straight—don't let them curl up or hang back and down during the movement.
4. Inhale as you bring your hands toward your shoulders, stopping just before your forearms touch your biceps.
5. Exhale as you slowly lower your hands to the initial position.
6. Repeat 12 to 15 times.

## WATER BREAK

A British study found that drinking large amounts of water could reduce the risk of breast cancer by 70 percent and colon cancer by 45 percent, which is probably due to water's ability to flush toxins from the body.

## ENERGY LIFT
### Stairs to nowhere

This stair climbing will not only raise your heart rate, burn fat, and increase circulation, it will firm and tone the fronts of your legs and your buttocks, making you feel more energetic.

1. Stand up straight and place your feet hip distance apart. Bend your knees slightly, lift your chest, contract your abdominals, press your shoulders back and down, align your head and spine, and face forward. Hold on to the back of a chair for balance.
2. Pretend you are climbing stairs. Lift your knees as high as you would if you were climbing a flight of stairs. Do 1 to 2 minutes or until you feel your breathing accelerate.
3. Or find a flight (or two or three) of stairs and climb it once or twice. Add a flight each week.

## WATER BREAK

How do you know if you are hydrated? Check your urine. If it is clear, you are drinking enough water. If your urine is dark and has a strong odor, you need more water.

## ENERGY BALANCE SNACK
### Mushroom Pita Pizza

1 small piece whole-grain pita bread
2 tablespoons tomato sauce
2 to 3 ounces chicken or turkey
2 sliced mushrooms
1 ounce shredded low-fat Monterey Jack cheese

1. Lightly toast the pita bread.
2. Place the pita bread on a small plate and spread it with the tomato sauce.
3. Add the chicken and mushrooms and sprinkle with the cheese.
4. Place in toaster oven and heat until the cheese is melted and bubbly.

| CORE FOUR APPROXIMATE BREAKDOWN | PROTEIN ➤ chicken or turkey: 12 to 18 grams CARBOHYDRATE ➤ pita bread: 12 to 15 grams | FAT ➤ cheese: 2 grams FIBER ➤ pita bread: 1 to 2 grams |
|---|---|---|

## TAKE 10
### Chest and shoulder stretch

This stretch will open up your rib cage and increase your capacity to breathe more deeply.

1. Stand up straight and place your feet hip distance apart. Bend your knees slightly, lift your chest, contract your abdominals, press your shoulders back and down, align your head and spine, and face forward.
2. Place both hands behind your back. Interlace your fingers with your palms facing upward. Press your shoulder blades together and feel the stretch in the fronts of your shoulders and your chest.

**3.** Hold for as long as comfortable and then release.

**4.** Take a deep breath and repeat 3 times.

# ENERGY BALANCE DINNER

## DINING IN

### Chicken, Lean Steak, or Shrimp Waldorf Salad

4 to 6 ounces chicken, lean steak, or grilled shrimp

3 cups field greens

1/2 apple, finely chopped

1/2 ounce raisins

1 small tomato and lots of vegetables

2 tablespoons chopped walnuts

2 tablespoons Parmesan cheese

2 tablespoons poppy seed dressing or balsamic-vinegar and olive oil dressing

Mix together all of the ingredients and enjoy!

## DINING OUT

Order a protein-rich appetizer, such as a shrimp cocktail or a cheese plate, a glass of wine, a dinner salad with dressing on the side, and another protein rich appetizer. Finish with a decaf cappuccino or latte.

➤If you want a larger meal: Finish with 2 to 3 ounces of your favorite ice cream. If you can't have just 2 to 3 ounces yet, don't tempt yourself. Ice cream is a low-glycemic-index food because it enters the bloodstream slowly due to its balance of protein, fat, and sugar. Always choose real ice cream over the low-fat, high-sugar alternatives because when fat is removed more sugar is added to make it taste good. This high-sugar ice cream causes more of an insulin response and increases fat-storing capacity.

### CORE FOUR APPROXIMATE BREAKDOWN

| PROTEIN | FAT |
|---|---|
| ➤ chicken, lean steak, or shrimp: 20 to 25 grams | ➤ walnuts, dressing, cheese: 10 grams |
| ➤ ice cream: 6 to 8 grams | ➤ ice cream: 10 to 15 grams |
| **CARBOHYDRATE** | **FIBER** |
| ➤ field greens, apple: 15 grams | ➤ field greens, apple, walnuts: 10 grams |
| ➤ ice cream: 15 to 20 grams | |

# WATER BREAK

Ideally, you should never feel thirsty. By the time your body tells your mind it wants a drink, your body is already becoming dehydrated.

# ENERGY BALANCE SNACK

### Cheesy Soup

1 cup tomato or any low-carbohydrate soup

1 1-ounce stick string cheese

### CORE FOUR APPROXIMATE BREAKDOWN

| PROTEIN | FAT |
|---|---|
| ➤ string cheese: 6 grams | ➤ string cheese: 7 grams |
| **CARBOHYDRATE** | **FIBER** |
| ➤ tomato soup: 17 grams | ➤ tomato soup: 2 grams |

# STRETCH, RELAX, AND SLEEP

**1.** Chest/posture stretch

**2.** Neck and upper spine stretch

**3.** Lower spine stretch

# STRESS RELIEF TIP

There is a magic formula for banishing the blues: Make 30 minutes of exercise a part of your everyday activities. Moderate exercise accesses endorphins and reduces stress hormones, giving you a temporary high that puts your emotions back on a balanced plane.

# Tennis Anyone?

J UST AS HITTING A TENNIS BALL can be a great stress releaser, so can lying on top of one!

A tennis ball has just the right flexibility to give a little when you press on it (don't try this with a golf ball!) yet enough oomph to press into those tired sore muscles along your spine. Right before you go to bed, stretch out on the floor and place a tennis ball between your shoulder blade and spine. Slowly lean into the ball until you feel that "good sore" feeling. Gently roll back and forth over the ball, working out those knots you accumulated throughout the day. I like to stretch my arm across my chest to lengthen the muscles between my spine and shoulder blade. Ahhhh . . . Continue this until you've massaged the entire length of your back.

Repeat on the other side and expect an especially good night's sleep. Remember the following guidelines whenever you're giving yourself a tennis ball massage or receiving one from a friend or massage therapist.

➤ **AVOID PAIN:** For the best stress release, keep the pressure firm but not so hard that it's painful. Pain is your body's way of saying "Stop!" Listen to this message or you'll do yourself more harm than good.

➤ **BREATHE DEEPLY:** Stress release is enhanced through breathing, so as you receive your massage, focus on a regular and deep breathing rhythm. If you're holding your breath, you're probably in pain and the pressure is too deep.

➤ **BE GENTLE:** Don't be fanatic about getting rid of all your knots. It probably took more than a few minutes to create all those tight spots of tension throughout your muscular system, so please don't try to release them all in one massage session. Let go of the ones that are ready and leave the others for another time.

# More from Chores

URN YOUR HOUSEWORK or yard work into a mini workout routine with the following tips. For each task, follow the safety cues and, when possible, work up a sweat.

## STANDING CHORES

Washing dishes, cooking, or any activity where your torso and lower back are stabilized and there is moderate movement of your arms and shoulders can turn into strengthening exercise with a knee bend. This combined movement works your abdominals, lower back, front of thighs, and buttocks.

1. Stand with your feet hip distance apart, toes pointing out. Bend your knees slightly, lift your chest, contract your abdominals, press your shoulders back and down, align your head and spine, and face forward.
2. If possible, look in a mirror to ensure proper alignment of your spine and torso.
3. Hold on to a countertop or sink with one hand for balance.
4. Inhale while bending your knees over your heels (make sure your knees do not go past your toes!), and lower your buttocks toward the floor.
5. Hold for two seconds while slightly squeezing your buttocks.

Exhale as you return to a standing position. Repeat 10 times.

## REACHING OUTWARD CHORES

Chores such as clearing dinner dishes from the table can be used as an opportunity to work the entire body, especially the front of the arm, shoulder, chest, and the large back muscles.

1. Stand with your feet hip distance apart, toes pointing out. Bend your knees slightly, lift your chest, contract your abdominals, press your shoulders back and down, align your head and spine, and face forward.
2. Clear the dishes that are the furthest away from you first, using your right arm and stretching a little beyond your reach.
3. Take the dishes to the sink and return, repeating the movement with the left arm.
4. Continue clearing with a little more speed than normal, which will help to burn a few more calories.

## REACHING UPWARD CHORES

Reaching chores, which include cleaning windows and mirrors, mainly work the upper body, arms, shoulders, and the rotator cuff muscle group, which is comprised of four small muscles that attach the upper arm and shoulder joint together. This muscle group allows the shoulder joint its range of movement and, as we age, often becomes tender and fragile. The following exercise will help to strengthen this area.

1. Stand up tall, lift your chest, contract your abdominals, press your shoulders back and down, and align your head and spine.

# MORE FROM CHORES

**2.** Inhale and slowly squat. Sit back as far as you can, making sure your knees are over your heels, not your toes.

**3.** Hold for two seconds while slightly squeezing your buttocks.

**4.** Exhale as you return to a standing position.

**5.** Now reach up as far as your arms allow, stretching the entire side of the waist.

**6.** Squat again as you change the dusting cloth to the other hand and reach up again.

**7.** Repeat movement, alternating hands, until the chore is done.

## PUSH-AND-PULL CHORES

Chores that use equipment, such as vacuuming, mopping, hoeing, raking, and mowing, if done properly and combined with a lunge, can work the entire body.

**1.** Stand with your knees slightly bent, lift your chest, contract your abdominals, press your shoulders down and back, and align your head and spine. Place your feet so that your right heel supports most of your weight.

**2.** As you push the equipment forward, extend your left leg straight behind you, toes on the floor and heel lifted.

**3.** Keep your right knee over your right heel— don't let it drift over your toes.

**4.** Bend both knees as you lower your body slightly. The combined movement will be a small lunge, like a fencer's lunge.

**5.** Thrust and retreat reaching out as far as comfortable. Make sure to alternate sides with every 10 repetitions.

## SHOVELING CHORES

Clearing dirt or snow can be great exercise but form is important. With the proper alignment, a task as simple as shoveling the driveway can work the legs, buttocks, lower back, shoulders, forearms, biceps, and chest.

**1.** Stand facing what you are going to lift, with your feet hip distance apart. Bend your knees slightly, lift your chest, contract your abdominals, press your shoulders back and down, align your head and spine, and face forward.

**2.** Push the shovel down into the dirt or snow with your right foot and swing to the right to empty the shovel load.

**3.** Do not twist or turn the body while still holding a heavy load. Instead, move your feet so you are facing the direction where you are planning to empty the load.

**4.** Repeat this movement four times, and then change sides. This will help to prevent you from using one side more than the other and will balance out use of the back.

**5.** Breathe deeply and take breaks, as shoveling quickly raises your heat rate and can overload the cardiovascular system.

## POLISHING CHORES

Dusting furniture, wiping a table, or any polishing chore can easily turn into a calorie burner. With an added bicep curl, you will work your shoulder, rotator cuff, chest, back, and front and back of your arm.

1. As you move around the table, increase your pace. Polish with one hand for ten turns, switch hands, and then take the following weight-training break:

2. Stand with feet a little more than shoulder width apart, lift your chest, contract your abdominals, press your shoulders back and down, align your head and spine, and face forward.

3. Hold 3- to 5-pound weights or two books of the same weight in your hands with your palms facing upward. Keep your shoulder blades down and back throughout the movement.

4. Glue your elbows to your waist, with a slight bend in your elbows, and your wrists rigid and straight—don't let them curl up or hang back and down during the movement.

5. Inhale as you bring your hands toward your shoulders, stopping just before your forearms touch your biceps.

6. Exhale as you slowly lower your hands to the original position.

7. Repeat 12 to 15 times.

## KNEELING CHORES

When you are on your knees doing chores such a cleaning the bathtub and making the bed, you are putting extra pressure on the lower back. Take a break between these chores and do a lower back stretch releaser.

1. Stand with your upper body leaning slightly forward from your hips, with your feet hip distance apart. Bend your knees slightly, lift your chest, contract your abdominals, press your shoulders back and down, align your head and spine, and face forward with your hands on the fronts of your thighs.

2. Exhale as you contract and pull in your abdominals and round your back toward the ceiling like a cat. Allow your shoulders to round forward, stretching the upper and back. If you do this movement correctly, you will look as if you were hit in the midsection with a large ball.

3. Hold for a few seconds and release back to the original position. If your back is strong and flexible, release into a slight arch, which will make the stretch more pronounced.

4. Repeat 3 times.

# MORE FROM CHORES

## LIFTING AND TWISTING CHORES

Picking up a laundry basket or taking heavy objects in and out of a car or shopping cart can cause strain to the lower back. When lifting a heavy object, be particularly careful about how you pick it up. Most back injuries occur when things are lifted at an odd angle. Here are a few safety tips.

1. Make sure your hips are parallel to the object being lifted.
2. Feet should be a little more than hip distance apart, your knees should be slightly bent, and your abdominals contracted.
3. Bend your legs at the knees so you are in a semi-squat position.
4. Lift with your legs, not your lower back, and straight up, not to the side
5. Never twist something heavy out of a car trunk or off a lower shelf. Pull the object onto a higher shelf or the edge of the trunk and then lift straight up and out from there.
6. Use the same two-step motion when you are putting something into your car trunk—from cart to edge of trunk, then slide it into the trunk well.

7. When lifting a small child, pick the child up waist height with your thighs and knees braced against a chair or couch, then pull the child straight up into your arms.
8. When carrying a child, don't lean back and arch your lower back. Make sure you keep your abdominals contracted and your lower back in a neutral position.

You can strengthen your lower back using a movement in yoga called the cobra.

1. Lie face down on the floor with your forehead on a small pillow, arms flat against the floor and your palms facing up.
2. Inhale as you slowly lift your head off of the pillow until you feel a slight tightening in your lower back.
3. Exhale as you lower your head back to the pillow and relax.
4. Repeat as many times as comfortable, working up to 8-10 repetitions.

# DAY 6

## WAKE-UP AFFIRMATION

"The secret of success is constancy of purpose."

—*Benjamin Disraeli, British prime minister
and novelist*

## WAKE-UP WORKOUT

**1.** Let body slowly wake up
**2.** Take several deep breaths
**3.** Full-body tighten and release
**4.** Pelvic tilts
**5.** Pillow sit-ups
**6.** Hamstring stretch
**7.** Hands and knees yoga stretch

## CORE FOUR

**1.** Push-up
**2.** Sit-up
**3.** Sit and stand
**4.** Posture squeeze/biceps curl

## PORTION CONTROL TIP

Avoid overdoing it when topping a piece of bread or a bagel with cream cheese or butter by spreading the topping thinly enough so that you can see the bread through it.

## ENERGY BALANCE BREAKFAST

### Muffin Treat

1/2 bran muffin, toasted
2 tablespoons cinnamon-walnut cream cheese

➤ If you want a larger meal: Add 1 scrambled egg and 2 egg whites. Eat a whole small bran muffin.

Drink water with lemon or 4 ounces of juice and 6 ounces of water, plus decaffeinated tea or coffee, if desired. Add low-fat creamer to taste.

| CORE FOUR APPROXIMATE BREAKDOWN | PROTEIN ➤ cream cheese: 14 grams ➤ whole egg and 2 egg whites: 13 grams CARBOHYDRATE ➤ 1/2 muffin: 15 grams ➤ whole small muffin: 25 to 30 grams | FAT ➤ 1/2 muffin: 3 to 5 grams ➤ whole small muffin: 6 to 10 grams ➤ egg yolk: 5 grams FIBER ➤ 1/2 muffin: 2 to 3 grams ➤ whole small muffin: 3 to 5 grams |
|---|---|---|

## TAKE 10

### Eyes wide open

These simple movements will help relieve tension in your face and eyestrain by enhancing circulation. Do these movements whenever you need a break from staring at your computer screen.

**1.** Raise your eyebrows and open your eyes as wide as possible. Now close as tightly as possible.
**2.** Repeat 2 to 4 times.
**3.** Open your mouth as wide as possible to stretch the muscles around your nose and chin and then stick out your tongue as far as you can.
**4.** Hold for 5 seconds and repeat 2 times.

## SIT AND BE FIT
### Hamstring stretch

This stretch will not only relax the backs of your thighs, it will also release tension in your lower back, which increases flexibility.

1. Sit in a chair, lift your chest, contract your abdominals, press your shoulders back and down, align your head and spine, and face forward. Your knees should be directly over your heels.
2. Slide your right leg forward, keeping your heel on the floor, until your right knee is straight but not locked, with your toe pointing upward toward the ceiling.
3. Slide your hands down the extended leg until you feel a slight tightening in the back of your thigh. How far down your leg you go depends upon your flexibility. Keep your back flat and your chest and abdominals lifted.
4. Hold for 15 to 20 seconds and release.
5. Repeat on the other side and begin again, for a total of 3 sets.

## WATER BREAK

Some sodas are dehydrating due to the high amount of caffeine they contain. Caffeine is a diuretic, which will make your kidneys work harder and release more water than is healthy.

## ENERGY BALANCE SNACK
### Roast Turkey Wrap

1/2 piece small whole-grain pita bread or 1/2 tortilla
Low-fat mayonnaise or honey mustard
2 or 3 slices roast turkey breast
1 ounce hard cheese (such as cheddar or swiss)
2 lettuce leaves
1 slice tomato

1. Spread out the tortilla or pita bread.
2. Spread a small amount of mayonnaise or honey mustard on the pita bread.
3. Place the turkey, cheese, lettuce, and tomato on the pita bread.
4. Roll it up.

| CORE FOUR APPROXIMATE BREAKDOWN | PROTEIN ➤ turkey breast: 15 grams  CARBOHYDRATE ➤ pita bread or tortilla: 15 grams | FAT ➤ cheese: 6 grams ➤ low-fat mayonnaise: 4 grams  FIBER ➤ pita bread or tortilla: 1 gram |
|---|---|---|

## WATER BREAK

Drinking water can help alleviate bloating by flushing sodium from your tissues. Avoid taking a diuretic unless prescribed by your doctor, because it can cause the loss of two important minerals: potassium and magnesium.

## ENERGY LIFT
### Standing cat stretch

This stretch will strengthen your abdominals and lower back without placing any strain on your mid-section, which makes it especially good for anyone who can't do standard floor sit-ups.

1. Stand with your upper body leaning slightly forward from your hips, with your feet hip distance apart. Bend your knees slightly, lift your chest, contract your abdominals, press your shoulders back and down, align your head and spine, and face forward with your hands on the fronts of your thighs.
2. Exhale as you contract and pull in your abdominals and round your back toward the ceiling like a cat. Allow your shoulders to round forward, stretching the upper and back. If you do this movement correctly, you will look as if you were hit in the midsection with a large ball.
3. Hold for a few seconds and release back to the original position. If your back is strong and flexible, release into a slight arch, which will make the stretch more pronounced.
4. Repeat 3 times.

## ENERGY BALANCE LUNCH

### DINING IN
### Tuna and Apple Salad

　　3 ounces water-packed tuna

　　1 medium apple

　　2 to 3 tablespoons low-fat mayonnaise or salad
　　　　dressing

　　1 slice whole-grain bread

1. Drain water from the tuna and mash it with a fork into a fine consistency.
2. Core and chop the apple into small pieces.
3. Toss the apple and tuna with the mayonnaise and serve with bread.

### DINING OUT

Order a tuna salad and ask for a chopped apple on the side. If they don't have an apple, have a piece of fresh fruit with your salad.

➤If you want a larger meal: Have two cookies and a decaf coffee.

| CORE FOUR APPROXIMATE BREAKDOWN | PROTEIN ➤ tuna: 20 grams CARBOHYDRATE ➤ apple: 20 grams ➤ bread: 12 grams | FAT ➤ mayonnaise: 2 to 3 grams FIBER ➤ apple: 2 grams |
|---|---|---|

## SIT AND BE FIT
### Roll away fatigue

This movement seems easy, but after a few repetitions, you will feel it strengthening your hands, wrists, and forearms, the area most often injured in tennis or golf or through repetitive office work.

1. Sit in a chair, lift your chest, contract your abdominals, press your shoulders back and down, align your head and spine, and face forward.
2. With both arms, hold the top of a full-length towel in front of your chest, with your hands shoulder width apart and your palms facing the floor, elbows slightly bent. Keep your shoulder blades down and back throughout the movement.
3. Holding your body steady and breathing evenly, roll up the towel in your hands until you have rolled it into a large tubular shape.
4. Unfurl it to its original position and roll it up 2 more times.

## WATER BREAK

Tiny filters, called nephrons, regulate the flow of water through the kidneys. As you age, concentrations of minerals, salts, and protein cause these filters to wear out more quickly. Drinking lots of water helps postpone or relieve kidney problems by cleaning out these filters.

# ENERGY LIFT
Chair straddle

This energy lift will not only help improve your balance and torso stability, it will also firm and tone your thighs and buttocks. Repetition of this exercise will make walking or any other aerobic activity easier due to the improved balance and strength in your lower body.

1. Straddle the seat of a chair, standing with your toes turned out and your hands on the back of the chair, looking straight ahead.
2. Throughout the movement, keep your abdominals and buttocks contracted, and your rib cage lifted, and make sure your knees don't go past your toes.
3. Inhale as you bend your knees, almost as if you were going to sit down.
4. Gently touch the chair seat with your buttocks and exhale as you stand back up.
5. Repeat 10 to 15 times.

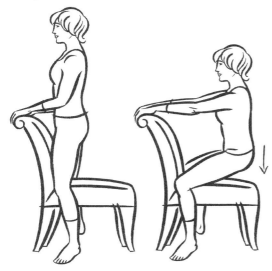

# WATER BREAK
Puffiness around your eyes is a good indication that you need to drink more water.

# ENERGY BALANCE SNACK
Cantaloupe and Beef Jerky

1 ounce beef jerky
1/2 cup cantaloupe chunks

| CORE FOUR APPROXIMATE BREAKDOWN | PROTEIN ➤ beef jerky: 11 grams CARBOHYDRATE ➤ cantaloupe: 5 grams | FAT ➤ beef jerky: 1 to 2 grams FIBER ➤ cantaloupe: 1 to 2 grams |
|---|---|---|

# TAKE 10
Cross-triceps extension

This exercise will tone the backs of your arms, working the muscle group involved in all pushing movements.

1. Sit in a chair, with your feet flat on the floor, your chest lifted, your abdominals contracted, your shoulders pressed back and down, your head aligned with your spine and looking straight ahead.
2. Place your right hand on your left shoulder, with your right elbow pointing outward a little higher than your chest.
3. Exhale as you extend your arm straight out, feeling a gentle tightening in the back of it.
4. Make sure to keep your elbow slightly bent when your arm is fully extended.
5. Inhale as you return to the starting position.
6. Repeat 10 to 15 times.
7. Repeat on the left arm.
8. When this movement is easy, hold a 3- to 5-pound weight for more resistance.

# WATER BREAK
A recent Harvard study found that drinking at least 6 to 8 glasses of water a day lowers the risk of bladder cancer by 51 percent.

# ENERGY BALANCE DINNER

## DINING IN

### Lemon Chicken Piccata

1 teaspoon butter

1 4- to 6-ounce chicken breast

Lemon-pepper and seasoning salt to taste

1/2 lemon, peeled, sliced

1 teaspoon capers

1/2 cup dry white wine

1. Melt the butter in a nonstick skillet over medium heat.
2. Add chicken, lemon pepper, and seasoning salt and cook for 3 to 4 minutes, turning once. Transfer to a plate.
3. Add lemon slices and capers to skillet; cook 1 minute.
4. Increase heat under skillet to high, stir in wine, and simmer 2 minutes.
5. Return chicken to pan; cook for 1 minute or until chicken is no longer pink in the middle.
6. Serve with 1/2 baked potato or yam, topped with 1 tablespoon low-fat sour cream or butter, and a large green salad with 2 tablespoons low-fat dressing.

## DINING OUT

Order the Chicken Piccata with the sauce on the side. Use just enough to make the chicken taste good. Order a small Caesar salad and go easy on the dressing. Add a small glass of wine if you want.

➤If you want a larger meal: Start with a protein-rich appetizer, like a shrimp cocktail or 1 ounce of cheese.

| CORE FOUR APPROXIMATE BREAKDOWN | PROTEIN ➤ chicken breast: 20 to 25 grams CARBOHYDRATE ➤ 1/2 baked potato: 15 grams ➤ salad: 3 grams | FAT ➤ dressing and butter: 10 to 15 grams FIBER ➤ salad and potato skin: 2 to 5 grams |
| --- | --- | --- |

# ENERGY BALANCE SNACK

### Yogurt Fruit Parfait

1/2 cup low-fat cottage cheese

1/2 cup plain yogurt

1/3 cup unsweetened apple-sauce

1/2 cup strawberries, raspberries, or blueberries

Sprinkle of cinnamon and nutmeg

Sprinkle of sliced almonds

1. Layer the first four ingredients in a bowl or parfait glass.
2. Sprinkle with cinnamon, nutmeg, and almonds.

| CORE FOUR APPROXIMATE BREAKDOWN | PROTEIN ➤ cottage cheese: 7 grams ➤ yogurt: 2 grams CARBOHYDRATE ➤ cottage cheese, yogurt, and berries: 10 grams | FAT ➤ almonds: 7 grams FIBER ➤ almonds and berries: 2 to 3 grams |
| --- | --- | --- |

# STRETCH, RELAX, AND SLEEP

1. Chest/posture stretch
2. Neck and upper spine stretch
3. Lower spine stretch

# STRESS RELIEF TIP

Caffeinated drinks, such as coffee, cola, tea, and hot chocolate, should be avoided for at least 3 hours before you go to bed because they will make it harder for you to fall asleep. Caffeine will also affect your blood sugar levels, which can make you wake up the next morning tired and craving sugar.

# Reject a Quick Fix

W HAT'S THE DIFFERENCE between dangerous energy and healthy energy? Dangerous energy is much easier to obtain than healthy energy—at least in the short run. Rather than make the effort to eat well so our bodies grow strong, it's tempting to try "quick fix" solutions such as grabbing a cup of coffee or relying on the sugar high of a candy bar. A burst of adrenaline may get you through the afternoon, and it may be more convenient than making sure you have a full night's sleep or including regular movement in your daily routine, but eventually misusing your body's hormones will leave you depleted and susceptible to a myriad of illnesses. And there's nothing convenient about cancer, ulcers, or heart disease.

Look beyond this moment to the entirety of your life. Regularity and repetition may seem boring, but in the long run, you'll run longer and stronger by practicing healthy habits daily.

# DAY 7

## WAKE-UP AFFIRMATION

**"Self-esteem comes from being able to define the world in your own terms and refusing to abide by the judgments of others."**

—*Oprah Winfrey, talk show host*

## WAKE-UP WORKOUT

1. Let body slowly wake up
2. Take several deep breaths
3. Full-body tighten and release
4. Pelvic tilts
5. Pillow sit-ups
6. Hamstring stretch
7. Hands and knees yoga stretch

## CORE FOUR

1. Push-up
2. Sit-up
3. Sit and stand
4. Posture squeeze/biceps curl

## PORTION CONTROL TIP

If you want to indulge in a dessert at a restaurant, plan to split your portion with a partner, and when ordering your meal, keep it low in carbohydrates. For example, start with a high-protein appetizer and a salad, and for a main course order fish or poultry and lots of steamed vegetables. Have one glass of wine and a decaf cappuccino or latte. Then split a dessert.

## ENERGY BALANCE BREAKFAST

### Oat Bran Breakfast

  1 tablespoon protein powder (Use a protein powder that contains less than 1 gram carbohydrate and dissolves easily in water.)
  1/2 cup water
  1/4 cup oat bran
  1/4 cup nonfat milk
  1 tablespoon raisins
  1 teaspoon cinnamon
  1 packet artificial sweetener

1. In a microwavable bowl, whisk the protein powder in water.
2. Stir in oat bran and microwave on high for 45 seconds to 1 minute.
3. Stir in milk, raisins, cinnamon and sweetener.
4. Serve with 1 scrambled egg or 4 slices of turkey bacon or any other small protein source.

➤ If you want a larger meal: Double the above recipe.

Drink water with lemon or 4 ounces of juice and 6 ounces of water, plus decaffeinated tea or coffee, if desired. Add low-fat creamer to taste.

| CORE FOUR APPROXIMATE BREAKDOWN | PROTEIN ➤ protein powder: 10 grams ➤ egg and turkey bacon: 12 grams CARBOHYDRATE ➤ oat bran, raisins, and nonfat milk: 25 grams | FAT ➤ egg yolk: 5 grams FIBER ➤ oat bran: 3 grams |
|---|---|---|

# TAKE 10
## Balance practice

This movement will help strengthen your ankles, while improving your balance and posture.

1. Stand up straight, and place your feet hip distance apart. Bend your knees slightly, lift your chest, contract your abdominals, press your shoulders back and down, align your head and spine, and face forward.
2. Place the toe of your right foot on top of your left foot, with your heel resting on the front of your shin.
3. Hold this position for 15 to 20 seconds. If you start to lose your balance, hold on to something to regain your balance and then try it again without a brace.
4. Change legs and repeat.

# SIT AND BE FIT
## Posture in line

Gravity is pulling your body toward the floor all day long, so slouching is a natural result of its pull combined with weak muscles. Since you can't stop gravity, you can work on building up your abdominals, midback, and lower back muscles instead.

1. Sit in chair or car seat with your upper body slightly away from the back of the chair.
2. Lift your rib cage and slightly contract your abdominals. Take a deep breath and then exhale.
3. Note the way your shoulders and head seem to fall into a straight line when the rib cage is lifted and your shoulder blades fall into their natural position and aid in supporting the torso. This is what good posture feels and looks like.

Standing in your good-posture position is the same as when seated, only with your knees unlocked and a natural curve in your lower back. Maintaining correct posture takes effort and awareness. Make an effort all day to think tall and lifted, which will keep your muscles doing their job without too much effort.

# WATER BREAK

A study at the University of Kansas found that drinking four cups of green tea a day supplies enough antioxidants to reduce cancer risk by up to 70 percent.

# ENERGY BALANCE SNACK
## Baked Apple

    1/2 apple
    1 tablespoon raisins
    1/2 cup cottage cheese or ricotta cheese
    1/2 cup vanilla low-fat yogurt
    Sprinkle of walnuts
    Sprinkle of nutmeg
    Sprinkle of cinnamon

1. Core the apple and halve it lengthwise (you can save the other half for another snack).
2. Place the apple cut side up in a small microwavable dish.
3. Place the raisins in the middle and microwave on high for 3 to 5 minutes.
4. Mix together the cottage cheese, yogurt, walnuts, and spices.
5. When the apple is cooked, place the mixture in the middle of the apple and enjoy.

CORE FOUR APPROXIMATE BREAKDOWN

**PROTEIN**
➤ cottage cheese or ricotta cheese: 7 grams

**CARBOHYDRATE**
➤ apple, raisins, and yogurt: 20 grams

**FAT**
➤ walnuts: 6 grams

**FIBER**
➤ apple and walnuts: 2 grams

## WATER BREAK

Water is the core ingredient of the fluid that lubricates the joints. Drinking enough water can significantly ease pain for up to 80 percent of back and joint pain sufferers.

## ENERGY LIFT

### 15-minute walk

Time to see the world.

Walking tip: If it is hard to find time in your day to walk, wear your walking clothes, such as a T-shirt and shorts, to bed at night. Place your shoes next to the bed, and the first thing after your Wake-up Workout, put on your shoes, grab a quick Energy Balance snack, and head for the door. Don't stop to think about it; just do it!

## ENERGY BALANCE LUNCH

### DINING IN

### Chicken Waldorf Salad

    1/4 cup diced celery

    1/4 cup diced apple

    1/2 cup chopped walnuts

    10 grapes, halved

    1/2 cup chopped cooked chicken breast or turkey

    1 tablespoon low-fat mayonnaise

Lightly toss ingredients together and serve.

### DINING OUT

Order a Waldorf salad with a side of chicken or turkey.

➤If you want a larger meal: Eat more chicken or turkey. Have a decaf cappuccino or latte.

| CORE FOUR APPROXIMATE BREAKDOWN | PROTEIN ➤ turkey or chicken: 20 to 25 grams  CARBOHYDRATE ➤ fruit salad: 25 to 30 grams | FAT ➤ walnuts: 9 grams  FIBER ➤ fruit salad: 3 to 5 grams |
|---|---|---|

## SIT AND BE FIT

### Do the monkey

1. Sit on the edge of your chair with your feet flat on the floor, your chest lifted, your abdominals contracted, your shoulders pressed back and down, your head in alignment with your spine, and looking straight ahead.
2. Your arms should be hanging at your sides, palms facing inwards, elbows slightly bent, and your wrists in a neutral position (in a straight line with your arm).
3. Bring one arm up in front of you to chest height (no higher) and then return to the starting position. Alternate lifting and lowering each arm.
4. Breathe evenly as you do this exercise.
5. When this movement is easy, add 3- to 5-pound weights.
6. Repeat 10 times with each arm.

## WATER BREAK

Water provides support for your cells and cushions your organs, acting as a shock absorber to help minimize damage to your organs.

# ENERGY LIFT
## Get up and dance!

Put on your favorite music and dance up your heart rate. Even 10 minutes of shaking your groove thing will strengthen your heart and lungs and burn fat, but try to keep dancing for a half hour.

# WATER BREAK

Water helps maintain blood volume, which is the amount of blood circulating in your body at any given time. Blood is made up of many different parts: white and red blood cells, platelets, and plasma. Plasma, the liquid portion of blood, is about 92 percent water, and the average person's blood volume should be around 4 to 5 quarts. When it is not, fatigue and other effects of dehydration can occur.

# ENERGY BALANCE SNACK
## Celery and Peanut Butter

4 or 5 large stalks celery

2 tablespoons peanut butter

Stuff the celery with peanut butter and enjoy.

| CORE FOUR APPROXIMATE BREAKDOWN | PROTEIN ➤ peanut butter: 8 grams | FAT ➤ peanut butter: 14 grams |
| --- | --- | --- |
| | CARBOHYDRATE ➤ peanut butter: 8 grams | FIBER ➤ celery: 1 to 2 grams |

# TAKE 10
## Shoulder rotation

The purpose of this movement is to increase the range of motion in the rotation of your shoulder joints, strengthen your rotator cuffs, and improve stability.

**1.** Sit in a chair that has arms.

**2.** Lean to the right supporting your head with your hand, and place your right elbow on the arm of the chair.

**3.** Bend your left elbow at a 45 degree angle and press it against the side of your body with your hand in a loose fist.

**4.** Inhale as you rotate your forearm in toward your body and then away from your body so that your palm faces out.

**5.** Exhale as your return to the starting position.

**6.** Repeat on each side 8 to 10 times.

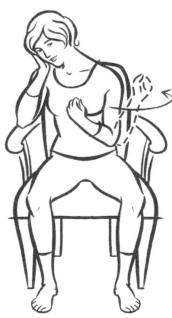

# WATER BREAK

Water balances electrolytes (minerals such as sodium and potassium), which help regulate body temperature and blood pressure.

# ENERGY BALANCE DINNER

## DINING IN

### Pasta Bowl

6 to 8 ounces cooked turkey or turkey sausage (usually two large links), chopped

1/2 cup cooked whole wheat pasta

1/2 cup tomato sauce

1 fresh tomato

1 1/2 cups sautéed vegetables (such as onions, peppers, and artichoke hearts)

Mix together all ingredients and serve with a large green salad with low-fat dressing.

## DINING OUT

To start, order a dinner salad with dressing on the side. Then order a chicken pasta dish with a red sauce. Eat only half the pasta. Finish with a decaf cappuccino or latte.

➤ If you want a larger meal: Add another link of sausage.

| CORE FOUR APPROXIMATE BREAKDOWN | PROTEIN<br>➤ sausage:<br>20 to 25 grams<br>CARBOHYDRATE<br>➤ pasta: 30 grams<br>➤ salad and vegetables:<br>5 grams | FAT<br>➤ sausage: 18 grams<br>FIBER<br>➤ pasta, salad, and<br>vegetables:<br>5 to 10 grams |
| --- | --- | --- |

# ENERGY BALANCE SNACK

### Fruit Plus

1/2 fruit plus one of the following:

2 slices chicken or turkey

1 hard-boiled egg

8 ounces nonfat milk or vanilla soy milk

| CORE FOUR APPROXIMATE BREAKDOWN | PROTEIN<br>➤ cheese: 6 grams<br>➤ chicken or turkey:<br>10 grams<br>➤ egg: 6 grams<br>➤ milk: 8 to 10 grams<br>CARBOHYDRATE<br>➤ fruit: 12 to 15 grams<br>➤ milk: 10 grams | FAT<br>➤ cheese: 6 grams<br>➤ egg: 5 grams<br>FIBER<br>➤ fruit: up to 1 gram |
| --- | --- | --- |

# STRETCH, RELAX, AND SLEEP

**1.** Chest/posture stretch

**2.** Neck and upper spine stretch

**3.** Lower spine stretch

# HELPFUL HINT

Sleeping conditions and positions that protect your lower back:

**1.** A firm mattress is better than a soft one.

**2.** If you sleep on your back, place a pillow under your knees to keep your lower back pressed into the mattress and stress-free.

**3.** If you sleep on your side, try placing a pillow between your knees to keep your hips in alignment. This will prevent your top leg from pulling on your lower back and alleviate pressure on your lower back.

**4.** To rise from bed, lie on your side with both knees bent and drop your knees over the side of the bed as you push with both arms to sit up. Scoot to the edge of the bed and position your feet under your buttocks. Stand up while keeping your knees bent and your back in a neutral position. Take a deep breath and start your day.

# Feel Good and Then Tackle Your Problems

W HEN AN UPSETTING SITUATION comes into our lives, most of us focus our attention on solving the problem and then on feeling good again. We assume that until the difficulty is resolved, we're bound to feel hurt or angry or confused. However, quite the opposite is true. When we're upset, adrenaline races through our bloodstreams causing our hearts to race, our breathing rates to increase, and our minds to be less effective in finding creative solutions. Exactly when we need our problem solving abilities the most is the time we are least able to access them.

To maximize your problem solving abilities, follow these simple steps:

**STEP ONE: Close your eyes and take a deep, deep breath.**

Since you're stressed, this first breath probably will not go very deeply into your lungs and will show itself by the slight rising of your breasts. Remember, chest breathing is not deep breathing.

**STEP TWO: Wiggle your toes, make a funny face, and stick your finger in your ear.**

Your thoughts are probably sneaking back to the problem situation, aren't they? It's important to disrupt this anxiety pattern and one way to do this is to act silly. If you are in public and don't want to draw attention to yourself, mentally sing one chorus of a childhood song, such as "I'm a Little Teapot."

**STEP THREE: Repeat steps one and two until you see your tummy expanding when you inhale.**

Until you're breathing from your diaphragm, you're still too agitated to tackle your situation. Once you are breathing and balanced, you'll be ready to take care of whatever comes into your life. And you'll probably discover that the challenge isn't quite as ominous as it seemed a few minutes ago.

# Core Four Cardio

As YOU BECOME stronger and have more energy you may want to increase your level of activity. A good walking program strengthens your cardiovascular system and burns fat. And because there is no real right or wrong way to walk, it is easy to get started. Here are a few pointers that can make your walks more enjoyable and productive:

➤ To begin a walking program, keep in mind that you should not expect immediate results. A walking program is a slow and steady way of building health.

➤ Forget heart-rate checks and overexaggerated movement—initially just walk at a comfortable pace, a little faster than a stroll.

➤ Depending on your time constraints and fitness level, fit in a 10-, 15-, 20-, or 30-minute walk whenever possible.

➤ Walk slowly for the first five minutes, then pick up the pace.

➤ Don't worry about distance; just use time as your measurement.

➤ Try to walk at least three to five times a week. However, if all you can do is one or two times, it's better than none.

➤ To make walking a habit, you need to make a commitment and make it fun. Try to go first thing in the morning before you get caught up in other things. Or make it a social occasion—find a walking buddy and pick a fun destination, such as a coffee shop.

➤ Music can make walking alone more interesting. Make sure your music is not so loud that you can't hear the surrounding traffic and other sounds that could warn you of impending danger. One way to ensure safety is to wear only one earphone at a time.

➤ What to wear: You really need a comfortable pair of walking shoes. Go to a sporting shoe store and try on a variety of shoes. Ask the trained sales person to fit your foot for comfort. Choose a pair with a firm heel cup for stability, a rocker sole to enhance a smooth heel-to-toe motion, and plenty of room for toes so they can spread out as they push off. Wear the socks you are planning to use when trying on shoes. But outside of wearing comfortable clothing, there are no fashion do's and don'ts when it comes to exercise.

Here are a few guidelines to proper walking:

1. **POSTURE** Lean slightly forward from your ankles, not your waist. Leaning from your waist will only tire your back and make breathing harder. Keep your chest lifted, your head in alignment with your spine, your chin up, and your shoulders pressed back and down. Check your posture every once in a while. Are your shoulders creeping up toward your neck? Are you starting to slouch as you get a little more tired? If so, shake it out, roll your shoulders, and return to your original correct posture.

2. **ARM SWING** Keep your elbows firmly bent at a 90-degree angle and swing your arms from your shoulders. Your hands should end their forward swing at chest height. On the backswing, your upper arm should be almost parallel to the ground.

3. **STRIDE** Make sure your stride is natural and smooth. Don't overstride—taking unusually long strides will make you tired sooner. When you are walking with someone who is taller than you are and can take longer strides, don't try to keep up.

**4. FOOT PLACEMENT** Strike the ground with your heel, and let your foot roll forward naturally. Rotate your hips slightly and tighten your abdominals, and as you are pushing off with your toes, squeeze the buttock of the same leg. This helps draw the leg back, which increases your speed and firms your buttocks.

**5. BREATHING** Use your breathing as an indicator of the intensity of your walk. If you are out of breath, you are walking too fast and too hard. Try to aim for a breathing pattern that is what is called a sighing breath, where you are breathing deeply but you can still carry on a conversation.

**6. COOL-DOWN STRETCHES** Try the following stretches, which can be found in the Index:
➤ Front of thigh stretch
➤ Back of thigh stretch
➤ Calf and lower leg stretch

## Benefits of walking to fitness

Medical professionals have long advocated the benefits of walking for the following medical conditions:
➤ Heart disease
➤ Hypertension
➤ Diabetes
➤ Arthritis
➤ Aging

Walking will also:

➤ Lower cholesterol
➤ Improve muscle coordination and strength
➤ Improve psychological well-being by reducing depression, tension, and anxiety
➤ Elevate mood to a higher and more joyful plane
➤ Burn fat for energy and reduce body-fat percentages
➤ Elevate your metabolism for hours after a moderate walk
➤ Increase energy through improved circulation and oxygen delivery
➤ Allow for sounder and deeper sleep
➤ Level blood sugar, which helps to decrease appetite and reduce sugar cravings

## Safety Alert

Don't walk with arm or ankle weights. They can irritate your joints and eventually cause knee problems. When you push off with your rear leg and swing it forward to take another step, a weight around your ankle will create added momentum. This added momentum could cause your knee to hyperextend and place a great deal of stress on your knee joint and the surrounding tendons and ligaments.

If you wear weights on your wrists, the same thing can happen. Weights are to be used in a gym or home, not out on a walk. Walking with weights doesn't do that much to tone the legs and arms anyway.

If you want to create more resistance as you become stronger, walk a little faster, walk hills, or strap on a fanny pack with a 32-ounce bottle of water inside. As you walk, take a few sips. As you get a little more tired, the weight will decrease right when you need it, and you will be hydrating yourself at the same time.

Using home cardiovascular fitness equipment such as treadmills and stair steppers offers the same benefits as walking in the open air. The main ingredient in every system and program is consistency. Without a consistent, enjoyable way to be fit, you won't reap the benefits.

The most important part of any fitness program is looking forward to the next time. This means you are having fun. So make music tapes, find a buddy or a beautiful trail—whatever it takes to have fun!

# DAY 8

## WAKE-UP AFFIRMATION

**"Learning to live in the present moment is part of the path of joy."**

—*Sarah Ban Breathnach, author*

## WAKE-UP WORKOUT

**1.** Let body slowly wake up
**2.** Take several deep breaths
**3.** Full-body tighten and release
**4.** Pelvic tilts
**5.** Pillow sit-ups
**6.** Hamstring stretch
**7.** Hands and knees yoga stretch

## CORE FOUR

**1.** Push-up
**2.** Sit-up
**3.** Sit and stand
**4.** Posture squeeze/biceps curl

## PORTION CONTROL TIP

Eating slowly gives your brain a chance to send the message that you are full. One way to slow down when eating is put down the fork while chewing.

## ENERGY BALANCE BREAKFAST

Balanced Energy Drink

> 8 ounces 1 or 2 percent milk or vanilla soy milk
>
> 1/2 cup frozen berries (such as strawberries or blueberries)
>
> 1/4 banana
>
> 2 tablespoons protein powder with less than 1 gram of carbohydrate
>
> 4 ice cubes

**1.** Combine all the ingredients in a blender.
**2.** Blend until creamy and enjoy.

➤If you want a larger meal: Add 4 strips turkey bacon or 2 ounces turkey jerky.

Drink water with lemon or 4 ounces of juice and 6 ounces of water, plus decaffeinated tea or coffee, if desired. Add low-fat creamer to taste.

| CORE FOUR APPROXIMATE BREAKDOWN | **PROTEIN** ➤ protein powder: 20 grams **CARBOHYDRATE** ➤ 1 or 2 percent milk: 8 grams ➤ soy milk: 10 grams | **FAT** ➤ 1 or 2 percent milk: 3 to 5 grams ➤ soy milk: 3 grams **FIBER** ➤ berries: 1 gram |
| --- | --- | --- |

## TAKE 10

Buttocks lift

Because your buttock muscles support your spine, you can protect your lower back by keeping them strong and toned. This gentle movement will stretch the tops of your thighs and your buttocks. If at any time you feel pressure in your lower back, don't continue with the exercise, and check your position before resuming.

1. With your knees about hip distance apart, kneel on a pillow or exercise mat behind a chair.
2. Keep your shoulders over your hips and place your hands on the back of the chair.
3. Point your toes, lift your chest, contract your abdominals, press your shoulders back and down, and put your lower back in a neutral position (i.e., don't arch).
4. Lift one knee off the pillow or mat (keep your stationary leg bent at a 90-degree angle) behind your hip. Lower and repeat 10 to 20 times.
5. Repeat with other leg.
6. Gently sit back and stretch the tops of your thighs. Be careful not to sit back too far, as this will place stress on your knees.

## SIT AND BE FIT

Lower back stretch

This stretch relieves pressure and tension in your lower back while stretching your buttocks.

1. Seated in a chair, place your left arm under your left knee and bring your knee to your chest.
2. Curl your body into a tucked position, with your head down as close to your knee as possible, and hold for 20 to 30 seconds.
3. Change legs and repeat.

## WATER BREAK

Your body uses water, via the blood, to help transport protein, minerals, and the vitamins B and C.

## ENERGY BALANCE SNACK

Hummus and Pita Bread

2 tablespoons any flavor hummus
1 small piece whole-grain pita bread, sliced into strips

| CORE FOUR APPROXIMATE BREAKDOWN | PROTEIN ➤ hummus: 7 grams CARBOHYDRATE ➤ pita bread: 15 grams | FAT ➤ hummus: 6 grams FIBER ➤ pita bread: 1 to 2 grams |
|---|---|---|

## WATER BREAK

Eight ounces of cola contains 40 mg. of caffiene, iced tea contains 50 mg., and coffee contains 350 mg., but water doesn't contain any!

## ENERGY LIFT

Arm circles

This movement is an isometric contraction that will wake up your upper body and help strengthen your shoulder girdle area.

1. Sit in a chair, lift your chest, contract your abdominals, press your shoulders back and down, align your head and spine, and face forward.
2. Hold your arms out to your sides at shoulder level, with your elbows slightly bent.
3. Making small circles, slowly move your arms inward, keeping them at the same height, and move them together in front of your chest at chest level.
4. Hold for one second and then circle back to the starting position.
5. Drop your arms, shake them out, and repeat 4 more times or until you become tired.

## ENERGY BALANCE LUNCH

DINING IN

Salmon Salad Sandwich

3 ounces water-packed salmon
1 to 2 tablespoons low-fat mayonnaise
1/4 cup combined chopped celery and onion
1 piece whole-grain pita bread
1 1-ounce stick string cheese

1. Drain the salmon and mix it with the mayonnaise, celery, and onion.
2. Place the salad in the pita bread. Top with the string cheese.
3. If you want, add a selection of chopped vegetables, such as carrots, cucumber, red, yellow, and green bell peppers, and jicama.

## DINING OUT

Order a tuna sandwich with as little mayonnaise as possible. Add a small green salad.

➤ If you want a larger meal: Have more vegetables with a low-fat, low-sugar dip.

**CORE FOUR APPROXIMATE BREAKDOWN**

**PROTEIN**
➤ tuna: 18 grams
➤ string cheese: 6 grams

**CARBOHYDRATE**
➤ pita bread: 26 grams
➤ There is a small amount of carbohydrate in the vegetables but not enough to count. Eat all you want.

**FAT**
➤ mayonnaise: 2 to 5 grams
➤ string cheese: 7 grams

**FIBER**
➤ pita bread: 2 to 5 grams
➤ vegetables: 5 to 10 grams

## SIT AND BE FIT
### Side stretches

This stretch will increase your ability to bend to the side and open up your shoulder joints. When you have a greater range of motion in your waist, you will take pressure off your lower back.

1. Sit in a chair, lift your chest, contract your abdominals, press your shoulders back and down, align your head and spine, and face forward. Place your feet flat on the floor and keep your arms hanging by the sides of your chair.
2. Bring your the left arm up and over your head and reach for the ceiling, with your palm facing inward. Rest your right hand on the edge of your chair.
3. Gently lean to the right and slowly turn your head to look up at your extended arm. Keep your hips glued to the chair and press your weightbearing shoulder down.
4. Breathe easily and evenly as you do this stretch.
5. Hold for 20 to 30 seconds or as long as comfortable.
6. Slowly turn your head forward. Return to the starting position and repeat on the other side.

## WATER BREAK

Water is a significant source of trace minerals, such as magnesium, cobalt, and copper.

## ENERGY LIFT
### Kick out the stress

This heart-rate-raising, stress-relieving activity will not only help condition your cardiovascular system; it will bring circulation from your lower extremities to your upper body and brain, helping you think more clearly.

1. Stand up straight and place your feet hip distance apart. Bend your knees slightly, lift your chest, contract your abdominals, press your shoulders back and down, align your head and spine, and face forward. Hold on to the back of a chair for balance.
2. Kick left with your left foot and then right with your right foot. Keep your kicks low and try to move at a good pace. Make sure you kick out far enough to the side that you don't kick the chair.
3. Don't snap your knees; let them stay slightly bent at the full extension.
4. Kick away all the stress and keep kicking until you feel a slight heart-rate response.

## WATER BREAK

Water in the blood transports essential nutrients to your skin's surface, making it more healthy.

# ENERGY BALANCE SNACK
### Banana Bites

    1 small ripe banana
    2 tablespoons granola
    1 teaspoon peanut butter
    1 teaspoon honey
    1/4 teaspoon unsweetened cocoa

1. Slice banana in half lengthwise.
2. Combine the remaining ingredients and stir well.
3. Spread the mixture over one half of the banana and top with the other half.
4. Cut into three sections.

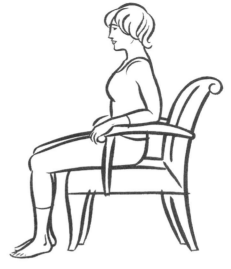

| CORE FOUR APPROXIMATE BREAKDOWN | PROTEIN<br>➤ peanut butter: 2 grams<br>CARBOHYDRATE<br>➤ banana and granola: 18 grams | FAT<br>➤ peanut butter and granola: 3 grams<br>FIBER<br>➤ granola and banana: 2 grams |
| --- | --- | --- |

# TAKE 10
### Armchair lifts

These dips firm and tone the backs of your arms and the large muscles of your back. You are also firming your buttocks and abdominals when your muscles contract to stabilize your torso during the movement.

1. Sit in a stable chair with arms. Lift your chest, contract your abdominals, press your shoulders back and down, align your head and spine, and face forward.
2. Scoot forward to the edge of the chair and place both hands on the chair's arms facing out.
3. Exhale as you lift your body with your arms until they are fully extended, but keep your elbows slightly bent.
4. Keep your abdominals and buttocks contracted.
5. Repeat the exercise 10 to 15 times or as many times as comfortable.
6. If you feel strain on your wrists, do only 2 or 3 until your wrists are flexible and strong enough to support your weight.

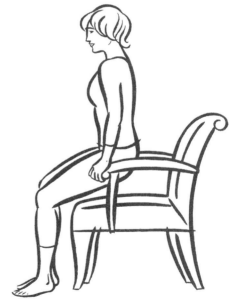

# WATER BREAK

Infants and toddlers have a poorly developed thirst mechanism and might not know when their body needs fluids. Make sure they get enough to drink throughout the day.

# ENERGY BALANCE DINNER

### DINING IN

Almond-Crusted Turkey Cutlets

1 tablespoon ground or finely chopped almonds

3 tablespoons Parmesan cheese

1/2 teaspoon each dried salad herbs and paprika

Salt to taste

1 6- to 8-ounce turkey cutlet (If turkey cutlets are not available, use a turkey breast and slice it into thinner portions.)

1 tablespoon butter

1 tablespoon olive oil

1 cup white wine

1 teaspoon lemon juice

Lemon slices optional

1. Mix the almonds with the Parmesan cheese, herbs, paprika, and salt on a flat surface.
2. Dip the cutlets into the mixture, coating both sides.
3. Heat the butter and oil in a nonstick skillet over medium heat.
4. Add the cutlets and cook until browned (approximately 4 minutes per side), turning once.
5. Remove them to heated serving platter.
6. Pour the wine and lemon juice into the pan.
7. Increase heat until the mixture boils rapidly and thickens slightly.
8. Spoon over the cutlets and garnish with lemon slices (if using).
9. Serve with 1/2 baked potato, 1 cup green vegetables, and a green salad with 2 tablespoons low-fat dressing.

### DINING OUT

Order roasted turkey with a little gravy and stuffing. Start with a large green salad and finish with a decaf cappuccino or latte.

➤If you want a larger meal: Add a small dinner roll.

| CORE FOUR APPROXIMATE BREAKDOWN | PROTEIN<br>➤ cutlets:<br>20 to 25 grams<br>CARBOHYDRATE<br>➤ potato: 15 grams<br>➤ salad and vegetables:<br>5 to 10 grams | FAT<br>➤ low-fat dressing,<br>Parmesan cheese,<br>butter, and olive oil:<br>18 grams<br>FIBER<br>➤ almonds, salad,<br>and vegetables:<br>5 to 10 grams |
| --- | --- | --- |

# ENERGY BALANCE SNACK

Cheesy Veggies

1 cup mixed vegetables topped with 1 ounce melted grated cheese

| CORE FOUR APPROXIMATE BREAKDOWN | PROTEIN<br>➤ cheese: 6 to 8 grams<br>CARBOHYDRATE<br>➤ vegetables:<br>5 to 10 grams | FAT<br>➤ cheese: 6 to 7 grams<br>FIBER<br>➤ vegetables:<br>2 to 4 grams |
| --- | --- | --- |

# STRETCH, RELAX, AND SLEEP

1. Chest/posture stretch
2. Neck and upper spine stretch
3. Lower spine stretch

# STRESS RELIEF TIP

Small amounts of alcohol may help you relax, but large amounts may increase stress, disrupt sleep, and cause hangovers. Too much alcohol also wreaks havoc with your blood sugar levels, causing them to fluctuate rapidly and putting them in fat-storing mode.

# Strong at Any Age

"**Y**OU CAN'T CONTROL your chronological age, but you can help determine your fitness age," says personal trainer Sandy Lewis, owner of Sierra Fitness in Southern California. "There's a level playing field after the age of 40. Everyone ages differently, but if you include regular movement in your life, you can increase strength, flexibility, and muscle mass."*

My experience confirms Sandy's claim. When I was in my 20s, exercise was a foreign concept. I ate poorly, rarely got a full night's sleep, and compulsively overworked. In 1985 I suffered a serious burnout that left me in physical, emotional, and spiritual despair. I slowly started adding movement into my life, little by little. Even though it's more than 15 years later, I now have significantly more stamina and strength in every area of my life. Remember, being strong and feeling fit is not reserved for the young. The joy of being strong is attainable at any age.

* From an interview with Sandy Lewis, A.C.E., A.F.A.A. (July 2001)

# DAY 9

## WAKE-UP AFFIRMATION

"Take each day as you find it. If things go wrong, don't mind it, for each day leaves behind it a chance to start anew."

—*Gertrude Ellgas, poet*

## WAKE-UP WORKOUT

1. Let body slowly wake up
2. Take several deep breaths
3. Full-body tighten and release
4. Pelvic tilts
5. Pillow sit-ups
6. Hamstring stretch
7. Hands and knees yoga stretch

## CORE FOUR

1. Push-up
2. Sit-up
3. Sit and stand
4. Posture squeeze/biceps curl

## PORTION CONTROL TIP

The best way to eat less food is to prepare less or, when in a restaurant, order less. If you are still hungry after you have eaten your meal, you probably didn't eat enough protein or fat. Before ordering more, try drinking a hot tea or decaf coffee with a little cream to see if that fills the hunger void. Remember, you can always have an Energy Balance snack a few hours later.

## ENERGY BALANCE BREAKFAST

### Cinnamon French Toast

1 egg and 4 egg whites (egg substitute equal to 20 grams of protein)
2 pieces whole-grain bread
1 tablespoon plus 2 teaspoons cinnamon
1/2 teaspoon vanilla extract
Vegetable oil spray
1 teaspoon trans-fat-free margarine
1 tablespoon low-sugar syrup

1. Whisk the egg and egg whites together with 1 tablespoon cinnamon and vanilla in a large bowl.
2. Allow the bread to soak in the egg mixture until well saturated.
3. Heat a large skillet that has been sprayed with vegetable oil over medium heat.
4. Place the bread in the skillet and pour the remaining egg mixture over the bread.
5. Increase heat to medium-high and cook until well-done.
6. Serve topped with margarine and syrup and a sprinkle of cinnamon.

➤If you want a larger meal: Add 2 slices of ham.

Drink water with lemon or 4 ounces of juice and 6 ounces of water, plus decaffeinated tea or coffee, if desired. Add low-fat creamer to taste.

| CORE FOUR APPROXIMATE BREAKDOWN | PROTEIN<br>➤ 1 egg and 4 egg whites: 20 grams<br>CARBOHYDRATE<br>➤ bread: 24 grams<br>➤ syrup: 5 grams | FAT<br>➤ margarine: 5 grams<br>➤ egg yolk: 5 grams<br>FIBER<br>➤ bread: 3 grams |
| --- | --- | --- |

# TAKE 10
## Sink push-up

This modified push-up is an excellent way to tone and strengthen the backs of your arms (triceps), the fronts of your shoulders, and the center of your chest. This exercise can place a lot of pressure on your wrists. If you have any pain, substitute a TAKE 10 exercise you liked from another day.

1. Place a folded towel on the edge of the sink.
2. Place your hands next to each other on the folded towel, shoulder width apart.
3. Walk your feet away from the sink until your body forms a diagonal line.
4. Keeping your body straight, gently lower your chest toward the sink while contracting your abdominals and tightening your buttocks.
5. Get as close to your hands as possible and then push back up to the starting position.
6. Start with 4 to 8 repetitions and work up to 12 to 15.

# SIT AND BE FIT
## Neck strengthener

This exercise will help strengthen the sides of your shoulders and upper neck, which, by helping support your head, will take pressure off your spinal column.

1. Sit in a chair, with your chest lifted, your abdominals contracted, your shoulders pressed back and down, and your head facing forward.
2. Your elbows should be bent at a 90-degree angle and pinned to your waist, with your hands in front of you in loose fists, palms facing down.
3. Exhale as you raise your elbows out to the sides, stopping at a little below shoulder height. Hold for 5 seconds.
4. Return to the original position and inhale.
5. Repeat 5 to 10 times or as long as comfortable.

# WATER BREAK

After the age of 65, we are more susceptible to dehydration, so keep drinking!

# ENERGY BALANCE SNACK
## Edamame

1 heaping cup edamame (boiled soybeans), a Japanese treat found wherever sushi is sold.

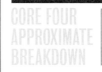

| CORE FOUR APPROXIMATE BREAKDOWN | PROTEIN<br>➤ 9 grams | FAT<br>➤ 5 grams |
|---|---|---|
| | CARBOHYDRATE<br>➤ 11 grams | FIBER<br>➤ 8 grams |

# WATER BREAK

Women who are pregnant should drink 2 glasses of water beyond the recommended 8 a day. Adequate water intake can decrease morning sickness.

# ENERGY LIFT
## Pace it out

Any time you are tired or stressed or both, get up and pace anywhere there is room to walk in circles. It doesn't matter where or when, as long as you are moving and increasing your circulation.

# ENERGY BALANCE LUNCH

### DINING IN
## Smoked Turkey Salad

8 ounces smoked turkey, cubed (Ask your deli for 1/2 pound as one thick slice.)
1 cup combined thinly sliced red onion, red and green bell pepper, and cucumber
2 to 3 cups lettuce
2 tablespoons low-fat peppercorn ranch dressing

1. Toss together all of the ingredients.
2. Add a latte with nonfat milk for dessert.

## DINING OUT

Order your favorite salad with protein and a variety of vegetables. Pick out half the croutons and ask for the dressing on the side. If you order a Chinese chicken salad, take off half the crispy noodles.

➤If you want a larger meal: Add 3 ounces turkey and increase the amount of lettuce.

| CORE FOUR APPROXIMATE BREAKDOWN | PROTEIN ➤ tuna: 18 grams ➤ string cheese: 6 grams CARBOHYDRATE ➤ whole-grain bread: 26 grams ➤ There is a small amount of carbs in the chopped veggies – not enough to count. Eat all you want. | FAT ➤ low-fat mayonnaise: 2 to 5 grams ➤ string cheese: 7 grams FIBER ➤ whole-grain bread: 2 to 5 grams ➤ veggies: 5 to 10 grams |
| --- | --- | --- |

## SIT AND BE FIT

### Isometric bicep curl

This exercise is an isometric hold, meaning you use your body weight against an immovable object to strengthen a muscle. Due to the tightening of all the muscles in your torso, it will also help tone the abdominals and back muscles.

1. Sit in a chair, lift your chest, contract your abdominals, press your shoulders back and down, align your head and spine, and face forward. Place your feet flat on the floor.
2. Slide your chair close to your desk.
3. With your elbows pinned to your waist, put your hands flat against the underside of your desk and try to lift it off the floor.
4. If you have a light desk, use a countertop or another surface that is impossible to lift.

5. Hold the contraction for as long as comfortable and release.
6. Repeat 8 to 12 times until you feel your muscles working.

## WATER BREAK

Even daily chores such as gardening, shopping, and cleaning make you perspire, increasing your body's need for water.

## ENERGY LIFT

### Doorknob knee bend

This exercise tightens the fronts of your thighs and your buttocks and stretches your back muscles.

1. Find a door on which you can hold on to the knobs on both sides at the same time.
2. Hold on to the doorknobs with both hands. Stand up straight, with your chest lifted, your abdominals contracted, your shoulders down and back, and your feet shoulder width apart.
3. Inhale as you bend your knees into a seated (squat) position, keeping your knees over your heels and your arms straight.
4. Hold at the bottom of the movement for 5 seconds or as long as comfortable.
5. Exhale, tighten your buttocks, and keep your knees slightly bent as you return to the starting standing position.
6. Repeat 8 to 12 times.

## WATER BREAK

Your skin receives moisture from the inside out, so drinking water keeps your skin plump and hydrated (a cheap alternative to lotion!).

# ENERGY BALANCE SNACK
Veggies, chips, and dip

2 cups vegetables
1/2 cup low-fat dip
1 cup ricotta cheese
10 chips

1. Chop the vegetables.
2. Mix the dip with the riccotta cheese.
3. Serve with chips. (Eat no more than 10! If you can't have just 10, then don't open a bag)
There should be about 1 1/4 cups of dip left over. Refrigerate the balance and save it for another time you want an Energy Balance snack.

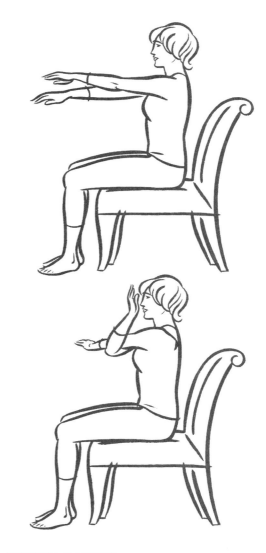

| CORE FOUR APPROXIMATE BREAKDOWN | | |
|---|---|---|
| **PROTEIN**<br>➤ ricotta cheese: 10 grams | **FAT**<br>➤ chips: 10 to 15 grams | |
| **CARBOHYDRATE**<br>➤ vegetables and chips: 15 grams | **FIBER**<br>➤ vegetables: 1 to 2 grams | |

# TAKE 10
Rotator cuff stretch

General stretching of this area will help increase energy and keep your shoulders and back limber. If you play tennis or golf, this movement will help relax your shoulders and rotator cuffs before and after your play.

1. Sit in a chair, with your feet flat on the floor. Lift your chest, contract your abdominals, press your shoulders back and down, align your head and spine, and face forward.
2. Hold both arms straight out in front of your body, chest level and palms facing the floor.
3. Cross your left arm under the right above your elbow, making an X with your arms. Your right arm will be resting in the crook of the your arm.
4. Keeping your shoulders facing forward and square, bend your left arm at the elbow until your palm is close to your face.
5. Squeeze your left arm until you feel a gentle stretch in your right rear shoulder and the right part of mid-back.
6. Hold for 20 to 30 seconds. Repeat the stretch on the other side.

# WATER BREAK
Diet colas are loaded with caffeine, which is a diuretic that dehydrates your system. Remember one of the side effects of dehydration is fatigue, which can counteract any energy you might get from the caffeine.

# ENERGY BALANCE DINNER

## DINING IN

### Grilled Salmon with Parmesan Broccoli

1 bunch broccoli, cut into florets
1 tablespoon olive oil
1 clove garlic, peeled and minced
2 tablespoons Parmesan cheese
1 tablespoon fresh lemon juice
Lemon-pepper or salt and pepper to taste
6 to 8 ounces grilled salmon

1. Steam the broccoli florets until tender and crisp. Remove to a heated serving dish and cover.
2. Heat the olive oil with the garlic in a small skillet over medium heat; remove the garlic after 3 to 4 minutes and discard.
3. Grill salmon over medium-high until just opaque in center, about 5 minutes per side.
4. Toss the broccoli in the garlic oil and sprinkle with cheese, lemon-pepper, or salt and pepper and lemon juice.
5. Serve immediately with the salmon and a small baked potato or 1/2 small yam (with trans-fat-free margarine) prepared ahead of time and kept warm.

The broccoli recipe will make about four portions, but broccoli is so nutritious you can eat all you want and save the rest for another meal.

## DINING OUT

Order salmon and broccoli, drizzle with a vinegar and olive oil dressing. Add a large green salad with a small dinner roll or one slice of sourdough bread with dinner.

➤ If you want a larger meal: Eat more salmon and broccoli. Add a decaf cappuccino or latte.

| CORE FOUR APPROXIMATE BREAKDOWN | PROTEIN ➤ salmon: 20 to 28 grams CARBOHYDRATE ➤ potato: 15 grams ➤ broccoli: 5 to 10 grams | FAT ➤ Parmesan cheese, margarine, and olive oil: 18 grams FIBER ➤ potato skin and broccoli: 5 to 10 grams |
| --- | --- | --- |

# ENERGY BALANCE SNACK

## Got Milk?

8 ounces 1 percent milk or vanilla soy milk

| CORE FOUR APPROXIMATE BREAKDOWN | PROTEIN ➤ 6 to 8 grams CARBOHYDRATE ➤ 8 to 10 grams | FAT ➤ 3 to 5 grams FIBER ➤ 0 grams |
| --- | --- | --- |

# STRETCH, RELAX, AND SLEEP

1. Chest/posture stretch
2. Neck and upper spine stretch
3. Lower spine stretch

# EXTRA, EXTRA

## Sit and stretch

1. If this is a comfortable position, sit on your bed with your legs crossed. If not, this stretch can also be done seated with the soles of your feet touching each other.
2. Extend your arms front of you as far as possible.
3. Bend forward from your waist gently and allow your lower back to stretch and relax.
4. Breathing evenly, drop your head forward while relaxing your entire spine. Hold for a few seconds and return to the original position.

# STRESS RELIEF TIP

Sometimes you need a mental health day. When the world seems overwhelming, take a day off from work or get a babysitter for the kids and do something your enjoy, whether it is gardening or reading or just staring off into space for a few hours. By taking a "sick" day when you are physically fine but are feeling stressed or overwhelmed, you may be saving yourself from actually getting ill.

# Pace Yourself

I'VE LOST COUNT of the rigorous exercise programs I've started with great enthusiasm, only to be laid up after a week or two. A good friend of mine finally said, "Has it occurred to you yet that you're putting too much stress on your body through exercise, or do you need to go through this one more time?" I hate to admit it hadn't occurred to me, and I thank God for good friends who speak the truth. The fact was, I assumed rigorous exercise wasn't stressful. But it can be stressful, and any stress, regardless of the source, can weaken our immune systems. Plus, doing too much too soon puts us at risk of injury.

You're now in the second week of this program and, hopefully, becoming more attuned to your body. Move in harmony with your body's needs. It may have taken years to get out of shape. It will take more than a few days to realize optimal health and stamina. So pace yourself and enjoy the process. Remind yourself that your goal is health, not a number on the scale.

# DAY 10

## WAKE-UP AFFIRMATION

"**Creativity is inventing, experimenting, growing, taking risks, breaking rules, making mistakes, and having fun.**"

—*Mary Lou Cook, activist and minister*

## WAKE-UP WORKOUT

**1.** Let body slowly wake up
**2.** Take several deep breaths
**3.** Full-body tighten and release
**4.** Pelvic tilts
**5.** Pillow sit-ups
**6.** Hamstring stretch
**7.** Hands and knees yoga stretch

## CORE FOUR

**1.** Push-up
**2.** Sit-up
**3.** Sit and stand
**4.** Posture squeeze/biceps curl

## PORTION CONTROL TIP

When you go to a restaurant, never look at the menu—before you go plan what you are going to eat. Once you have your head set on a dish, your fork will follow.

## ENERGY BALANCE BREAKFAST

### Through the Garden Omelette

1 egg and 4 egg whites
1 teaspoon chopped fresh parsley and tarragon
Lemon-pepper or salt and pepper to taste
1/2 cup each diced yellow, red, and green bell pepper and tomato
1/2 cup shredded low-fat cheddar cheese
1 green onion, chopped

**1.** Beat the egg and egg whites until frothy; stir in the parsley and season with lemon-pepper, salt, and pepper.
**2.** Place a nonstick skillet coated with olive oil cooking spray over medium heat.
**3.** Pour in the egg mixture and cook until the eggs begin to set.
**4.** Sprinkle in the remaining ingredients and flip over the omelette.
**5.** Cook a few more minutes until the eggs are set.
**6.** Serve with 1 piece whole-grain toast or 1/2 a large whole-grain bagel spread with low-fat cream cheese.

➤If you want a larger meal: Make the omelette with 2 whole eggs and 4 egg whites. Serve with 2 slices of toast or a large whole-grain bagel.

Drink water with lemon or 4 ounces of juice and 6 ounces of water, plus decaffeinated tea or coffee, if desired. Add low-fat creamer to taste.

**CORE FOUR APPROXIMATE BREAKDOWN**

| PROTEIN | FAT |
|---|---|
| ➤ egg and egg whites: 20 to 26 grams | ➤ 1 egg yolk: 5 grams |
| | ➤ cheese: 5 grams |
| **CARBOHYDRATE** | **FIBER** |
| ➤ bread: 13 grams | ➤ bread or bagel: 3 to 5 grams |
| ➤ 1/2 bagel: 13 grams | ➤ vegetables: 2 to 3 grams |

# TAKE 10
Neck massage

This movement not only relieves tension in your upper neck but also gives you a quick massage break, which reduces stress.

1. Sit in a chair, lift your chest, contract your abdominals, press your shoulders back and down, align your head and spine, and face forward.
2. Grab the back of your neck with the fingers of your right hand.
3. Place your thumb between your neck muscles and your collarbone.
4. Pull with your fingers while squeezing your upper neck with your thumb.
5. Massage this way for 10 to12 seconds and then do the other side.

# WATER BREAK

If you become thirsty during a workout, you have already passed out of the safe stage of hydration. When exercising or working in hot humid weather, your body needs 4 to 8 ounces of water every 20 minutes to replace water loss.

# SIT AND BE FIT
Wrist workout

The following exercise is beneficial for anyone who suffers from carpal tunnel syndrome, an injury caused by repetition, often from overuse of computer keyboards. If you don't currently have this condition, this exercise will also help prevent this problem.

1. **WRIST EXTENSION AND FLEXION** Lay your arm on its side across a tabletop with your hand in a fist. Slowly bend your wrist forward and back. To measure your progress, hold a pencil in your fist to trace on a piece of paper how far your hand extends in each direction.

2. **WRIST ADDUCTION AND ABDUCTION** Lay your arm on a tabletop, palm down with your hand in a fist. Keeping your arm flat, bend your wrist downward so that your knuckles touch the table, then return to the original position.
3. Repeat 4 times.

# WATER BREAK

Caffeine is addictive, and addiction can be mistaken for panic attacks. Try to avoid consuming more than two cups of coffee or one cola a day.

# ENERGY BALANCE SNACK
Salmon Snack Balls

    1 6-ounce can salmon
    1 8-ounce package low-fat cream cheese, softened
    1 tablespoon lemon juice
    2 teaspoons chopped green onion
    1 teaspoon prepared white horseradish
    1 teaspoon salt
    3 tablespoons chopped parsley

1. Drain the salmon and combine all the ingredients except the parsley and mix thoroughly.
2. Chill for several hours.
3. Shape the salmon mixture into balls and roll in the parsley.

Eat 5 salmon balls with 5 whole-grain crackers. Cover the remaining balls and refrigerate them for another snack.

| CORE FOUR APPROXIMATE BREAKDOWN | PROTEIN ➤ salmon: 10 to 15 grams | FAT ➤ cream cheese and salmon: 10 grams |
| --- | --- | --- |
| | CARBOHYDRATE ➤ crackers: 10 to 15 grams | FIBER ➤ crackers: 1 to 2 grams |

## WATER BREAK

Microorganisms such as bacteria grow quickly in bottled water that is left open in warm environments such as your car. Keep your water bottles closed and as cool as possible.

## ENERGY LIFT

### Twist and shout

Whenever your muscles are stiff and cramped, get up and twist again like you did last summer. Combined with a hip swing and wiggle, this movement will get your blood circulating and your energy flowing. If you have lower back problems, take it easy.

## ENERGY BALANCE LUNCH

### DINING IN

### Chicken Tabbouleh Salad

1/2 cup tabbouleh salad (found in the rice aisle of your supermarket)

4 to 6 ounces cooked chicken breast, diced

1/2 tomato, diced

3 tablespoons diced scallions

2 tablespoons sliced almonds

3 tablespoons cucumber yogurt sauce, if desired (See recipe following)

1. Prepare tabbouleh salad mix according to directions on the box.
2. Mix in the chicken, with the tabbouleh, tomato, scallions, and almonds.
3. Top with cucumber yogurt sauce (if using).

### CUCUMBER YOGURT SAUCE

1/2 cup plain nonfat yogurt

1 tablespoon onion, chopped

1 tablespoon cucumber, chopped

1/2 teaspoon minced garlic

1/4 teaspoon lemon juice

Salt and pepper to taste

Mix all of the ingredients together.

### DINING OUT

Make this lunch out an adventure and dine in a Greek or Middle Eastern restaurant. Order a chicken breast and side of tabbouleh.

➤ If you want a larger meal: Add a small whole grain pita bread with 2 tablespoons hummus on the side.

| CORE FOUR APPROXIMATE BREAKDOWN | PROTEIN<br>➤ chicken: 20 to 25 grams<br>CARBOHYDRATE<br>➤ tabbouleh: 20 to 25 grams<br>➤ pita bread and hummus: 15 grams | FAT<br>➤ tabbouleh with 1 tablespoon olive oil: 12 grams<br>➤ hummus: 2 grams<br>FIBER<br>➤ tabbouleh: 3 grams<br>➤ pita bread: 1 to 2 grams |
|---|---|---|

## SIT AND BE FIT

### Palm push

This isometric exercise will help strengthen your chest wall, improve muscle symmetry, and promote muscle awareness. Repetition will not only make you stronger but, as your muscles become conditioned, also make doing push-ups easier.

1. Sit in a chair, lift your chest, contract your abdominals, press your shoulders back and down, align your head and spine, and face forward.
2. Clasp your hands in front of you, raise your arms to just below shoulder height, and bend your elbows at a 90-degree angle.
3. Inhale as you push your hands against each other and hold for a few seconds. You will feel your chest and the fronts of your shoulders contract.
4. Exhale and release.
5. Repeat 8 to 12 times or as times many as you find comfortable.

# WATER BREAK

Watch for the following dangers in your tap water: chemical toxins, copper or lead from pipes or containers, and pesticide runoff. Check with your water company to find out how your water is treated and maintained for drinking.

# ENERGY LIFT

Shake with stretch

This exercise will not only help prevent fatigue but also increase flexibility in the muscles and tendons of your wrists, hands, and forearms.

1. Sit on a chair with your feet on the floor and lift your chest, contract your abdominals, press your shoulders back and down, align your head and spine, and face forward.
2. Shake your hands all around, up, down, and side to side, bringing circulation to your hands and forearms. Shake your hands above your head, to the sides, below your waist, and back to the center. Pause and repeat 4 times.
3. With your elbows pinned to your waist and your right palm facing the ceiling, place the fingertips of your left hand on top of the fingertips of your right hand. Gently press your right hand back until you feel a stretch in your palm and fingers.
4. Turn over your right hand and with your left hand gently push on the back of your right hand, stretching it.
5. Release and repeat the stretch on your left hand.
6. Repeat this stretch on both hands 2 times.

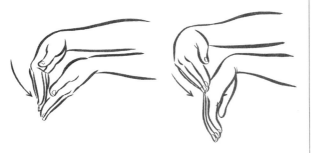

# WATER BREAK

Can you drink too much water? Yes, but it is rare. Drinking several liters of water a day (4 quarts) combined with excessive perspiring can lead to a condition called hyponatremia, which occurs when sodium levels are too low. Symptoms include anxiety, headaches, muscle twitching, and weakness. If you are suffering from any of these symptoms, see your doctor, drink a little less water, and make sure you are eating foods that contain natural sodium.

# ENERGY BALANCE SNACK

Peanut Butter and Cheese

1 slice whole-grain bread
1 tablespoon peanut butter
1/2 cup low-fat cottage cheese

Spread peanut butter on bread and top with cottage cheese.

CORE FOUR
APPROXIMATE
BREAKDOWN

**PROTEIN**
➤ peanut butter: 4 grams
➤ cottage cheese: 7 grams

**CARBOHYDRATE**
➤ bread: 13 grams

**FAT**
➤ peanut butter: 4 grams

**FIBER**
➤ bread: 3 to 5 grams

# TAKE 10

Wrist and forearm stretch

The more strength and flexibility you can give your hands, wrists, and forearms, the less likely you are to suffer from carpal tunnel syndrome.

1. Lay your arm palm down on a tabletop with your wrist just over the edge. Let your wrist bend down slowly and then straighten it.
2. Turn over your hand and forearm so your palm is facing up and repeat the movement.
3. Repeat with the other hand.

## WATER BREAK

Too many soft drinks are bad for your bones. Many soft drinks contain fizz-producing phosphoric acid, which can prevent your body from absorbing bone-building calcium. If you drink soda, try to consume more calcium-rich foods such as low-fat milk and soy milk. Also all women should be sure to take a calcium supplement of at least 1,000 to 1,500 milligrams a day.

## ENERGY BALANCE DINNER

### DINING IN

Grilled Fish with Tropical Salsa

> 1/2 cup each finely chopped mango, pineapple, papaya, tomato, cucumber, and red bell pepper
>
> 1 teaspoon diced cilantro
>
> 1 teaspoon lime juice
>
> 2 tablespoons canned black beans, drained, rinsed
>
> 6 to 8 ounces grilled red snapper, halibut, or any other fish

1. In a large bowl, combine 1/2 cup each of mango, pineapple, papaya, tomato, cucumber, and red bell pepper.
2. Gently stir in the cilantro, lime juice, and black beans. If you like a spicier version, add a small amount of diced jalapeño pepper. Cover and refrigerate until serving.
3. Grill fish on medium-high heat, about 5 minutes per side, and place the salsa on top of the fish. Serve with a large green salad with 2 tablespoons poppy seed dressing, a steamed green vegetable, and 1/2 small baked potato with a small amount of low-fat sour cream and chives.

### DINING OUT

Many restaurants have fish with salsa on the menu. If you don't like spicy salsa, ask for the salsa without the spice. If this isn't possible, ask for some fresh fruit on the side. Order a green salad and 1/2 baked potato. Finish with a decaf latte.

> If you want a larger meal: Have a larger piece of fish with more salsa and a larger green salad with lots of vegetables.

| CORE FOUR APPROXIMATE BREAKDOWN | | |
|---|---|---|
| **PROTEIN**<br>➤ fish: 20 to 25 grams<br>**CARBOHYDRATE**<br>➤ salsa: 10 to 15 grams<br>➤ 1/2 baked potato: 10 grams<br>➤ salad and vegetables: 5 to 10 grams | **FAT**<br>➤ poppy seed dressing: 10 grams<br>➤ sour cream: 5 grams<br>**FIBER**<br>➤ salsa: 2 to 5 grams<br>➤ salad, vegetables, and potato: 10 to 15 grams | |

## ENERGY BALANCE SNACK

Hot Chocolate

8-ounce glass of nonfat milk or vanilla soy milk
3/4 package low-fat instant hot chocolate mix
Sprinkle of cinnamon and/or nutmeg

Heat milk, stir in hot chocolate mix, top with cinnamon and nutmeg, and enjoy.

| CORE FOUR APPROXIMATE BREAKDOWN | | |
|---|---|---|
| **PROTEIN**<br>➤ 1 percent milk: 8 grams<br>➤ soy milk: 6 grams<br>**CARBOHYDRATE**<br>➤ 1 percent milk: 11 grams<br>➤ soy milk: 10 grams | **FAT**<br>➤ 1 percent milk or soy milk: 4 grams<br>**FIBER**<br>➤ 0 grams | |

## STRETCH, RELAX, AND SLEEP

1. Chest/posture stretch
2. Neck and upper spine stretch
3. Lower spine stretch

## HELPFUL HINT

Don't strike your computer keys too hard—the pressure can place stress on your nerves and can cause swelling and pain. When working at the computer, take frequent breaks and vary the position of your wrists, avoiding a bent position.

# Take a Break

NEARLY EVERY ASPECT OF OUR LIVES has been computerized—we shop online, keep in touch with our friends and family through e-mail, balance our checkbooks and pay our bills via computer, and relax with a computerized game of solitaire. Even if you don't make your living in front of a keyboard like I do, you probably spend some portion of your day typing away. It's easy to become so engrossed in a task that before you know it, you've been sitting in the same position for an hour or two. Combining a stationary posture with repetitive hand movements can cause pain and injury to your wrists and arms, contribute to water retention around your ankles, fatigue your back muscles, overstress your neck and shoulder muscles, and trigger tension headaches. Who knew sitting at a computer could be so detrimental to your health?

Author David Ruegg advises computer users to take regular breaks in order to prevent repetitive strain injuries. It doesn't take long to bring a little blood and oxygen to tense areas. Every ten minutes or so, look away from your monitor and stretch your arms, shoulders, fingers, and hands. Ruegg also recommends taking a stand-up break every half hour. Use it as an opportunity to get a glass of water, file some papers, or simply stretch. I've found that not only does my body benefit but my concentration is increased in the long run if I take short breaks at regular intervals—a genuine body-mind advantage.

David Ruegg , *Repetitive Strain Injury: A Handbook on Prevention and Recovery* (Largo, 1999)

# Taking a Break

SOME OF MY MOST relaxing moments have occurred in the bathtub. Here are some easy ways to de-stress with stretches while you soak.

➤ Fill your bathtub with herbal-scented bath salts; use formulas that relax tired muscles.

➤ Slowly slide into the water and rest your head against a bath pillow. As you are relaxing, envision the cares and worries of your day dissolving away. Replace these thoughts with daydreams of what you would like the future to hold. Breathing evenly and deeply, relax as long as you need—this is your time for yourself.

➤ While you are still soaking, place both hands behind the knee of your right leg and slowly bend the leg, pulling it up towards your chest. Make sure your left leg is braced against the foot of the tub to prevent you from slipping under the water. Hold this position for a few seconds, before straightening the right leg up to the ceiling as far as it is comfortable, keeping your knee slightly bent. Hold for a few seconds. Repeat this entire stretch with your left leg, alternate back and forth for two sets each. This exercise will release your hamstrings (back of the thigh) and your lower back, which feels especially great if you are desk bound most of the day.

➤ After you have finished relaxing in this prone position, slowly sit up and, with your legs straight out in front of you and your knees slightly bent, lean forward as if you were going to grab the faucet. Feel the stretch in the back of your thighs and lower back. Hold for a few seconds and release. Repeat two more times.

➤ Still sitting, bend both knees and put your feet flat on the tub's floor, grasping the toes of your left foot with your left hand. Slowly slide the left heel out in front of you until you feel a gentle tightness in the calf. Hold for a few seconds and release. Repeat the stretch with your right foot for two more sets. This exercise is ideal if you wear any kind of a heel, even only a few inches, because your calves become shortened and you need to stretch them in order to prevent injury to the Achilles tendon, which attaches your calf to the bottom of your heel.

➤ Relax back into the warm water and when ready slowly rise from your bath and dry off.

## Take a Meditation Break

Meditation allows you time to reflect on your life and how you are fulfilling your personal destiny. Meditation is not a time to solve problems, just allow your mind to turn your problems over to your soul and wait for the answer. You will be surprised how often the response you are seeking comes right when you need it.

## Meditation with the "Hamsa" Mantra:

The "Hamsa" Mantra, or mystical incantation, is a wonderful introduction to meditation.

➤ Sit comfortably—a quiet place is preferred, but not required.

➤ Close your eyes and breathe naturally. Sit for about one minute before you begin thinking the Hamsa mantra.

➤ Gently bring your attention to your breath and begin to think the mantra, gently and easily. Just let it come, don't force it. Think "ham" on the inhale and "sa" on the exhale. Allow yourself to be absorbed in the words.

➤ Let your thoughts and feelings come and go with detachment. Don't try to control them in any way. When you realize that you are not re-peating Hamsa, gently return to the mantra. Do not try to force yourself to think the mantra to the exclusion of all other thoughts. This breath-ing exercise may help you to experience a deep state of relaxation.

➤ Meditate in this way for 20 minutes (children for less time). Try to estimate the time spent be-cause the use of an alarm clock will jolt you out of the meditation.

➤ Take about a minute to slowly return to normal awareness.

# DAY 11

## WAKE-UP AFFIRMATION

*"I am only one; but still I am one. I cannot do everything, but still I can do something. I will not refuse to do something I can do."*

—*Helen Keller, author and public speaker*

## WAKE-UP WORKOUT

**1.** Let body slowly wake up
**2.** Take several deep breaths
**3.** Full-body tighten and release
**4.** Pelvic tilts
**5.** Pillow sit-ups
**6.** Hamstring stretch
**7.** Hands and knees yoga stretch

## CORE FOUR

**1.** Push-up
**2.** Sit-up
**3.** Sit and stand
**4.** Posture squeeze/biceps curl

## PORTION CONTROL TIP

Your greatest challenge when eating out at a restaurant is the often oversized portions. One way to eat less is to fill up on the vegetables first, then eat a hand-sized portion of the protein, and then the other carbohydrates and fat.

## ENERGY BALANCE BREAKFAST

Eggs Benedict Energy Balance Style

2 slices Canadian bacon
1 egg and 2 egg whites, poached
1 small whole-grain English muffin
1 tablespoon prepared hollandaise sauce (Can be made fresh or found in the deli department of your supermarket.)

**1.** Toast the muffin and heat the bacon in the microwave for 20 seconds.
**2.** Place the Canadian bacon and eggs on top of the English muffin.
**3.** Drizzle the hollandaise sauce on top.

➤ If you want a larger meal: Add 2 more slices Canadian bacon.

Drink water with lemon or 4 ounces of juice and 6 ounces of water, plus decaffeinated tea or coffee, if desired. Add low-fat creamer to taste.

| CORE FOUR APPROXIMATE BREAKDOWN | | |
|---|---|---|
| **PROTEIN**<br>➤ egg and egg whites: 12 grams<br>➤ Canadian bacon: 17 grams<br>**CARBOHYDRATE**<br>➤ English muffin: 30 grams | **FAT**<br>➤ egg yolk: 5 grams<br>➤ Canadian bacon: 5 grams<br>➤ hollandaise sauce: 10 grams<br>**FIBER**<br>➤ English muffin: 2 to 5 grams | |

# TAKE 10
## Heel raise and stretch

This combination lift and stretch is not only good for firming and toning your lower legs; it will increase circulation to the area and help prevent varicose veins. By doing this exercise you will also notice an improvement in your balance and the strength of your step.

1. Stand with your legs hip distance apart, holding on to the sink or the back of a chair.
2. Bend your knees slightly, lift your chest, contract your abdominals, press your shoulders back and down, align your head and spine, and face forward.
3. Lift your heels so that you are standing on the balls of both feet, hold for a second, and return to the starting flat-footed position. Repeat 10 to 15 times.
4. Stand with your feet side by side. Keeping your heel on the floor, slide your left foot back as far as it will comfortably go and hold for 20 to 30 seconds. You should feel a gentle stretch in the back of your calf and your Achilles tendon.
5. When you are doing this stretch, your toes and heels should be perfectly straight in alignment with each other. A common mistake is turning your heel inward. Also, your front knee should be over your heel, not your toes.
6. Step back to the starting position and repeat with your other leg.

# SIT AND BE FIT
## Neck warm-up and stretch

This neck stretch prevents or relieves a stiff neck. Your neck muscles are constantly supporting about 10 pounds (your head), so stretching can give your neck a much needed break from keeping your head and neck in a stiff position for long periods.

1. Sit in a chair, lift your chest, contract your abdominals, press your shoulders back and down, align your head and spine, and face forward.
2. Drop your head to your chest and slowly roll it toward your right shoulder and stop, then roll it to the left and stop. (Don't roll your head in a circle, which can put too much pressure on the vertebrae and disks in your upper neck.) Repeat 4 times.
3. Facing forward, place your left hand over your head and on your right ear.
4. Place your right arm behind your back with your elbow bent at a 90- degree angle.
5. Breathing gently and evenly, pull your head toward your left shoulder.
6. Hold for 20 to 25 seconds and repeat on the other side.

# WATER BREAK

Once you get used to drinking more water, you will find that your body craves it, a natural response to getting the life-sustaining fluid it needs.

# ENERGY BALANCE SNACK
## Energy Bar

Have 1/2 a balanced nutrition bar (see "Energy Balance Basics") and decaffeinated tea or coffee; add low-fat creamer to taste.

| CORE FOUR APPROXIMATE BREAKDOWN | PROTEIN<br>➤ 5 grams<br>CARBOHYDRATE<br>➤ 10 grams | FAT<br>➤ 3 grams<br>FIBER<br>➤ 1 gram |
|---|---|---|

# WATER BREAK

Water aids digestion and keeps food moving through your digestive tract, which will help to reduce indigestion and constipation.

# ENERGY LIFT

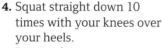

Marching knee bend

This combination uses the large muscles of your body to increase circulation and burn fat while strengthening and toning your buttocks and thighs.

1. Stand beside a chair, holding the back, with your feet hip distance apart. Bend your knees slightly, lift your chest, contract your abdominals, press your shoulders back and down, align your head and spine, and face forward.
2. Lift one knee as if you were marching down the street and return to the starting position, 10 times for each leg, alternating sides.
3. Place your legs hip distance apart with your toes turned slightly out to the sides.
4. Squat straight down 10 times with your knees over your heels.
5. Repeat this series of exercises 2 times.
6. Breathe deeply as your heart rate accelerates.

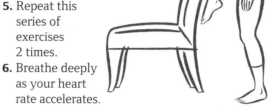

# ENERGY BALANCE LUNCH

## DINING IN

Barbecue Chicken Pizza

6 to 8 ounces chicken breast, grilled, chopped

2 teaspoons tomato-based barbecue sauce

1/4 cup tomato sauce

1 piece whole-grain pita bread

1/2 cup sautéed sliced Vidalia onions, roasted red bell peppers, and artichoke hearts

1/2 cup mozzarella cheese

1. Spread the tomato sauce on the pita bread.
2. Toss the chicken in the barbecue sauce.
3. Place the chicken and vegetables on the pita.
4. Sprinkle with the mozzarella cheese and toast on high until the cheese bubbles.
5. Serve with a large green salad with 2 tablespoons low-fat dressing.

## DINING OUT

Order one piece of barbecue chicken pizza. If you can only order a small one-person pizza, then eat half and take the rest home or back to the office and have a piece later for a snack. Ask for a light amount of cheese and extra vegetables and sauce. Order a large green salad with oil and vinegar dressing. For dessert order a decaf latte with nonfat milk.

➤If you want a larger meal: Fill up on 1/2 balanced energy bar with your decaf latte.

| CORE FOUR APPROXIMATE BREAKDOWN | PROTEIN<br>➤ chicken: 20 to 25 grams<br>**CARBOHYDRATE**<br>➤ pita bread or thin pizza crust: 25 to 30 grams | FAT<br>➤ cheese: 10 grams<br>➤ oil and vinegar dressing: 5 grams<br>FIBER<br>➤ salad and vegetables: 3 to 5 grams<br>➤ pita bread or whole-grain pizza crust: 3 to 5 grams |
|---|---|---|

# SIT AND BE FIT

Waist whittler

This whittler will help strengthen the sides of your waist, making your waistline appear smaller. It will also help strengthen your lower back and spine.

1. Sit in a chair, lift your chest, contract your abdominals, press your shoulders back and down, align your head and spine, and face forward.

2. Place your hands on the sides of your waist or behind your head.
3. Exhale as you pull your left shoulder toward your left hip, crunching the side of your waist (left oblique) muscles.
4. Return to center and repeat 10 to 15 times, then repeat to the right (right obliques).
5. If you feel any twinges of pain in your lower back, stop immediately.

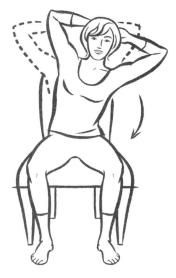

## WATER BREAK

Decaffeinated iced tea is a great summer refresher. Try mixing it with a small amount of low-calorie lemonade for an added treat.

## ENERGY LIFT

Front of thigh stretch

This exercise will not only stretch the fronts of your thighs but also help keep your knees flexible.

1. Stand with your feet hip distance apart. Bend your knees slightly, lift your chest, contract your abdominals, press your shoulders back and down, align your head and spine, and face forward. Hold on to the back of a chair for balance.

2. From behind, place your right hand on the toes of your right foot and pull it toward your buttocks, keeping your knees together. Don't arch your lower back. (If you are not flexible enough to reach your toes, wrap a towel around your foot and gently pull the ends of the towel toward your buttocks.)
3. Squeeze your buttocks and press your hips forward.
4. Bend your standing leg slightly to reduce stress on the lower back. Hold for 15 to 20 seconds and repeat the stretch with your left leg.

## WATER BREAK

To cut down on soda, try replacing it with flavored sparkling water combined with a little fruit juice.

## ENERGY BALANCE SNACK

Black Bean Soup

    1 cup canned black bean soup
    2 tablespoons low-fat sour cream
    2 teaspoons salsa
    Sprinkle of tortilla strips

1. Heat the soup.
2. Top with salsa, sour cream, and tortilla strips.

| CORE FOUR APPROXIMATE BREAKDOWN | PROTEIN<br>➤ black beans: 13 grams<br>CARBOHYDRATE<br>➤ black beans: 33 grams | FAT<br>➤ soup: 1 gram<br>FIBER<br>➤ soup: 11 grams |
|---|---|---|

## TAKE 10

Seated hamstring stretch

While stretching the backs of the thighs, this exercise will help release your lower back, making it more flexible.

1. Sit on the floor with your legs stretched out in front of your body.
2. Lift your chest with your abdominals contracted, your shoulders pressed back and down, and your head facing forward.

**3.** Slowly bend your upper body toward your knees, keeping your back flat and your knees slightly bent.

**4.** Stop when you feel a slight tightness in the backs of your thighs.

**5.** Hold for 20 to 30 seconds and release. Repeat 3 times.

# WATER BREAK

Squeeze a small amount of lemon, lime , or orange juice into your water, which will not only make the water taste better but also help slow your digestion and level your blood sugar.

# ENERGY BALANCE DINNER

## DINING IN

Chicken Walnut Pita

6- to 8-ounce chicken breast, broiled, diced
1 tablespoon chopped walnuts
1/2 cup shredded lettuce or spinach leaves
1/3 cup grated carrots
1 small dill pickle, chopped
1 tablespoon chopped olives
1/2 cup plain nonfat yogurt
1 tablespoon Parmesan cheese
1 tablespoon light mayonnaise
Pinch dill and pepper
1 large piece whole-grain pita bread, cut in half

**1.** In a large bowl, toss together the chicken, lettuce, walnuts, carrots, pickle, and olives.

**2.** In a small bowl, stir together the yogurt, cheese, mayonnaise, dill, and pepper until blended.

**3.** Fold the chicken mixture into the yogurt mixture and fill the pita bread halves with it.

**4.** Serve with a large green salad with low-fat dressing and melon chunks.

## DINING OUT

Order a bowl of vegetable, or chicken noodle soup and 1/2 turkey sandwich on whole-grain bread.

➤If you want a larger meal: Add a small green salad with oil and vinegar dressing.

| CORE FOUR APPROXIMATE BREAKDOWN | PROTEIN<br>➤ chicken: 20 to 25 grams<br><br>CARBOHYDRATE<br>➤ pita bread: 15 to 20<br>➤ soup and sandwich: 30 to 35 grams | FAT<br>➤ pita bread filling: 5 to 10 grams<br><br>FIBER<br>➤ pita: 5 grams<br>➤ small salad: 2 to 3 grams |
| --- | --- | --- |

# ENERGY BALANCE SNACK

Strawberry Shake

6 ounces low-fat milk or vanilla soy milk
5 strawberries and a small amount of melon
2 ice cubes
1 tablespoon low-carbohydrate protein powder

Mix all ingredients in a blender until smooth and drink slowly.

| CORE FOUR APPROXIMATE BREAKDOWN | PROTEIN<br>➤ protein powder: 10 to 12 grams<br><br>CARBOHYDRATE<br>➤ low-fat milk or soy milk: 6 to 8 grams | FAT<br>➤ low-fat milk or soy milk: 2 to 4 grams<br><br>FIBER<br>➤ strawberries and melon: 1 to 2 grams |
| --- | --- | --- |

# STRETCH, RELAX, AND SLEEP

**1.** Chest/posture stretch
**2.** Neck and upper spine stretch
**3.** Lower spine stretch

# STRESS RELIEF TIP

A growing body of evidence suggests that reducing stress is just a massage away. Doctors are now prescribing massage for everything from high blood pressure to asthma to anorexia, and some insurance companies will cover this treatment. Find a licensed massage therapist or bodywork professional and try to have a massage once or twice a month.

# Get in Touch

TOUCH IS NECESSARY FOR SURVIVAL. Ample research conducted with humans and animals has demonstrated that a lack of touch can be as fatal as starvation, suffocation, exhaustion, or exposure.

The bad news is that touch is often available only through sex, and even then touch may stimulate more than soothe, so many people today are touch deprived. The good news is that massage therapy is enjoying a high level of professionalism and widespread acceptance in our society. According to Laura Sibley in her article, "Therapeutic Massage," "some 25 million Americans make 60 million visits to 85,000 [massage] practitioners a year."* Not only is massage available in spas, health clubs, and resorts; the medical community is recognizing the benefits of therapeutic touch. Some hospitals even provide massage therapy before and after surgery as it aids in recovery. Dr. James Gordon of the Georgetown University School of Medicine, author of *Manifesto for a New Medicine* claims that "touch is medicine." **

Every cell in our bodies benefits when our skin is touched in a nurturing and safe context. Massage can strengthen our immune systems by activating our lymphatic systems and decreasing our production of stress hormones. Even our brains are affected in various ways, including the stimulation of the vagus nerve that impacts digestion and the absorption of nutrients. Heart rate, blood pressure, and adrenaline are reduced while serotonin, endorphins, and blood flow are increased. Perhaps the best result is that we feel so much better emotionally after a massage, a benefit that defies quantification by any scientific study.

Massage can benefit anyone who is not suffering from a specific condition that is aggravated by muscle stimulation, such as certain forms of cancer, recent injuries, skin ailments, colds, or flus. Check with your doctor if you have any questions.

* Laura Sibley, "Therapeutic Massage" (Online article, 2000)
** Dr. James Gordon, *Manifesto for a New Medicine* (Addison-Wesley, 1996)

# DAY 12

## WAKE-UP AFFIRMATION

*"What really matters is what you do with what you have."*

—*Shirley Lord, author*

## WAKE-UP WORKOUT

**1.** Let body slowly wake up
**2.** Take several deep breaths
**3.** Full-body tighten and release
**4.** Pelvic tilts
**5.** Pillow sit-ups
**6.** Hamstring stretch
**7.** Hands and knees yoga stretch

## CORE FOUR

**1.** Push-up
**2.** Sit-up
**3.** Sit and stand
**4.** Posture squeeze/biceps curl

## PORTION CONTROL TIP

Sometimes overindulgence results from boredom. Variety is the spice of life, especially when it comes to food, so be creative with your meals and snacks.

## ENERGY BALANCE BREAKFAST

*Cantaloupe Cooler*

> 1/2 cup low-fat cottage cheese or ricotta cheese
> 1/2 cup low-fat, low-sugar yogurt
> 1/2 fresh cantaloupe, seeded
> Dollop fat-free whipped topping
> Small amount of pecans or almonds

**1.** Combine the cottage cheese and yogurt.
**2.** Place the cottage cheese and yogurt mixture in cantaloupe half or on top of diced cantaloupe.
**3.** Add the whipped topping.
**4.** Sprinkle the nuts on top.

➤ If you want a larger meal: Increase both the cottage cheese and the yogurt by 1/4 cup.

Drink water with lemon or 4 ounces of juice and 6 ounces of water, plus decaffeinated tea or coffee, if desired. Add low-fat creamer to taste.

| CORE FOUR APPROXIMATE BREAKDOWN | PROTEIN ➤ cottage or ricotta cheese: 7 grams ➤ yogurt: 2 grams CARBOHYDRATE ➤ cantaloupe: 5 grams ➤ yogurt: 6 grams | FAT ➤ nuts: 5 to 7 grams FIBER ➤ cantaloupe: 1 to 2 grams |
|---|---|---|

## TAKE 10

*Reverse stationary lunge*

This exercise will strengthen and tone your thighs and buttocks and give your torso better support, making walking and other lower body activities easier.

**1.** Stand beside a chair with your right hand on the back for balance and your left hand hanging at your side. Lift your chest, contract your abdominals, press your shoulders back and down, align your head and spine, and face forward.

2. Shift so the heel of your right foot supports most of your weight. Slide your left leg back, with your knee bent and heel lifted, placing half your weight on your left toes.

3. Inhale as you lower your body toward the floor while keeping your right knee aligned over your right heel.

4. Exhale and push down on the right heel while rising from the lunge position and squeeze your buttocks as you return to the starting position.

5. Repeat 5 times alternating sides.

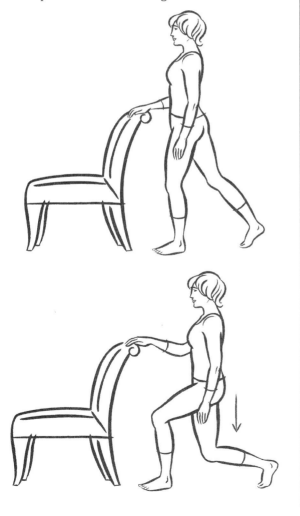

# SIT AND BE FIT

Besides improving posture, relieving tension, and aiding deep breathing, this movement stretches your entire torso. It can be done anywhere and any time you feel the day pushing down on you.

1. Sit in a chair, lift your chest, contract your abdominals, press your shoulders back and down, align your head and spine, and face forward.

2. Reach overhead with both arms, trying to touch the ceiling, and stretch as far as you can.

3. Look up and breathe deeply. Hold for 10 to 15 seconds and release. Repeat 3 times.

# ENERGY BALANCE SNACK

1/2 sliced apple
1 hard-boiled egg
1 handful soy nuts

| | PROTEIN | FAT |
|---|---|---|
| | ➤ egg: 6 grams | ➤ egg yolk: 5 grams |
| | ➤ soy nuts: 6 grams | ➤ soy nuts: 6 grams |
| | **CARBOHYDRATE** | **FIBER** |
| | ➤ apple: 12 grams | ➤ apple: 2 grams |
| | | ➤ soy nuts: 2 grams |

# ENERGY LIFT

If you're a dancer, you know this standard step. If you're not, this movement is a fun way to take a break and get yourself dancing.

1. Stand up straight with your feet together. Bend your knees slightly, lift your chest, contract your abdominals, press your shoulders back and down, align your head and spine, and face forward. Hold on to the back of a chair for balance.

2. Step forward with your left foot and place your weight on that foot.

3. Pick up your right foot and cross it over your left and transfer your weight to your right foot.

4. Step back with your left foot and place your weight on that foot.

5. Now, pick up your right foot and place it beside the left. You are back to the starting position and you have done a box step.

6. Do it again 4 times and then go the other way, beginning with your right foot.

Keep practicing until you no longer have to think to move. This energy lift will not only give you more energy through lower body circulation; it will be a new dance step for your repertoire. When you have mastered it, put on some music and try it out.

## ENERGY BALANCE LUNCH

### DINING IN

Tuna Cheese Spread

> 3 ounces water-packed tuna
> 1 ounce cream cheese, softened
> 2 tablespoons low-fat mayonnaise
> 1/2 tablespoon lemon juice
> Dash curry powder and salt
> 1 green onion, finely diced

1. Drain the tuna, put it into a bowl, and mash it with a fork.

2. Mix in the cream cheese and mayonnaise.

3. Add the lemon juice, curry powder, and salt. Mix well.

4. Stir in the onion.

5. Chill for 1 hour to allow flavors to blend.

6. Serve spread on whole-grain crackers or pita bread with carrots, radishes, and cherry tomatoes.

### DINING OUT

Order a tuna sandwich or tuna salad with lots of vegetables and low-fat dressing.

➤ If you want a larger meal: Add a decaf espresso, cappuccino, or low-fat latte with one cookie for dessert.

| CORE FOUR APPROXIMATE BREAKDOWN | PROTEIN ➤ tuna: 20 grams CARBOHYDRATE ➤ crackers or pita bread: 15 to 20 grams | FAT ➤ cream cheese and mayonnaise: 10 to 15 grams FIBER ➤ crackers or pita bread: 3 to 5 grams |
| --- | --- | --- |

## SIT AND BE FIT

Toe taps

By strengthening your shins with this exercise, you will prevent the often painful condition known as shin splints, an injury in which, through overuse, the muscle lifts away from the bone.

1. Sit in a chair with your chest lifted, your abdominals contracted, your shoulders pressed back and down, and your head facing forward.

2. Kick off your shoes and tap the toes of both feet 10 to 20 times, keeping your heels on the ground.

3. Repeat 2 or 3 times, pausing between sets.

## WATER BREAK

Drinking cool water is better than drinking water at room temperature, because cool water leaves your stomach faster, hydrating your system more quickly. This is especially important if you are exercising in hot weather.

## ENERGY LIFT

Roll-down/roll-up

This is not only a good spine and back of the thigh stretch, it is an excellent way to bring circulation to your brain, which will enable you to think more clearly.

1. Stand with your hands on your knees, which are bent as if you are going to sit down. Your abdominals are contracted, your back is slightly arched, and your head is relaxed as you look at the floor.

2. Inhale and run your hands down your shins toward your ankles. When you reach as close to your ankles as comfortable, hold for a few seconds, breathing evenly.

**3.** Gently straighten your legs as much as comfortable. Hold for a few seconds and then bend your knees back to the starting position.

**4.** Hold for a few seconds and gently run your hands back up your shins to your knees.

**5.** Arch your back like a cat and roll your spine up one vertebra at a time to a standing position.

**6.** Repeat 4 times.

# WATER BREAK

To lessen the bloated feeling in your lower part of your abdomen, drink more water and stay away from carbonated beverages.

# ENERGY BALANCE SNACK

Ploughman's Snack

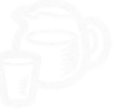

   1 apple, sliced
   5 water crackers
   2 ounces cheese
   1 large stalk celery
   2 ounces fat-free cream cheese

**1.** Place the apple slices on the crackers and melt the cheese on top.

**2.** Serve with the celery stuffed with the cream cheese.

| CORE FOUR APPROXIMATE BREAKDOWN | PROTEIN<br>➤ cheese: 15 grams<br>CARBOHYDRATE<br>➤ crackers: 10 to 15 | FAT<br>➤ cheese: 1 to 2 grams<br>FIBER<br>➤ celery: 1 to 2 grams |
|---|---|---|

# TAKE 10

Mini-vacation deep breathing

This meditation will relax and calm your mind, giving you the chance to set a goal and figure out how to get it accomplished.

**1.** Sit on the edge of a couch or comfortable chair with your chest lifted, your abdominals relaxed, your shoulders gently pressed back and down, your feet flat on the floor, and your palms facing the ceiling.

**2.** Close your eyes and think of a vacation you would like to take. Think of all the details, from where you would like to go to what you would like to wear. Try to get in touch with the joyful feeling of stepping on the plane and the excitement of landing and seeing different people and vistas. Are you alone, with friends, or on a romantic holiday with your love? Are you walking on the beach or biking through France? Create a haven in your mind that you can run away to whenever you are tired and stressed.

**3.** Another way to de-stress is to try to think of nothing. Choose your lucky number or favorite color and place it in front of your mind's eye, hold it there, and begin to breathe. The point of this exercise is to stop your mind from wandering and to allow it to empty out.

**4.** Stay in this peaceful place as you breathe in deeply through your nose, expanding your rib cage, and exhale through your mouth, collapsing your rib cage and tightening your abdominals.

**5.** Sit for at least 10 minutes, breathing and relaxing. If you begin to feel light-headed, just breathe normally.

# WATER BREAK

Many of the health problems associated with inadequate water intake, such as bladder and kidney disease, do not appear for years or even decades.

# ENERGY BALANCE DINNER

## DINING IN

Chicken Stuffed with Spinach
and Ricotta Cheese

1/2 cup finely chopped spinach, either fresh or
frozen

1/2 cup low-fat ricotta cheese

2 tablespoons goat cheese

Fresh minced garlic to taste

Dash salt, pepper, and nutmeg

1 large chicken breast, grilled

1. Steam the spinach until well-done and drain
thoroughly.
2. In a small bowl, mix the spinach with the
cheeses, garlic, salt, pepper, and nutmeg.
3. Slice open the chicken breast and place it in a
shallow pan or bowl. Fill the chicken with the
stuffing and heat it under the broiler for a few
minutes to melt the cheese.
4. Serve with a large green salad with low-fat
dressing and a small whole-grain dinner roll.

## DINING OUT

Order a spinach salad with dressing and a chicken
breast, vegetables, and roasted potatoes. Eat only
half the potatoes. Add a small dinner roll and a
small decaf latte.

➤ If you want a larger meal:
  **DINING IN** Double the recipe and eat until
  you're full. Save the rest for a snack tomorrow.
  **DINING OUT** Order 1/2 chicken.

| CORE FOUR APPROXIMATE BREAKDOWN | PROTEIN ➤ chicken: 20 to 25 grams  CARBOHYDRATE ➤ spinach, salad, vegetables, potatoes, and roll: 25 to 30 grams | FAT ➤ cheeses and salad dressing: 10 to 15 grams  FIBER ➤ spinach, vegetables, salad, and roll: 10 to 15 grams |
| --- | --- | --- |

# ENERGY BALANCE SNACK

Peanut Butter and Something

1 tablespoon peanut butter on
one of the following:
  1/2 apple
  2 stalks celery
  1 piece whole-grain bread
  1/2 banana
Or on a spoon right out of the jar.

| CORE FOUR APPROXIMATE BREAKDOWN | PROTEIN ➤ peanut butter: 4 grams  CARBOHYDRATE ➤ apple: 12 grams ➤ banana: 12 grams ➤ bread: 12 grams ➤ celery: 2 grams | FAT ➤ peanut butter: 7 grams  FIBER ➤ apple: 3 to 5 grams ➤ bread: 3 to 5 grams |
| --- | --- | --- |

# STRETCH, RELAX, AND SLEEP

1. Chest/posture stretch
2. Neck and upper spine stretch
3. Lower spine stretch

# STRESS RELIEF TIP

Is worry keeping you awake? Ninety percent of
what we worry about never happens! Action is the
antidote for worry, so try the following action plan.

1. Before bed, list your worries in your journal.
2. Promise yourself you will look at this list first
thing tomorrow.
3. When you wake up, take each worry one at a
time and decide if you can do something about
it today.
4. If not, put it on list to brainstorm about with a
friend, your spouse, or a professional therapist.
Often a concern will either disappear or a solution is found in the light of trusted opinions.

# Replace Worry with Action

JANETTE IS THE KIND OF PERSON who is always planning for the future—planning for the worst possible future, that is. "What if this happens?" and "What if that doesn't happen?" are her constant questions. Since there are unlimited possibilities, she can't even begin to worry about every future event, let alone develop a realistic plan to cope with what could actually happen. But she tries.

For many of us, worry does not lead to action. We are so busy obsessing that we fail to prepare realistically for what most of us might reasonably face. Have you fallen into this trap? Do you worry about getting breast cancer but put off getting a mammogram? Do you fret over losing flexibility as you age but fail to stretch out at least once a day? Do you medicate your tension headaches instead of actively decreasing the stress in your life?

Although it's true that anything could happen, don't waste your time and energy worrying about anything or everything. Instead, invest in becoming the healthiest, most optimistic person possible. Then, no matter what happens, you'll be at your best to confront whatever comes your way.

# DAY 13

## WAKE-UP AFFIRMATION

"A happy woman is one who has no cares at all; a cheerful woman is one who has cares but doesn't let them get her down."

—*Beverly Sills, opera singer*

## WAKE-UP WORKOUT

1. Let body slowly wake up
2. Take several deep breaths
3. Full-body tighten and release
4. Pelvic tilts
5. Pillow sit-ups
6. Hamstring stretch
7. Hands and knees yoga stretch

## CORE FOUR

1. Push-up
2. Sit-up
3. Sit and stand
4. Posture squeeze/biceps curl

## PORTION CONTROL TIP

Try to leave a little food on your plate at every meal, even if it's just one bite. This will help get you into the habit of not automatically eating everything that is served to you and focusing instead on whether you are hungry enough to eat it.

## ENERGY BALANCE BREAKFAST

### Parmesan Egg Bagel Sandwich

1/2 cup egg substitute

1/2 teaspoon Parmesan cheese

1 small whole-grain bagel or 1 large whole-grain bagel with the inside partially removed

1 ounce low-fat or regular cream cheese

1. In a frying pan over medium heat, scramble egg substitute with cheese until cooked.
2. Spread bagel with cream cheese and eggs on one half of bagel.
3. Cover with other half of bagel and eat like a sandwich.

➤ If you want a larger meal: Add 1/2 cup fruit with 1/2 cup nonfat yogurt.

Drink water with lemon or 4 ounces of juice and 6 ounces of water, plus decaffeinated tea or coffee, if desired. Add low-fat creamer to taste.

| CORE FOUR APPROXIMATE BREAKDOWN | PROTEIN ➤ egg substitute: 18 to 20 grams CARBOHYDRATE ➤ bagel: 25 to 30 grams | FAT ➤ egg substitute: 5 grams ➤ cream cheese: 9 grams FIBER ➤ bagel: 3 to 5 grams |
| --- | --- | --- |

# TAKE 10
## Reach for the floor

This movement exercises your obliques (sides of the waist), and when your obliques are toned, you have better support for your back, which comes in handy for anyone who plays golf or tennis.

1. Stand with your knees slightly bent and your toes turned out slightly to the sides. Lift your chest, contract your abdominals, press your shoulders back and down, align your head and spine, and face forward.
2. With a stick such as a golf club or a broom handle in your right hand and your left hand on your left hip, bend to the right while sliding the stick out to the side as far as comfortable.
3. Hold for a few seconds and return to the starting position.
4. Repeat 3 times.
5. Change sides and repeat on the left side.

# SIT AND BE FIT
## Hand squeeze and release

Besides loosening up your wrists and fingers, this exercise will increase circulation to your hands.

1. Sit in a chair, lift your chest, contract your abdominals, press your shoulders back and down, align your head and spine, and face forward.
2. Interlace your fingers in front of your chest and squeeze your hands tightly together.
3. Release and press your palms flat against each other, in a prayer position. Bend your fingers back as far as they will go.
4. Repeat the squeeze and release 4 times.
5. Interlace your fingers and circle your wrists to the right 5 times, stop in the center, and repeat to the left.

# WATER BREAK

The caffeine in two or more cups of coffee or tea a day is enough to impair your kidneys' absorption of calcium.

# ENERGY BALANCE SNACK
## Jicama Chips with Fruit Salsa

2 ripe mangoes, peeled, chopped into small pieces
1 kiwifruit, peeled, chopped
1/2 red bell pepper, finely chopped
1 tablespoon lime juice
1 tablespoon snipped fresh cilantro, parsley, or basil
1 tablespoon ginger
Dash ground red pepper (optional)
1 to 2 slices fresh turkey
1 jicama
1 1-ounce stick string cheese

1. Combine fruit, bell pepper, lime juice, and spices in a bowl. Cover and chill 1 hour or overnight.
2. Peel the jicama and cut it into large bite-size pieces.
3. Place turkey on top of the jicama and top with fruit salsa.
4. Serve with a 1-ounce stick of string cheese.

This recipe makes more fruit salsa than you need for this snack (about 2 cups). Keep it on hand for other snacks and to put on top of fish or chicken entrées.

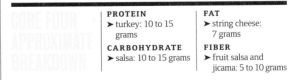

| CORE FOUR APPROXIMATE BREAKDOWN | **PROTEIN** ➤ turkey: 10 to 15 grams **CARBOHYDRATE** ➤ salsa: 10 to 15 grams | **FAT** ➤ string cheese: 7 grams **FIBER** ➤ fruit salsa and jicama: 5 to 10 grams |
|---|---|---|

# WATER BREAK

The general rule is to drink 64 ounces of water a day; however, you should drink an extra 10 ounces of water for every 25 pounds you are over your recommended weight.

# ENERGY LIFT
Shake, shake, shake your booty

This exercise is not only a mood lifter, it is a way to get the blood flowing to all parts of your body, burn fat, and laugh.

1. Put on your favorite music that's uplifting and makes you want to move.
2. Start with your hands and shake them up to the ceiling, out to the sides, and back down to the floor. Do this 10 times.
3. Shake your shoulders and your booty (buttocks) for 1 minute. Get it all going on together.
4. Add your hands, arms, and booty together. Shake it up, baby!
5. Take a kick break and kick your feet out in front of you for 3 minutes.
6. Go back to the booty shake for a few more minutes.
7. Keep this going as long as you feel good. Try to get your heart rate up a little and take deep breaths.
8. Have fun, look silly, and lift your spirits.

# ENERGY BALANCE LUNCH

## DINING IN
Turkey and Smoked Gouda Sandwich

  1 tablespoon honey mustard
  2 slices rye bread
  6 ounces turkey
  2 ounces smoked gouda cheese
  Lettuce, tomato, and sprouts

1. Spread the honey mustard on the bread.
2. Layer the turkey and cheese on top of the bread.
3. Top with lettuce, tomato, and sprouts.

## DINING OUT
Order a turkey sandwich with cheese and honey mustard. Eat a large green salad with low-fat dressing on the side.

➤ If you want a larger meal: Increase turkey and cheese by 2 ounces or finish off your meal with a decaf cappuccino or latte.

| CORE FOUR APPROXIMATE BREAKDOWN | PROTEIN ➤ Turkey and cheese: 35 grams CARBOHYDRATE ➤ bread and vegetables: 20 to 25 grams | FAT ➤ cheese: 16 grams FIBER ➤ bread and vegetables: 5 to 10 grams |
|---|---|---|

# SIT AND BE FIT
Bear hug

This exercise releases tension in your back and protects you, especially if you golf, from muscle sprain and strain.

1. Sit in a chair, lift your chest, contract your abdominals, press your shoulders back and down, align your head and spine, and face forward.
2. Try to grab your left shoulder blade with your right hand and your right shoulder blade with your left hand, as if you were hugging yourself.
3. Drop your chin toward your chest and lean forward as you take a deep breath.
4. Hold this position, breathing deeply, for 20 to 30 seconds and release.
5. Repeat 3 times.

# WATER BREAK

Make sure your child has plenty of water when he or she plays sports. The body, like a car, needs water to regulate its cooling system, and it can overheat just as easily.

# ENERGY LIFT
Standing kickbacks

Although this exercise looks like a windmill, it actually strengthens the backs of your thighs while raising your heart rate and burning fat.

1. Stand up straight and place your feet hip distance apart. Bend your knees slightly, lift your chest, contract your abdominals, press your shoulders back and down, align your head and spine, and face forward.
2. Lift your arms out to the sides, parallel with the floor, at shoulder height.
3. Place your weight on left foot as you kick your right foot toward your left hand, trying to touch your left hand to your right toes.
4. Place your weight on your right foot while kicking the left foot toward your right hand, trying to touch your right hand to your left toes.
5. Kick back and forth like this 10 to 20 times.

## WATER BREAK

Pay special attention to water's sodium content, which can be high in many bottled brands.

## ENERGY BALANCE SNACK

Vegetables and Dip

1/2 cup low-fat dip
1/2 cup low-fat sour cream
1/2 cup low-fat cottage cheese
Plate of your favorite raw vegetables
10 to 15 pita chips

1. Mix the dip with the sour cream and cottage cheese.
2. Serve with the vegetables and the chips.

This dip makes 3 servings, so save the balance for other snacks.

CORE FOUR
APPROXIMATE
BREAKDOWN

**PROTEIN**
➤ sour cream and cottage cheese: 10 to 15 grams
**CARBOHYDRATE**
➤ vegetables: 5 grams
➤ chips: 10 to 15 grams

**FAT**
➤ dip: 5 grams
➤ chips: 10 grams
**FIBER**
➤ vegetables: 2 to 5 grams

## TAKE 10

Standing hamstring stretch

This movement stretches the backs of your thighs and your lower back.

1. Stand up straight and place your feet hip distance apart. Bend your knees slightly, lift your chest, contract your abdominals, press your shoulders back and down, align your head and spine, and face forward.
2. Place one leg on a low chair or couch, your toes facing the ceiling and knee unlocked.
3. Bend the standing knee slightly to take pressure off your knee joint and lower back.
4. Place your hands together on the top of the extended leg.
5. Contract your abdominals and slowly bend your upper body over the leg on the chair.
6. Take the stretch to the point of comfort and hold for 20 to 30 seconds.
7. Release and repeat on the other leg.
8. Repeat 3 times on each leg, alternating legs.

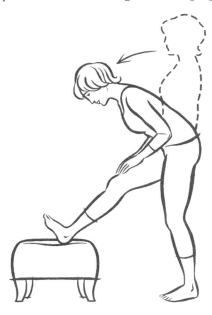

# WATER BREAK

Drinking water helps raise your energy level by transporting vital nutrients to organs and muscles.

# ENERGY BALANCE DINNER

## DINING IN

Orange Shrimp

> 1 teaspoon olive oil
> 6 large shrimp, peeled, deveined
> 1/2 large clove garlic, minced
> 2 tablespoons orange juice
> 1/2 teaspoon marjoram
> 1/2 teaspoon snipped fresh or dried oregano
> Salt and pepper to taste

1. Heat the olive oil in a nonstick skillet over medium heat.
2. When warm, add the shrimp and garlic and stir often until the shrimp turn pink.
3. Add the orange juice and bring to a boil over medium-high heat.
4. Stir and cook until the juice is slightly thickened.
5. Remove the skillet from heat and stir in the marjoram and oregano.
6. Serve with 1/2 cup brown rice with chopped vegetables and a large green salad with olive oil and balsamic vinegar.

## DINING OUT

Order lightly sautéed shrimp and a side of rice and vegetables. The rice usually comes in a dome in small bowl. Eat only the top of the dome, which is about 1/2 cup of rice. Have a large green salad with oil and vinegar to start.

> ➤ If you want a larger meal: Increase number of shrimp to 8 to 12.

| CORE FOUR APPROXIMATE BREAKDOWN | PROTEIN ➤ shrimp: 20 to 25 grams CARBOHYDRATE ➤ rice: 25 to 30 grams | FAT ➤ olive oil: 5 grams ➤ salad dressing: 6 to 9 grams FIBER ➤ vegetables: 10 to 15 grams ➤ salad: 5 to 10 grams |
|---|---|---|

# ENERGY BALANCE SNACK

Graham Cracker Treat

> 1/2 cup nonfat yogurt
> 1/2 cup low-fat cottage cheese
> 2 small graham cracker blocks

1. Mix the yogurt and cottage cheese.
2. Serve on top of the graham crackers.

| CORE FOUR APPROXIMATE BREAKDOWN | PROTEIN ➤ yogurt: 4 grams ➤ cottage cheese: 7 grams CARBOHYDRATE ➤ yogurt: 11 grams ➤ graham crackers: 5 grams | FAT ➤ total: 5 grams FIBER ➤ graham crackers: 1 gram |
|---|---|---|

# STRETCH, RELAX, AND SLEEP

1. Chest/posture stretch
2. Neck and upper spine stretch
3. Lower spine stretch

# HELPFUL HINT

According to the University of Florida College of Medicine, fruit pectin, which is found abundantly in apples, is shown to reduce cholesterol, help prevent colon cancer, and blunt the appetite. Eating two or three apples a day can reduce bad cholesterol by up to 20 percent in just one month.

# Become a Collector

ONE OF MY PET PEEVES is friends who don't collect anything. I always know what to get collectors for birthdays, Christmas, and other celebrations. But those folks who don't delight in minia-ture cows in their kitchens, first-edition children's books in their libraries, or Hawaiian holiday ornaments swinging from their trees are usually the very same ones who answer "Oh, I don't know" when asked what they'd like for a gift. I love giving presents, especially when I know I've located the perfect present. But it's no fun at all when it's time to give gifts to people who don't know how to receive.

Try this experiment. Exhale all the air from your lungs. Exhale again. And again. And again. Can't keep it up for too long, can you? Of course not. We're made to exhale and inhale, to give and receive. For our bodies, our spirits, and our relationships to be healthy, we need to take turns focusing on other people and focus-ing on ourselves. If you're always the giver, you ruin anyone else's chances of having the joy of giving. Worse yet, you'll wind up depleted, like a person trying to survive solely on exhaling. Make sure you're as good a receiver as a giver, as good at inhaling as your are at exhaling. And if you ever want to get a gift from me, start collecting something!

# DAY 14

## WAKE-UP AFFIRMATION

"Why not seize the pleasure at once? How often is happiness destroyed by preparation?"

—*Sojourner Truth, civil rights leader*

## WAKE-UP WORKOUT

**1.** Let body slowly wake up
**2.** Take several deep breaths
**3.** Full-body tighten and release
**4.** Pelvic tilts
**5.** Pillow sit-ups
**6.** Hamstring stretch
**7.** Hands and knees yoga stretch

## CORE FOUR

**1.** Push-up
**2.** Sit-up
**3.** Sit and stand
**4.** Posture squeeze/biceps curl

## PORTION CONTROL TIP

Appetizers are often the yummiest part of a meal. Take advantage of their size by ordering one as a main course with a large green salad. Or order a children's meal, which often is enough to fill you up.

## ENERGY BALANCE BREAKFAST

*Strawberry Omelette*

1 egg and 4 egg whites or 1/2 cup egg substitute
1 teaspoon cinnamon
1/2 cup crushed fresh or frozen strawberries
Low-fat whipped topping

**1.** Stir together the eggs and cinnamon
**2.** Pour the egg and egg whites into an oil-sprayed skillet that has been preheated over medium heat. Cook the eggs into a flat omelette, set all the way through.
**3.** Add the strawberries as filling and top with the whipped topping.
**4.** Fold over and serve with more strawberries on top and another dollop of whipped topping.
**5.** Add 1 slice whole-grain toast with butter.

➤ If you want a larger meal: Add a small portion of roasted potatoes.

Drink water with lemon or 4 ounces of juice and 6 ounces of water, plus decaffeinated tea or coffee, if desired. Add low-fat creamer to taste.

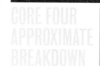

| CORE FOUR APPROXIMATE BREAKDOWN | PROTEIN ➤ Egg and egg whites and/or egg substitute: 20 grams CARBOHYDRATE ➤ toast: 13 grams | FAT ➤ butter: 10 grams FIBER ➤ strawberries: 2 grams ➤ toast: 2 to 5 grams |
| --- | --- | --- |

# TAKE 10
## One-arm fly

Strong chest muscles are part of a well-supported torso and correct posture. This exercise works the muscles in the front of your chest and the fronts of your shoulders, helping lift and firm the chest muscles that support your breasts.

1. Lie on your back on the edge of your bed with your head pointed toward the headboard, your right arm hanging over the side, and a 3- to 5-pound weight next to your hand.
2. Bend your knees, placing your feet flat on the bed and pressing your lower back into the bed.
3. Pick up the weight in your right hand and raise it straight toward the ceiling, keeping your elbow unlocked but fixed.
4. Inhale and slowly lower your arm until it is level with the bed.
5. Exhale and slowly raise it back toward the ceiling.
6. Repeat 12 to 15 times.
7. Turn around so your head is pointing toward the foot of the bed and repeat the exercise on the other arm.

# SIT AND BE FIT
## Chest stretch

One cause of poor posture is tight chest muscles that pull your shoulders forward. Strong back muscles and flexible chest muscles help keep your shoulder blades in place. If you sit a lot during the day and feel your posture sagging, do this stretch throughout the day to lift your spirits and energy.

1. Sit in a chair with your chest lifted, your abdominals contracted, your shoulders back and down, and your head facing straight ahead.
2. With your arms straight but your elbows unlocked, place your palms on the back of the chair.
3. Lean your upper body as far forward as you can while keeping your hands on your chair.

You should feel a gentle stretch across your shoulders and chest.
4. Breathing deeply and easily, hold for 20 to 30 seconds and release.

# WATER BREAK

Water provides an environment for your body's chemical reactions to occur. Without enough water, your body chemistry is knocked out of balance, which can cause dizziness or mood swings.

# ENERGY BALANCE SNACK
## Salty and Sweet

2 ounces beef jerky
1 piece fresh fruit

| CORE FOUR APPROXIMATE BREAKDOWN | PROTEIN ➤ beef jerky: 24 grams  CARBOHYDRATE ➤ fruit: 20 to 25 grams | FAT ➤ beef jerky: 5 grams  FIBER ➤ fruit: 3 to 5 grams |
|---|---|---|

# WATER BREAK

Water acts as a lubricant, lessening the wear and tear on your joints and surrounding tissue.

# ENERGY LIFT
## Wall sit and hold

This exercise will not only strengthen the fronts of your thighs, it will also help tone your abdominal wall and improve your posture. This intense isometric exercise is done by a lot of skiers to strengthen the fronts of their thighs for the grueling downhill trauma the thighs undergo when skiing.

1. Stand with the small of your back and your hips pressing into a wall and your feet shoulder width apart a few feet from the wall.
2. Bend your knees and lower your body down the wall while pushing with your lower back.

**3.** Your knees should be positioned over your ankles, not your toes, and at no more than a 90-degree angle.

**4.** Hold this position as long as you can. Work up to 30 seconds, then 1 minute.

**5.** Release and walk around for a few seconds and then try it 1 more time.

# ENERGY BALANCE LUNCH

## DINING IN

### Low-Fat Ham Sandwich with Fruit Salad

1 to 2 teaspoons Dijon-style mustard
1 tablespoon low-fat mayonnaise
2 slices whole-grain bread
3 or 4 slices of low-fat or turkey ham
Lettuce, tomato, and onion
Sliced dill pickle

**1.** Spread the mustard and mayonnaise on the whole-grain bread.

**2.** Pile the bread with the turkey, lettuce, tomato, onion, and pickles.

**3.** Serve with 1 cup fresh fruit salad and enjoy.

## DINING OUT

Order a ham sandwich with the works. Ask for fresh fruit on the side instead of potato salad or chips.

➤ If you want a larger meal: Add a small green salad with olive oil and vinegar dressing.

| CORE FOUR APPROXIMATE BREAKDOWN | PROTEIN<br>➤ ham: 15 to 20 grams<br>CARBOHYDRATE<br>➤ bread: 25 grams | FAT<br>➤ ham: 5 to 8 grams<br>➤ mayonnaise:<br>  3 to 4 grams<br>FIBER<br>➤ bread: 6 to 10 grams<br>➤ fruit: 2 to 5 grams |
|---|---|---|

# SIT AND BE FIT

### Leaning-over triceps extension

Who couldn't use a little help toning the backs of her arms (triceps)? Beyond lessening the flab factor, this exercise will help improve your posture because you use your entire torso to stabilize the movement.

**1.** Sit in a chair with your chest lifted, your abdominals contracted, your shoulders back and down, and your head facing forward.

**2.** Lean your upper body forward, keeping your arms in line with your torso and your elbows slightly bent.

**3.** Inhale and squeeze your shoulder blades together.

**4.** Exhale as you straighten and lift your arms toward the ceiling.

**5.** Hold a moment, release, and return to the starting position.

**6.** Repeat 4 times.

Hint: Try to keep your shoulders down and the tension out of your neck. If you feel the movement going into your upper neck muscles, raise your torso to a sitting position and do the movement from there.

# WATER BREAK

Water works like a shock absorber inside your eyes and spinal cord.

# ENERGY LIFT

### Overhead triceps stretch

This movement stretches the backs of your arms, while helping open up your shoulder area.

**1.** Sit in a chair, lift your chest, contract your abdominals, press your shoulders back and down, align your head and spine, and face forward.

**2.** Place both hands behind your head on the lower part of the back of your neck with your right palm on top of your left hand.

**3.** Your elbows should be pointing toward the ceiling. If you are not flexible in the shoulder or triceps area, your elbows may be pointing toward the front wall a little bit. This position will become easier as you become more flexible.

**4.** Hold for 20 to 30 seconds and repeat 2 times.

# WATER BREAK

In the human body, water serves as a solvent for minerals, vitamins, amino acids, glucose, and many other chemical processes.

# ENERGY BALANCE SNACK

## Pear Sandwich

    1 small pear
    2 ounces Canadian bacon
    1 ounce low-fat cheese

**1.** Slice the pear into large thin pieces.

**2.** Heat the Canadian bacon in a toaster and place small pieces of bacon and cheese between the pear slices.

| CORE FOUR APPROXIMATE BREAKDOWN | PROTEIN<br>➤ Canadian bacon: 15 grams<br>**CARBOHYDRATE**<br>➤ pear: 15 to 20 grams | **FAT**<br>➤ Canadian bacon: 5 grams<br>➤ cheese: 3 to 5 grams<br>**FIBER**<br>➤ pear: 3 to 5 grams |
|---|---|---|

# TAKE 10

## Hip and back balancer

This movement helps release lower back tension and stretch your hip flexors (front of hip muscles), which become shortened from sitting too much, which pulls the pelvis out of line.

**1.** Lie on your back on the floor with your left leg bent so it lies on the seat of a chair and your right leg lying on the floor beside the chair. Your buttocks should be against the legs of the chair so that your left knee is directly over your hip.

**2.** Bend your right leg and place a towel under your right foot. The use of the towel will keep

your lower back and your hip flat, and you won't be tempted to arch your lower back.

**3.** Straighten your right leg while holding on to the towel and hold this position, breathing evenly from your diaphragm, for at least 1 minute.

**4.** Change legs and repeat on the other side.

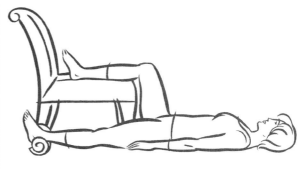

# WATER BREAK

Although adults are comprised of about 60 percent water, children's bodies contain even more. Make sure your children are drinking plenty of fluids during the day (sodas don't count).

# ENERGY BALANCE DINNER

### DINING IN

## Baked Turkey-Stuffed Tomato

    1 very large beefsteak tomato
    1/2 tablespoon butter
    1/2 tablespoon flour
    1/2 cup milk
    1/2 cup diced cooked turkey
    2 tablespoons finely diced celery
    1 tablespoon sliced green onion
    2 tablespoons chopped salted almonds or cashews
    3 tablespoons low-fat sharp cheddar cheese
    Salt and pepper to taste

**1.** Slice off the top of the tomato and scoop out the pulp from the center.

**2.** Sprinkle the inside of the tomato with a little salt and turn it upside down to drain.

3. In a small saucepan, melt the butter and stir in the flour. Cook over low heat until bubbly.

4. Take the pan off the heat and stir in the milk. Put it back on the burner and stir until the sauce is smooth and thickened.

5. Stir in the turkey, celery, onions, nuts, 2 tablespoons cheese, salt, and pepper.

6. Fill the tomato shell with the turkey mixture.

7. Place in a shallow baking dish and sprinkle with 1 tablespoon cheese.

8. Bake at 375° for 10 to 15 minutes or until golden brown on top.

9. Serve with a large green salad and a small whole-grain dinner roll.

### DINING OUT

Start with a small green salad with olive-oil-and-vinegar dressing. Order a turkey dinner with yams or mashed potatoes, stuffing, and cranberry sauce. Eat 1/2 the stuffing, potatoes, and cranberry sauce. Ask for the gravy on the side and drizzle a small amount over the turkey. Finish with decaf tea or coffee with sweetener and cream.

➤ If you want a larger meal:

**DINING IN** Make 2 servings.

**DINING OUT** Wait a few minutes and let your stomach signal your brain that you are full. If you are still hungry, have a decaf coffee, cappuccino, or latte.

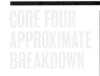
CORE FOUR
APPROXIMATE
BREAKDOWN

| PROTEIN | FAT |
|---|---|
| ➤ turkey: 20 to 25 grams | ➤ nuts, butter, and cheese: 10 to 15 grams |
| **CARBOHYDRATE** | ➤ restaurant meal: 20 grams |
| ➤ turkey and tomato stuffing: 5 grams | **FIBER** |
| ➤ salad and roll: 20 grams | ➤ tomato: 3 to 5 grams |
| ➤ restaurant meal: 30 grams | ➤ restaurant meal: 2 to 3 grams |

# ENERGY BALANCE SNACK

Gelatin Sundae

   1/2 cup sugar-free gelatin
      (You can buy it premade or make it yourself.)
   1/2 cup cottage cheese
   1/2 cup nonfat yogurt
   Small amount of low-fat whipped topping
   Sprinkle of chopped walnuts

1. Put gelatin into a small bowl.

2. Stir in cottage cheese and yogurt.

3. Top with walnuts and whipped topping.

CORE FOUR
APPROXIMATE
BREAKDOWN

| PROTEIN | FAT |
|---|---|
| ➤ cottage cheese: 14 grams | ➤ walnuts: 3 to 5 grams |
| **CARBOHYDRATE** | **FIBER** |
| ➤ yogurt: 7 grams | ➤ 0 grams |

# STRETCH, RELAX, AND SLEEP

1. Chest/posture stretch
2. Neck and upper spine stretch
3. Lower spine stretch

# STRESS RELIEF TIP

A recent study claims that harboring grudges and mentally reliving painful events can damage your health. Even briefly imagining a painful event and rehearsing your feelings can raise your blood pressure and heart rate. Forgiveness, however, offers an unexpected gift: more positive emotions and a decrease in stress levels, says researcher Charlotte van Oyen Witvliet, a psychology professor at Hope College in Holland, Michigan. So take a moment today to let go of your anger and pain.

# Check In

"**M**Y BOSS IS A PAIN IN THE NECK!" one of my massage clients told me. Sure enough, when I started working on her I found a huge knot in her neck. Often our bodies reflect our feelings—anxiety may show itself through butterflies in our stomachs, resentment through clenching our jaws. If you're falling in love, you may feel like dancing on air! It's impossible to separate emotional from physical states.

At least once a day, check in with your body, not only to discern how you feel physically but to discover in-depth information about the way how you feel emotionally. Every system in your body reveals your emotional states, including points of muscle tension, gastrointestinal functioning, and breathing patterns. Get to know your body's unique code. This valuable information will help you make decisions about all areas of your life. For example, your body can help you determine which relationships are beneficial and those that drain you of life energy or jobs that spark into your creativity and jobs that deplete you. Your body can guide you toward both physical fitness and emotional health.

# Core Four Upper Body

THIS routine is designed to build on your basic Core Four program. However, if you get tired or are in any pain, stop immediately. Don't push yourself too hard.

## Lying arm press with a wrist cross

This exercise strengthens the fronts of your shoulders and backs of your arms.

1. Lie on your back on the floor with a pillow under your head, contract your abdominals, and bend your knees, so your feet are flat on the floor.
2. Pick up either a 3- to 5-pound weight or a 1-liter water bottle in each hand.
3. Rest your bent elbows on the floor with your hands up at right angles and the weights parallel to the floor.
4. Inhale and then exhale as you push the weights straight up.
5. Cross your wrists at the top of the movement, keeping your elbows soft and unlocked.
6. Hold for a second and return to the starting position.
7. Repeat 12 to 15 times for 2 more sets. Take a 10-second rest between sets.

## Standing biceps curl

1. Stand, holding 3- to 5-pound weights or two books of the same weight in your hands with your palms facing up. Keep your shoulder blades down and back throughout the movement.
2. Glue your elbows to your waist as if holding folders under your arms. Your arms should be parallel to your thighs, with a slight bend in your elbows, and your wrists should be rigid and straight—don't let them curl up or hang back and down during the movement.

3. Inhale as you bring your hands toward your shoulders, stopping just before your forearms touch your biceps.
4. Exhale as you slowly lower your hands to the initial position.
5. Repeat 12 to 15 times.

## Triceps kickback

1. Stand with 3- to 5-pound weights or 1-liter water bottles in your hands, and lean forward from your hips, not your waist.
2. Keep your head and spine aligned without arching your lower back.
3. Bend your elbows slightly behind your waistline while pulling your shoulder blades together. Keep your shoulders pressed down (don't allow them to creep up toward your ears). Your elbows do not move during this exercise.
4. Exhale as you slowly straighten your arms toward the ceiling, tighten the backs of your arms, and hold for 1 second.
5. Return to the starting position, but do not allow the elbows to move from their stabilized position.
6. Repeat 12 to 15 times.

## Side of the shoulder raise

1. Stand with your palms facing your thighs, holding 3- to 5-pound weights or 1-liter water bottles.
2. Keep your elbows slightly bent.
3. Exhale and raise the weights to your sides, stopping just below shoulder level. Do not go higher than your shoulders, as it will tighten your neck muscles and place too much tension in the area.
4. Hold for 1 second and lower to the initial position.
5. Repeat 12 to 15 times for 2 sets.

## Sink pull

This exercise will strengthen your large back muscles.
1. Stand facing a kitchen or bathroom sink.
2. Contract your abdominals and lift your chest.
3. Hold on to the sink and let your body sit back into a squat position.
4. Exhale and pull yourself up to a standing position.
5. Don't let your legs do the work; let the fronts of your arms and your large back muscles do most of the pulling.
6. When you come back to the standing position, squeeze your buttocks, release, and sit back down into the squat.
7. Repeat 12 to 15 times and do 2 more sets, or until you feel tired. I don't recommend doing more than 3 sets.

## Rotator cuff raise

This exercise will strengthen the four small muscles that attach your arm and shoulder bones. These muscles allow your shoulder joint to rotate, reach up and down, and make circles. If you have a rotator cuff injury, consult with your doctor before you do this exercise.
1. Stand holding 3- to 5-pound weights or 1-liter water bottles in your hands and let them hang down by the sides of your body.
2. Turn your palms to face behind you with your thumbs touching your thighs.
3. Exhale and lift your arms to your sides just below shoulder height.
4. Hold for 1 second and release.
5. Repeat 12 to 15 times for 3 sets.

# STRETCHING EXERCISES

## Chest stretch

1. Standing, place your hands behind you in the small of your lower back.
2. Squeeze your shoulder blades together and feel a gentle stretch in your chest and the fronts of your shoulders.

## Triceps and biceps stretch

1. Standing, place your hands behind your head on the back of your neck.
2. Point your elbows toward the ceiling and hold for 20 to 30 seconds. This is a triceps stretch.
3. Lower your hands and extend your right arm in front of your thigh, palms facing your thigh.
4. Gently pull on your right wrist with your left hand and feel a stretch in the front of your arm. This is a biceps stretch.
5. Change hands and repeat the stretch on the other side.

## Back and shoulder stretch

1. Lift your chest, contract your abdominals, and wrap your hands around your opposite shoulders as far as they will go.
2. Drop your head forward and hold for 20 to 30 seconds before releasing.

## Rotator cuff stretch

1. Extend both arms out in front of you at shoulder height.
2. Place your left arm under your right arm.
3. Bend your left arm and cradle your right arm in the crook of your left elbow, pulling your right arm across your chest.
4. Hold for 5 seconds. Repeat on the other side.

# DAY 15

## WAKE-UP AFFIRMATION

*"You don't stop laughing because you grow old; you grow old because you stop laughing."*
—*Michael Pritchard, youth activist*

## WAKE-UP WORKOUT

**1.** Let body slowly wake up
**2.** Take several deep breaths
**3.** Full-body tighten and release
**4.** Pelvic tilts
**5.** Pillow sit-ups
**6.** Hamstring stretch
**7.** Hands and knees yoga stretch

## CORE FOUR

**1.** Push-up
**2.** Sit-up
**3.** Sit and stand
**4.** Posture squeeze/biceps curl

## PORTION CONTROL TIP

Most restaurants drown your food in sauce, so ask for the sauce on the side. A tasty sauce drizzled sparingly on your meal can add to a pleasurable dining experience without adding unnecessary fat.

## ENERGY BALANCE BREAKFAST

Breakfast Hash

1 red potato, diced
Pinch diced onion
1 stalk celery, diced
4 turkey sausage links, sliced
1 red bell pepper, finely chopped
1 yellow bell pepper, finely chopped
2 teaspoons chopped parsley
Salt and pepper to taste

**1.** Coat a skillet with olive oil or cooking spray and cook the potato, onion, and celery over medium heat until tender (about 5 to 10 minutes).
**2.** Stir in the remaining ingredients.
**3.** Reduce heat and cook for another 5 minutes, stirring occasionally.
**4.** Press mixture into the skillet creating a hashlike consistency.
**5.** Reduce heat and cook until a crust forms on the bottom; do not stir.
**6.** Remove to a warm plate and serve with low-sugar applesauce.
**7.** Add 1 slice whole-grain toast with 1 tablespoon trans-fat-free margarine.

➤ If you want a larger meal: Add 1 or 2 turkey sausage links on the side.

Drink water with lemon or 4 ounces of juice and 6 ounces of water, plus decaffeinated tea or coffee, if desired. Add low-fat creamer to taste.

CORE FOUR APPROXIMATE BREAKDOWN

**PROTEIN**
➤ turkey sausage: 15 to 20 grams

**CARBOHYDRATE**
➤ potato: 5 grams
➤ toast: 13 grams
➤ vegetables: 2 to 3 grams

**FAT:**
➤ turkey sausage: 5 grams
➤ margarine: 2 to 3 grams

**FIBER**
➤ toast and vegetables: 8 to 10 grams

# TAKE 10
Walk and stretch

Take a ten-minute walk. After your walk, do this front of the thigh stretch, which promotes a greater range of motion in the fronts of your thighs and decreases the chance of injury.

1. Stand with your feet hip distance apart. Bend your knees slightly, lift your chest, contract your abdominals, press your shoulders back and down, align your head and spine, and face forward. Hold on to the back of a chair for balance.
2. From behind place your right hand on the toes of your right foot and pull them up to your buttocks, keeping your knees together. Don't arch your lower back. (If you are not flexible enough to reach your toes wrap a towel around your foot and gently pull the ends of the towel toward your buttocks.)
3. Squeeze your buttocks and gently press your hips forward.
4. Bend your standing leg slightly to reduce stress on the lower back. Hold for 15 to 20 seconds and repeat the stretch with your left leg.

# SIT AND BE FIT
Chair pull and push

This exercise tones the large muscles in your back , as well as the muscles in the fronts of your arm.

1. Sit in a chair with rollers, lift your chest, contract your abdominals, press your shoulders back and down, align your head and spine, and face forward.
2. Grasp the edge of your desk with your hands and pull yourself forward. Try to get as close to the desk as possible.
3. Retaining the same position, gently push away as far as you can and then pull forward once again.
4. Inhale as you push away and exhale as you pull forward. Repeat 5 to 10 times, working up to 20.

# WATER BREAK

On average we lose about 2 quarts of water a day, which is one reason your weight fluctuates during the day. Because it is often just water weight, losing 2 to 5 pounds in the first few days of any reducing program is common. It takes at least a week to lose 1 to 2 pounds of real fat.

# ENERGY BALANCE SNACK
Repeat

Have a favorite snack from any of the other days.

| CORE FOUR APPROXIMATE BREAKDOWN | PROTEIN ➤ 10 to 15 grams | FAT ➤ 10 to 15 grams |
|---|---|---|
| | CARBOHYDRATE ➤ 15 to 20 grams | FIBER ➤ 2 to 5 grams |

# WATER BREAK

To determine how much more water you need if you exercise and perspire profusely, weigh yourself before and after you exercise. Any difference reflects your fluid loss from sweating. For each pound lost, you should replenish with 2 to 3 cups of water.

# ENERGY LIFT
Upper back lat stretch

1. Stand with your feet shoulder width apart, your knees bent slightly, and your toes pointing straight ahead.
2. Reach forward with both arms straight, grasping your left wrist with your right hand.
3. Round your back into an arch and hold.
4. Without turning your upper body, keep your left arm extended and pull it across to the right side of your body.
5. Feel the stretch along the back of your left arm and the left side of your upper back.
6. Keep your breath even and regular.

7. Change hands and repeat the stretch on the other side.
8. Do 3 sets, alternating side to side.

# ENERGY BALANCE LUNCH

## DINING IN

### Falafel with Cucumber Salad

1 package falafel mix
2 medium cucumbers, seeded and diced
1 teaspoon salt
1 small green bell pepper, diced
2 green onions, thinly sliced
1 cup low-fat plain yogurt
2 tablespoons fresh lemon juice
1 tablespoon olive oil
1 clove minced or pressed garlic
2 tablespoons chopped mint leaves
Crisp lettuce leaves

1. Prepare the falafel into 4 to 6 patties.
2. Sprinkle the cucumbers with the salt and let stand for 15 minutes on a paper towel. Rinse and drain well. Blot off excess water.
3. Mix the cucumbers with the green bell pepper, onions, yogurt, lemon juice, olive oil, garlic, and chopped mint. Cover and chill to blend flavors.
4. Place the cucumber salad on top of the lettuce.

This recipe makes about 4 servings. Eat 1 serving with 2 falafel and save the rest for a snack or a side dish for dinner or tomorrow's lunch.

## DINING OUT

Most Middle Eastern restaurants have some kind of cucumber salad. Order a large portion and eat with falafel. Add 1 small piece pita bread and a cup of herbal tea.

➤ If you want a larger meal: Have more cucumber salad and falafel.

| CORE FOUR APPROXIMATE BREAKDOWN | PROTEIN ➤ falafel: 12 grams CARBOHYDRATE ➤ falafel: 34 grams ➤ cucumber salad: 5 grams | FAT ➤ olive oil: 3 to 5 grams ➤ falafel: 12 grams FIBER ➤ falafel: 7 grams ➤ cucumber salad: 5 to 10 grams |
|---|---|---|

# SIT AND BE FIT

### Posture fix

As we age, our posture suffers as a result of the downward pull of gravity. This movement will firm and tone the backs of your shoulders and improve your posture.

1. Sit on the edge of a chair with 3- to 5-pound weights on the floor in front of you.
2. Bend forward, resting your upper body on a pillow on your knees for support.
3. Pick up the weights in both hands with your palms facing the floor.
4. Inhale as you lift the weights up and out to the side, keeping a slight bend in the elbows.
5. At the top of the movement, the weight should be straight out and parallel with your shoulders.
6. Hold for 1 second and then exhale as you return to the starting position.
7. Repeat 12 to 15 times for 3 sets.

# WATER BREAK

It can be difficult to realize your fatigue may be caused by dehydration, which can occur over the course of many days.

## ENERGY LIFT
Overhead stretch

This series will not only stretch your back and the sides of your waist but also open up your shoulder area, allowing for easier movement.

1. Sit in a chair, lift your chest, contract your abdominals, press your shoulders back and down, align your head and spine, and face forward.
2. Clasp your hands together in front of your chest with your arms straight.
3. Raise your arms over your head and place your elbows next to your ears.
4. Hold for 1 second and return to initial position.
5. At the starting position, push your hands out in front of you as far as you can. You will feel a gentle stretch in your mid-back.
6. Repeat this stretch 3 or 4 times or until you feel more energized.

## WATER BREAK

Caffeinated beverages dehydrate your body, which can lead to low potassium and electrolyte levels. When your body is low on minerals, especially potassium, leg cramps can occur. For a drink that will quickly relieve low-potassium leg cramps, mix 2 teaspoons apple cider vinegar and 1 tablespoon honey with a glass of warm water.

## ENERGY BALANCE SNACK
Pineapple Cottage Cheese

1 cup low-fat cottage cheese topped with 1/2 cup of pineapple and a sprinkle of chopped walnuts

CORE FOUR
APPROXIMATE
BREAKDOWN

| **PROTEIN** | **FAT** |
|---|---|
| ➤ cottage cheese and pineapple: 28 grams | ➤ walnuts: 10 grams |
| **CARBOHYDRATE** | **FIBER** |
| ➤ cottage cheese and pineapple: 17 grams | ➤ pineapple: 1 gram |
| | ➤ walnuts: 1 gram |

## TAKE 10
Buttocks lift

This exercise will lift, firm, and tone your buttocks, which will improve your balance and stabilize your lower back.

1. Stand on your right leg with your hip and toes slightly turned out to the side, bend your left knee and place your left foot slightly behind your right ankle on the floor.
2. Hold on to a chair for balance while lifting your chest and contracting your abdominals. Be careful not to arch your lower back. Keep your shoulders back and down, with your head forward and aligned with your spine.
3. Lean slightly forward from your hips and exhale as you lift your left leg straight back until you feel a tightening in your buttocks. You should not, however, feel a tightening in your lower back. If you do, substitute this exercise with one that will tone your abdomen, which will strengthen your lower back.
4. Return the leg to the starting position and repeat 5 times, working up to 15 to 20 times.
5. Change legs and repeat on the other side.

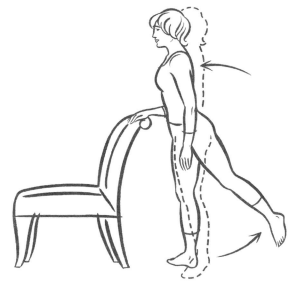

## WATER BREAK

Proper hydration is critical during pregnancy because in the mother's womb water carries life-sustaining nutrients to the embryo, as well as helping carry waste out of the mother's body.

## ENERGY BALANCE DINNER

### DINING IN

Spinach Filled Salmon

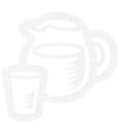

8-ounce salmon fillet

Salt and pepper to taste

1 cup baby spinach, coarsely chopped

2 tablespoons prepared pesto

1 tablespoon chopped sun-dried tomatoes

1 tablespoon pine nuts

1. Heat oven to 400° F.
2. Make a slit 2/3 of the way down the salmon, but do not cut through it.
3. Season the salmon with the salt and pepper.
4. In a bowl, combine the spinach, pesto, sun-dried tomatoes, and pine nuts.
5. Spoon 1/3 cup of the mixture into the slit salmon.
6. Place the salmon on a broiler pan coated with cooking spray.
7. Roast 8 to 10 minutes or until the spinach mixture is heated through.
8. Serve with a large green salad with lots of vegetables and 1/2 cup brown rice. Use low-fat salad dressing.

### DINING OUT

Order a salmon fillet with light pesto sauce. Add vegetables and a small amount of roasted potatoes or a small baked potato with light sour cream and chives. Have a small Caesar salad with dressing on the side. Dip your fork into the dressing and then into the salad to lessen the fat content. Drink decaf tea, coffee, or latte.

➤ If want a larger meal: Have 2 ounces more salmon, salad, and vegetables.

| CORE FOUR APPROXIMATE BREAKDOWN | PROTEIN | FAT |
|---|---|---|
| | ➤ salmon: 20 to 25 grams | ➤ salmon and filling: 15 to 20 grams |
| | **CARBOHYDRATE** | ➤ salad dressing: 3 to 5 grams |
| | ➤ salad and vegetables: 10 grams | ➤ light sour cream: 3 to 5 grams |
| | ➤ potato: 10 to 15 grams | **FIBER** |
| | ➤ rice: 10 to 15 grams | ➤ entire meal: 10 to 15 grams |

## ENERGY BALANCE SNACK

Frozen Fruit

1 frozen fruit bar

1 cup low-fat yogurt

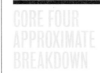

| CORE FOUR APPROXIMATE BREAKDOWN | PROTEIN | FAT |
|---|---|---|
| | ➤ yogurt: 4 grams | ➤ yogurt: 2 to 3 grams |
| | **CARBOHYDRATE** | **FIBER** |
| | ➤ fruit bar: 10 grams | ➤ 0 grams |

## STRETCH, RELAX, AND SLEEP

1. Chest/posture stretch
2. Neck and upper spine stretch
3. Lower spine stretch

## STRESS RELIEF TIP

Eighty percent of illnesses are suspected to be stress related. Massage therapy is recommended to relieve stress and bolster the immune system. By lowering anxiety levels, massage decreases the production of the stress hormone cortisol.

# Make Peace with Gravity

MANY OF US ASSUME aches and pains are unavoidable as we age. In fact, the majority of our moans and groans are not due to our chronological age but come from problems we have created through poor posture. Our bodies are designed to work with gravity—each section of our physique is meant to be in balance with the rest so that the pull of gravity helps us stand upright and move easily. If we're out of alignment, however, gravity and our bodies are in conflict. We must exert extra effort to perform the simple tasks of standing in line, walking across a parking lot, or reaching for items on market shelves. No wonder so many of us prefer to sit on our fannies rather than fight the earth's pull.

Our muscles and fascia primarily determine our posture by positioning and holding our bones in place. If you want to realign your posture, realign your muscles—something you are already doing by participating in this program. In addition, try this simple exercise.* Lie on the floor or on a bed with a firm mattress. Relax your arms at your sides. One by one, starting at the base of your skull and working to your tailbone, slowly flatten each vertebra against the floor or mattress. Take a deep breath and hold for a count of ten. Repeat this five times and then lie still for a few moments to let your body absorb this realignment. Expect to feel lighter and freer when you stand up.

* Julia Busch, "Straighten Your Back to Lift Your Face" (Internet article, 2000).

# Balance Ball Workout

A GOOD WAY TO INCREASE your activity level is with a Balance Ball workout, which is a highly effective and safe way to exercise. Although it looks like a toy and appears to be a novelty, the Balance Ball is based on sound scientific principles that maximize muscle coordination, strength, and flexibility. This program delivers results you can feel and see.

Balance Ball exercise was started in the 1950s in Switzerland to restore patients' motor skills after serious injuries. Today the exercises are recommended by personal trainers and physical therapists to strengthen the torso stabilizer muscles in the back, abdomen, legs, and buttocks.

These balls are available at sporting goods stores, home exercise equipment stores, and specialty back stores. I recommend the 65-centimeter ball for the following exercises. This size ball is best used as a desk chair for most people.

Please follow the safety tips listed below before beginning this fun and very effective program.

1. Inflate your ball until it is firm.
2. Sit on the ball. You should have approximately a 90-degree angle at both your hips and your knees.
3. Make sure you have plenty of room to exercise. Look to see if there are any objects around that could be dangerous if you rolled into or onto them.
4. Take it easy. Don't bounce too high, stretch back too far, or work too hard.
5. Use the Balance Ball as a piece of equipment that will relax you as well as work you out.
6. Give your body time to adapt to this new way of exercising—take it slow!
7. Take care to exercise at your level of fitness. Don't push or try to do any exercise that feels difficult. Remember that exercise should always be fun and easy.
8. No special clothes are required. Many of my clients use the Balance Ball in their street clothing. However, if you are going to do a full workout, you will want to change into something that will allow free movement. Wear flat, nonskid shoes or go barefoot.
9. Place your Balance Ball on carpet (not wood or stone floors) and away from furniture, walls, and stairs, unless the directions call for you to use a chair for balance or a wall for positioning.
10. Children should use the Balance Ball only with an adult present.

THE BALANCE BALL IS FOR EXERCISE ONLY. IT'S NOT A TOY. PLEASE READ ALL INSTRUCTIONS PRIOR TO USE AND USE ONLY AS INSTRUCTED.

## BALANCE BALL EXERCISES
### Basic sitting position

Just by sitting on the Balance Ball, you are already on your way to stronger and flatter abdominals, because your muscles must constantly contract and release to help keep you balanced. The stronger your body gets, the easier it will be to do each exercise.

1. Sit in the middle of the ball, lift your chest, contract your abdominals, press your shoulders back and down, align your head and spine, and face forward.
2. At first you may feel a little unsteady, so hold on to a chair, couch or desk for better balance. Place your feet as wide apart as possible.

3. Maintain a neutral posture while sitting on the ball; keep your spine between an arched and a flat-back position.

4. Sit on your Balance Ball for 10 to 15 minutes a day while watching TV or any other seated activity.

## Desk sit

This desk chair alternative improves the core muscle strength structure while giving your upper neck, hands, and arms a break.

1. Sit in the middle of the ball, lift your chest, contract your abdominals, press your shoulders back and down, align your head and spine, and face forward.

2. Sit on the ball instead of your desk chair for 10 to 15 minutes, then take a break and return to your regular chair.

3. Take another Balance Ball break for 10 minutes and go back and forth all day.

4. At the end of the day, without realizing it, you have strengthened your abdominals and lower back and improved your posture—easily!

## Bounce the stress and day away

This stress-easing bounce will not only raise your mood; it will help release the ever-present stress hormones that flood our muscles all day long.

1. Sit in the middle of the ball, lift your chest, contract your abdominals, press your shoulders back and down, align your head and spine, and face forward.

2. Begin bouncing, but do not bounce so high that your buttocks leave the ball.

3. For a more of an aerobic, fat-burning workout, bounce for 10 minutes using the fronts of your thigh muscles. Make your thighs do most of the lifting and try to control the momentum of the bounce of the ball.

4. If you get out of breath, slow down and go back to an easy bounce.

5. When you have caught your breath, take your breathing and heart rate up again by using the larger muscles of your thighs.

6. Continue on this back and forth until you want to stop, then bounce gently to bring down your heart rate.

7. Once your heart rate has returned to normal, lean forward over your knees and allow your lower back to stretch and relax.

8. Hold for a few seconds and slowly roll up one vertebra at a time to a seated position.

**NOTE:** If you have lower back considerations, don't bounce too vigorously. This is exercise and you can overstress your back. Take it easy and strengthen your lower back with the abdominal and lower back exercises listed below.

## One-foot balance

This movement strengthens your core midsection stabilizer muscles (abdominals and back) and strengthens your thighs, the fronts of the hips (hip flexors), and your ankles. When these muscles are strong, your balance is improved.

1. Sit in the middle of the ball, lift your chest, contract your abdominals, press your shoulders back and down, align your head and spine, and face forward.

2. Hold on to a chair for balance.

3. Place your feet together.

4. Pick up one foot, extend your leg, tighten your knee slightly, and hold for as long as comfortable.

5. As you feel your balance improving, let go of the chair and hold both arms out to the sides, palms facing the ceiling.

6. Hold for as long as comfortable. Change sides.

7. Repeat 3 times, alternating legs.

## Sides of the waist (obliques)

This exercise will condition the sides of your waist and increase the flexibility of your spine.

1. Sit in the middle of the ball with your feet wider than hip distance apart. Lift your chest, contract your abdominals, press your shoulders back and down, align your head and spine, and face forward.
2. Lift your arms over your head, palms facing inward.
3. Move your hips to the left and then to the right. Do not move your shoulders. The ball will follow the movement of your hips. If your arms become tired, relax and rest your hands on your thighs or the sides of the ball.
4. Do this for a few minutes and then move on to the next exercise.

## Relax the back

While stretching and relaxing your back, this exercise will increase blood flow and circulation to your head and brain because your head is resting lower than your chest.

1. Face the ball in a kneeling position and bring the ball under your belly.
2. Your toes are tucked under, your feet are flexed, and your hands are on the sides of the ball.
3. Gently roll your body over until you are relaxing on top of the ball. As you roll onto the ball, allow your hands to rest on the floor in front of the ball.
4. Let your body hang in a relaxed position and allow the tension of the day to drain away.
5. Stay in this position as long as comfortable.

## Lower back lift

This exercise will strengthen your back muscles.

1. Assume the same position as the prior exercise, Relax the back. Place your hands on the floor and relax over the ball.
2. Gently lift your upper body until your spine is straight. Don't arch your back; keep it tabletop straight. Hold for a few seconds and then relax.

If you are not used to doing exercises for the lower back, do 1 set of 6 repetitions. Work up to 3 sets of 12 repetitions.

## Reverse roll abdominal toner

This toner will not only safely firm and tone your abdominal wall, it will help strengthen your lower back and improve balance, strength, and posture.

1. Sit in the middle of the ball with your feet wider than hip distance apart, lift your chest, contract your abdominals, press your shoulders back and down, align your head and spine, and face forward. Hold on to a chair or desk for balance.
2. Gently roll the ball forward with your hips as you lean back slightly, feeling your abdominals tighten. Hold for 30 seconds.
3. Return to the starting position. Begin with 3 sets of 5 repetitions, working up to 3 sets of 20 repetitions.

## Abdominal stretch

This stretch is not only good for the front of your body, it will help keep your spine flexible, too.

1. Assume the same position as in the previous exercise, th abdominal toner, and walk your feet out a little further in front of your body while rolling your spine down the ball to the middle of your back.

**2.** Hold on to a chair or your desk for balance and place one hand behind your neck to support your head.

**3.** Relax your back on the ball and allow your head to hang slightly over the top of the ball. Extend your legs in front of you a little further, until you feel a gentle stretch all along the front of your body.

**4.** Hold as long as comfortable.

## Inner thigh squeeze

While this exercise firms and tones your inner thighs, it will also stretch your entire spine all the way down to your lower back if you relax your chest on top of the ball during the exercise.

**1.** Sit on a chair or couch and hold the ball between your legs with your chest lifted, your abdominals contracted, your shoulders pressed back and down, and your head facing straight ahead.

**2.** Place both hands on top of the ball for support, or lower the ball enough that you can relax your torso on top of it.

**3.** Squeeze your thighs together. Hold for 1 second and release.

**4.** Work up to 3 sets of 20 repetitions; rest 30 seconds between each set.

## Wall squat

This exercise will strengthen the fronts of your thighs and your buttocks, helping protect your lower back from injury. Keep your knees in proper alignment to ensure less pressure on your knee joints, ligaments, and tendons.

**1.** Place the Balance Ball in the middle of your lower back and against a wall.

**2.** Place your feet hip distance apart. Move them out in front of you until you are a little off balance. (You will have to lean against the ball in order not to fall.)

**3.** Bend your knees and roll down the wall until your thighs are parallel to the floor.

**4.** Keep your knees over your heels, not your toes.

**5.** Hold at the bottom of the movement for a few seconds.

**6.** Roll back up to the starting position. Don't lock your knees.

**7.** Repeat. Work up to 3 sets of 20 repetitions; rest a few seconds between each set.

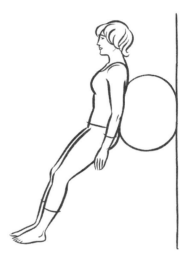

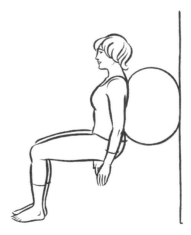

# DAY 16

## WAKE-UP AFFIRMATION

*"To handle yourself, use your head. To handle others, use your heart."*

—*Anonymous*

## WAKE-UP WORKOUT

**1.** Let body slowly wake up
**2.** Take several deep breaths
**3.** Full-body tighten and release
**4.** Pelvic tilts
**5.** Pillow sit-ups
**6.** Hamstring stretch
**7.** Hands and knees yoga stretch

## CORE FOUR

**1.** Push-up
**2.** Sit-up
**3.** Sit and stand
**4.** Posture squeeze/biceps curl

## PORTION CONTROL TIP

Remember that 4 tablespoons equals 1/4 cup. By keeping your measuring spoons handy, you'll easily use the correct portions.

## ENERGY BALANCE BREAKFAST

### Almond French Toast

2 thin slices whole-grain bread
1 egg and 2 egg whites
1 tablespoon milk
1 teaspoon cinnamon
2 tablespoons sliced almonds
1 teaspoon powdered sugar

**1.** In a small bowl, whisk together the egg, egg whites, milk, and cinnamon.
**2.** Dip the bread into the egg mixture until moist but not saturated.
**3.** Layer the almonds evenly onto the egg-coated bread, pressing until the almonds stick to the egg mixture.
**4.** Heat a skillet coated with cooking spray over medium heat.
**5.** Place the bread almond side down in skillet and cook until golden brown.
**6.** Flip the bread and cook until the second side is golden brown.
**7.** Serve immediately, dusted with powdered sugar.

➤ If you want a larger meal: Add a thick slice of cooked lean ham.

Drink water with lemon or 4 ounces of juice and 6 ounces of water, plus decaffeinated tea or coffee, if desired. Add low-fat creamer to taste.

| CORE FOUR APPROXIMATE BREAKDOWN | **PROTEIN**<br>➤ egg and egg whites: 13 grams<br>➤ ham: 15 grams<br>**CARBOHYDRATE**<br>➤ bread: 25 to 30 grams | **FAT**<br>➤ egg yolk: 5 grams<br>**FIBER**<br>➤ bread: 6 to 10 grams |
|---|---|---|

# TAKE 10
## Buttocks firmer

This isometric exercise will not only tone your buttocks and thighs, it will help improve your balance.

1. Stand a few inches behind a chair, with your back positioned a foot from wall. Lift your chest, contract your abdominals, press your shoulders back and down, align your head and spine, and face forward.
2. Place your hands on the top of the chair with your feet parallel to the legs of the chair.
3. Relax both knees slightly and lift your right foot off the floor, moving it slightly outward away from your hip.
4. Breathing evenly and naturally, lift your leg so your right foot is against the wall at knee level. Keep your hips level and facing forward.
5. Push your foot as hard as you can against the wall 10 times, gradually working up to 20 and then 30 repetitions.
6. With your foot still against the wall, lift your right hand off the chair and hold your balance for as long as comfortable.
7. Release and repeat on the other side. As you progress and become stronger, do 2 to 3 more sets.

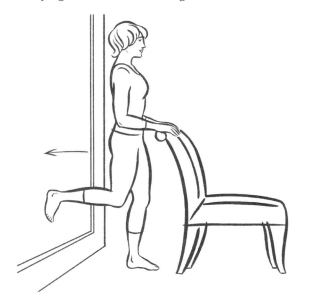

# SIT AND BE FIT
## Seated hamstring stretch

This easy thigh stretch is an effective complement to the last exercise.

1. Sit in a chair behind a desk. Lift your chest, contract your abdominals, press your shoulders back and down, align your head and spine, and face forward.
2. Kick off your shoes and move your chair back far enough so that you can place 1 foot on the top of your desk with your toes pointing towards the ceiling.
3. Keeping your knee slightly bent, slowly straighten your leg until you feel a gentle tightening in the back of your thigh. To increase the stretch, lean forward with a flat back from your hips.
4. Hold for 20 to 30 seconds and then repeat on the other leg.

This stretch can also be done sitting on a couch, using a chair instead of your desk.

# ENERGY BALANCE SNACK
## Peanut Butter Pretzel

10 peanut butter-filled pretzels

| CORE FOUR APPROXIMATE BREAKDOWN | PROTEIN ➤ 5 grams | FAT ➤ 6 grams |
|---|---|---|
| | CARBOHYDRATE ➤ 20 grams | FIBER ➤ 0 grams |

# WATER BREAK

An easy way to dress up water is to create flavorful ice cubes. Place diced lemons and limes in an ice tray half full of water and freeze. Now anytime you are thirsty, you will have a zesty way to chill your drink.

## ENERGY LIFT

### Pivot point knee bend

This exercise tones the fronts of your thighs and firms your buttocks.

1. Stand a few inches from a chair, bench, or couch with your abdominals contracted and your head aligned with your spine. Throughout the entire movement, keep your knees slightly bent.
2. Inhale and slowly sit back, as if you are going to sit down, with your hands on your knees and your elbows pointing out the sides. Touch the chair with your buttocks.
3. Exhale and stand back up to the starting position while tightening your buttocks and tucking them under with a slight squeeze.
4. Throughout the squat, keep your knees over your heels; don't let them drift over your toes. When your buttocks touch the chair, hold for a second and look down at your knees to see if they are directly over your heels. If not, then stand up and move your feet a little farther from the chair. Keep doing this until you are in the proper knees-over-heels position.
5. Do 10 and see how you feel. If you are out of breath, stop; the goal is to work up to 20 to 30 repetitions.

## ENERGY BALANCE LUNCH

### DINING IN

### Tuna Burger

2 tablespoons olive oil
1/2 cup eggplant, chopped
1/2 cup zucchini, chopped
1/2 cup red bell pepper, chopped
2 tablespoons balsamic vinegar
1 hard roll, hollowed out
1 tablespoon low-fat mayonnaise
1 8-ounce tuna steak, cooked

1. Heat the oil in a nonstick skillet over medium-high heat.
2. Add the eggplant, zucchini, and pepper to the skillet and sauté until cooked but still crisp.
3. Remove the vegetables from heat and toss them with the vinegar.
4. Spread the hard roll with the mayonnaise and top with tuna steak and vegetables.

### DINING OUT

Order grilled tuna with vegetables and eat 1/2 roll.

➤ If you want a larger meal: Add 2 ounces more tuna.

| CORE FOUR APPROXIMATE BREAKDOWN | PROTEIN ➤ tuna: 30 grams CARBOHYDRATE ➤ roll: 15 to 20 grams | FAT ➤ mayonnaise:10 to 15 grams FIBER ➤ vegetables: 5 to 10 grams |
|---|---|---|

## SIT AND BE FIT

### Stress releasing neck stretches

This stretch will not only release tension in your neck; it will help prevent headaches due to tight and tired neck muscles.

1. Sit in a chair, lift your chest, contract your abdominals, press your shoulders back and down, align your head and spine, and face forward.
2. Drop your head forward, stretching the muscles in the back of your neck, and hold 5 seconds. Return to the original position.
3. Place your hands behind your lower back and grab your right wrist with your left hand.
4. Drop your head to your left shoulder and at the same time pull down your right arm, stretching the neck from both ends. Hold 20 seconds.
5. Bring your head back up and repeat on the other side. Pull down your left arm as you drop your head to the right.
6. Alternate this stretch back and forth for 3 sets.

# WATER BREAK

Many women hate perspiring, thinking it unfeminine. But it's neither masculine nor feminine—it is your body's way of cooling itself through evaporation. Be sure to replace any water lost with a nice cool drink.

# ENERGY LIFT

Cat curl stretch

This exercise gives you energy, lengthens your spine, stretches the sides of your waist and back, and tightens your abdominals.

1. Stand a few feet from a chair, table, or sink counter.
2. Bend over from your hips and place your hands flat on the chair, table, or counter so your torso is parallel to the floor and your arms are extended as far from the chair as possible, with your elbows and knees bent slightly.
3. Inhale and slowly drop your head between your arms.
4. Hold this stretch for a few seconds, exhale, and slowly contract your abdominals and round your back to the ceiling like an arched cat. Hold for a few seconds and release to a flat back.
5. Repeat the flat back to cat arch 2 times.

# WATER BREAK

Body fluid (water) terms
➤ Intracellular fluid: fluid within cells
➤ Interstitial fluid: fluid between cells (a component of extracellular fluid)
➤ Extracellular fluid: fluid outside cells, includes interstitial fluid, plasma, and the water in skin and bones. Accounts for a third of the body's water.

# ENERGY BALANCE SNACK

Grapefruit Compote

   1/2 grapefruit, peeled, chopped into small pieces
   1/2 cup melon, any kind, chopped
   1/2 cup crushed sweetened strawberries
   1/2 cup honey-flavored nonfat yogurt
   Sprinkle of crushed almonds or walnuts

1. Mix the fruit with the yogurt.
2. Top with crushed almonds or walnuts.
3. Serve with 2 or 3 slices of deli turkey or chicken.

| CORE FOUR APPROXIMATE BREAKDOWN | PROTEIN<br>➤ turkey or chicken: 10 to 15 grams<br>CARBOHYDRATE<br>➤ grapefruit compote: 15 to 20 grams | FAT<br>➤ nuts: 5 to 10 grams<br>FIBER<br>➤ fruit and nuts: 3 to 5 grams |
|---|---|---|

# TAKE 10

Inner thigh stretch

This stretch helps to relax your entire body.

1. In a private place, lie on your back with a rolled-up towel or a pillow under your head.
2. With bent knees, place the soles of your feet together and hold. Don't press or help this stretch, but let gravity gently pull your knees toward the floor.
3. Breathe deeply and evenly, holding this relaxed stretch 30 seconds.

# WATER BREAK

Dehydration occurs when water output exceeds water input. Signs of dehydration include dry skin, dry mucous membranes, rapid heart beat, low blood pressure, and general weakness.

## ENERGY BALANCE DINNER

### DINING IN

Broccoli, Sausage, and Pesto Penne

1 tablespoon olive oil

1/2 cup fresh or frozen chopped broccoli

2 links soy, turkey, or nitrate-free Italian sausage, cooked, chopped

1/2 cup whole-grain penne, cooked al dente

2 teaspoons prepared pesto

Dash salt and pepper

1. Heat the olive oil in a skillet over medium heat. Sauté the broccoli until bright green (about 4 minutes).
2. Add the sausage and heat thoroughly.
3. Toss the penne with the pesto until coated, then add the sausage and broccoli.
4. Add salt and pepper to taste. Serve immediately or at room temperature.

### DINING OUT

Order a pasta dish with similar ingredients, but eat only 1/2 cup pasta. (You are bound to be served more.)

➤ If you want a larger meal: Add more sausage and broccoli.

| CORE FOUR APPROXIMATE BREAKDOWN | **PROTEIN** ➤ sausage: 20 to 25 grams **CARBOHYDRATE** ➤ penne: 25 to 30 grams ➤ vegetables: 5 grams | **FAT** ➤ sausage: 10 to 15 grams ➤ olive oil: 10 grams **FIBER** ➤ penne: 3 to 5 grams ➤ vegetables: 5 to 10 grams |
|---|---|---|

## ENERGY BALANCE SNACK

Oatmeal Delight

1/2 cup oatmeal

Sprinkle raisins and cinnamon

1/2 cup cottage cheese

Sprinkle walnuts, chopped

1. Make the oatmeal according to the directions on the package.
2. Add the raisins and cinnamon.
3. Stir in the cottage cheese and top with the walnuts.

| CORE FOUR APPROXIMATE BREAKDOWN | **PROTEIN** ➤ cottage cheese: 7 grams **CARBOHYDRATE** ➤ oatmeal: 15 grams | **FAT** ➤ walnuts: 5 grams **FIBER** ➤ oatmeal: 3 to 5 grams |
|---|---|---|

## STRETCH, RELAX, AND SLEEP

1. Chest/posture stretch
2. Neck and upper spine stretch
3. Lower spine stretch

## HELPFUL HINT

If you indulge in a high-calorie, high-fat food, it does not mean you've fallen out of the program but simply that you had a snack. But you can lessen the effects of that food on your body by supplementing it with an Energy Balancing food.

# Let Your Body Take Shape

**M**ORE THAN HALF the American female population is a size 14 or larger, yet car seats, airplane seats, theater seats, and nearly every other kind of seat are designed for behinds that are size 12 or smaller. If a larger woman didn't already have trouble with her self-esteem, she would as soon as she sat down nearly anywhere in public. Many of us who have struggled with weight have tried desperately to achieve the body society deems attractive—thin, muscular, and not a cell of fat in sight. Yet at least half the women in our country have failed, and most of the women I've talked with feel bad about themselves in proportion to their dress size.

I encourage you to give up your quest for the perfect body. Instead, invest yourself in two simple activities—move every day and eat well. That's all it takes for our bodies to naturally take the shape they were meant to be—strong, healthy, feminine bodies. The shapes will probably not be like the bone-thin models who populate magazine covers, and that's okay. Our bodies have immense wisdom, and when given what they need in terms of nutrition and exercise, they will develop muscle tissue, keep our hearts beating strong, help our immune systems grow powerful, and retain and discard fat as best suits our health. It's time we let our bodies inform our attitudes about desirable body size, not the other way around.

# DAY 17

## WAKE-UP AFFIRMATION

"**Many people will walk in and out of your life; friends will leave footprints on our heart.**"

—*Eleanor Roosevelt, first lady and social activist*

## WAKE-UP WORKOUT

**1.** Let body slowly wake up
**2.** Take several deep breaths
**3.** Full-body tighten and release
**4.** Pelvic tilts
**5.** Pillow sit-ups
**6.** Hamstring stretch
**7.** Hands and knees yoga stretch

## CORE FOUR

**1.** Push-up
**2.** Sit-up
**3.** Sit and stand
**4.** Posture squeeze/biceps curl

## PORTION CONTROL TIP

One of the benefits of using a prepared frozen meal is that it usually conforms to the proper portion size, which can be educational. With it, you can easily see the amount of food that makes up the protein, carbohydrate, and fat gram count. Perhaps the biggest surprise regarding size is the potato or pasta portion, which can be much smaller than anticipated. When you have the ability to spot the right amount of these high-sugar, high-carbohydrate foods, it will be a lot easier to stay in the Energy Balance range of 25 to 30 grams of carbohydrate per meal.

## ENERGY BALANCE BREAKFAST

Baked Potato and Poached Eggs

1/2 baked potato
1 teaspoon trans-fat-free margarine or butter
2 poached eggs
1 slice whole-grain toast

**1.** Mash the potato and spread with the margarine.
**2.** Place the eggs on top and season to taste.
**3.** Serve with lightly buttered toast.

➤ If you want a larger meal: Add 3 scrambled egg whites.

Drink water with lemon or 4 ounces of juice and 6 ounces of water, plus decaffeinated tea or coffee, if desired. Add low-fat creamer to taste.

| CORE FOUR APPROXIMATE BREAKDOWN | | |
|---|---|---|
| **PROTEIN**<br>➤ eggs: 12 grams<br>**CARBOHYDRATE**<br>➤ potato: 15 grams<br>➤ toast: 15 grams | | **FAT**<br>➤ egg yolks: 10 grams<br>➤ margarine or butter: 5 grams<br>**FIBER**<br>➤ potato and whole-grain toast: 3 to 5 grams |

# TAKE 10
### Away from the wall torso stretch

This stretch will not only make your torso more flexible; it will help improve your tennis serve or your golf swing by increasing the flexibility of your spine.

1. Stand a few inches from a wall with your back toward the wall and your feet hip distance apart. Bend your knees slightly, lift your chest, contract your abdominals, press your shoulders back and down, align your head and spine, and face forward.
2. Without moving your feet, slowly twist to your right and place both hands on the wall behind you. Hold a few seconds.
3. Return to the starting position, then slowly turn your torso to the left and touch the wall with both hands and hold.
4. Repeat this stretch 2 times on each side.

# SIT AND BE FIT
### Assisted chair stand

This exercise will lift and tone your buttocks, the backs of your arms, and the fronts of your thighs.

1. You will need a chair with arms for this exercise. Sit as far back in your chair as you can until your buttocks touch the chair's back support. and rest your hands lightly on the armrests.
2. Lift your chest, contract your abdominals, press your shoulders back and down, align your head and spine, and face forward.
3. Exhale as you slowly push yourself up and out of the chair with your arms. When you are at the top of the movement (arms almost fully extended), tighten your buttocks without arching your lower back. Lessen the support by your arms but do not let go of the armrests.
4. Hold 2 seconds and return to the starting position.
5. Do 10 times and work up to 15 and 20. Rest and then do 1 or 2 more sets.

**Note**: This exercise will place some strain on your wrists, as most of your weight will be on the backs of your arms and your wrists. If you experience any pain, stop the exercise and substitute it with one from another day.

# WATER BREAK

Caffeine is not all bad—research has shown that drinking a 6- to 8-ounce cup of coffee before a workout will aid endurance, release fatty acids into the bloodstream to be burned for energy, and raise exercise metabolism. This saves your muscle fuel, glycogen, to be used later when needed.

# ENERGY BALANCE SNACK
### Healthy Trails

1/4 cup raisins
1/2 cup unsalted peanuts
1/2 cup salted sunflower seeds
1/4 cup chocolate chips

Mix the ingredients together. This trail mix recipe makes about 6 servings of 4 tablespoons each. Save the balance for later snacks.

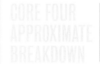

| CORE FOUR APPROXIMATE BREAKDOWN | PROTEIN ➤ 6 grams | FAT ➤ 11 grams |
| --- | --- | --- |
| | CARBOHYDRATE ➤ 17 grams | FIBER ➤ 2 grams |

# WATER BREAK

Here's the breakdown of water in some foods to help you meet your water intake requirements for the day.

➤ Fruits and vegetables: 90 to 99 percent water
➤ Fruit juice: 80 to 89 percent water
➤ Pasta, legumes, beef, and dairy products: 10 to 60 percent water

# ENERGY LIFT
## High and low march

This energy-lifting march strengthens your heart muscle, burns fat, and tones the fronts of your hips and thighs.

1. Stand up straight with your feet hip distance apart. Bend your knees slightly, lift your chest, contract your abdominals, press your shoulders back and down, align your head and spine, and face forward.
2. Hold on to the back of a chair or a doorway.
3. Lift your right knee as high as you can to the front, lower and lift left knee as high as you can. Then lift 10 times, alternating knees.
4. Exhale as you lift and inhale as you lower each of your legs.
5. Alternate lifting your knees to a very low height 10 times.
6. Go back to the high knee lifts.
7. Alternate the high and low lifts for 3 sets.

# ENERGY BALANCE LUNCH

## DINING IN
## Shrimp Salad

1/2 cup cleaned and cooked shrimp
1/2 cup chopped celery
1 hard-boiled egg white, chopped
3 tablespoons chickpeas
1/2 teaspoon finely chopped onion
2 tablespoons fat-free Thousand Island dressing
1 cup shredded romaine lettuce

1. In a large bowl, combine the shrimp, celery, egg white, chickpeas, and onions.
2. Add the dressing and toss until coated.
3. Cover and chill in refrigerator about 30 minutes.
4. Serve on top of lettuce with a small dinner roll.

## DINING OUT

Order a Caesar salad with a little dressing. Ask for shrimp on top. Finish with a nonfat decaf latte.

➤ If you want a larger meal: Add a cup of clear soup.

| CORE FOUR APPROXIMATE BREAKDOWN | PROTEIN ➤ shrimp and egg: 20 to 25 grams | FAT ➤ walnuts: 10 to 15 grams |
|---|---|---|
| | CARBOHYDRATE ➤ roll: 25 grams | FIBER ➤ vegetables: 3 to 5 grams |

# SIT AND BE FIT
## One leg at a time

This exercise will stretch your entire spine and the backs of your thighs, allowing for freer movement in your lower back.

1. Sit on the edge of a chair.
2. Place your right forearm securely under your right knee and pull your knee toward your chest as far as comfortable.
3. Round your upper body over to meet your knee.
4. Breathing deeply and evenly, hold 20 seconds and release.
5. Repeat this stretch with your left forearm under your left knee.

# WATER BREAK

The standard rule for most people is 6 to 8 glasses of water a day; however, the amount of water needed varies from person to person. Water intake is dependent upon body size, activity level, altitude, physical health, caffeine and alcohol consumption, air temperature, humidity, and the amount of fiber in your diet.

# ENERGY LIFT
Doorway push and stretch

This movement will strengthen your chest muscles and firm and tone the backs of your arms and fronts of your shoulders. Working these muscle groups will promote flexibility and help prevent common injuries.

1. Place your hands at shoulder level on a doorway with your elbows bent, your feet together, your body in a straight line (like a floor push-up), your heels together and pushed into the floor, and your knees unlocked.
2. Move your upper body forward keeping your elbows bent and close to your waist. Allow your chest to push through the doorway until you feel a comfortable stretch in your arms and chest.
3. Keep your chest and head up.
4. Hold 15 to 30 seconds and breathe easily.
5. Push back to the initial position. Repeat 4 times.

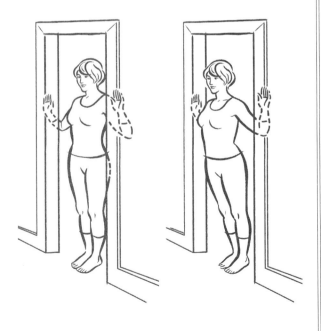

# WATER BREAK

You need water to regulate your metabolism and boost your immune system, both of which are essential for weight control and fat loss.

# ENERGY BALANCE SNACK
Peanut Butter from the Jar

1 tablespoon peanut butter right out of the jar

This is an excellent way to boost your blood sugar level when you don't have access to a balanced snack.

| CORE FOUR APPROXIMATE BREAKDOWN | PROTEIN ➤ 4 grams | FAT ➤ 7 grams |
|---|---|---|
| | CARBOHYDRATE ➤ 4 grams | FIBER ➤ 0 grams |

# TAKE 10
Reach for it . . . with a side stretch

By stretching the sides of your waist and your shoulders, you will increase blood flow to your heart and brain. Any time you lift your arms overhead, you raise your heart rate by 10 beats per minute.

### OVERHEAD ARM PUNCHES

1. Sit in a chair, lift your chest, contract your abdominals, press your shoulders back and down, align your head and spine, and face forward.
2. Punch arms overhead, left, right, left, right, continuously for 15 to 30 seconds. This will raise your heart rate and increase circulation to your upper neck area. If you suffer from any upper back or neck problems, punch straight out in front of your body instead of overhead.

### SIDE STRETCH

1. Let your heart rate come down.
2. Allow your right arm to hang down beside your chair.
3. Place your left hand on your waist and keep

your hips glued to your chair.

4. Raise your right arm straight up over your head with your elbow next to your ear.

5. Exhale and slowly lean to your left as far as comfortable so you can feel a stretch in the right side of your waist. Hold a few seconds and return to the starting position.

6. Change arms and repeat on the other side.

## WATER BREAK

To find the amount of water you should drink, divide your body weight by two. That gives you the number of ounces of water you should be drinking on a daily basis.

## ENERGY BALANCE DINNER

### DINING IN

Turkey Meat Loaf

6 ounces turkey meat loaf (from the deli or follow your regular meat loaf recipe and exchange the beef for ground turkey.)

1 cup broccoli

1 ounce shredded cheese

2 cups salad greens

1/4 cup combined walnuts, feta cheese, raisins, and small croutons (Don't overdo the extras. Use them for flavor.)

1. Place the meat loaf on a plate.

2. Steam the broccoli and top with the cheese.

3. Toss the salad greens with the walnuts, feta cheese, raisins, and croutons.

4. Serve the meat loaf, salad, and broccoli with 1 small dinner roll.

### DINING OUT

Order meat loaf. Have a small portion with roasted potatoes, vegetables sprinkled with Parmesan cheese, and a Caesar salad with a light amount of low-fat dressing.

➤ If you want a larger meal: Eat more meat loaf and add a decaf cappuccino or latte.

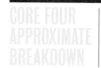

| CORE FOUR APPROXIMATE BREAKDOWN | PROTEIN ➤ meat loaf: 20 to 25 grams CARBOHYDRATE ➤ salad, broccoli, and roll: 25 to 30 grams | FAT ➤ whole meal: 15 to 20 grams FIBER ➤ salad and broccoli: 5 to 10 grams |
| --- | --- | --- |

## ENERGY BALANCE SNACK

Fruit Cocktail Surprise

1/2 cup canned light fruit cocktail

1/2 cup low-fat cottage cheese

Dollop nonfat whipped topping

Sprinkle of chopped walnuts

1. Combine the fruit and cottage cheese.

2. Top with the whipped topping and walnuts.

| CORE FOUR APPROXIMATE BREAKDOWN | PROTEIN ➤ cottage cheese: 14 grams CARBOHYDRATE ➤ fruit cocktail: 13 grams | FAT ➤ walnuts: 5 grams FIBER ➤ fruit cocktail: 1 to 2 grams |
| --- | --- | --- |

## STRETCH, RELAX, AND SLEEP

1. Chest/posture stretch

2. Neck and upper spine stretch

3. Lower spine stretch

## STRESS RELIEF TIP

Set aside time to play. By taking time to play and relax, you are improving your health and boosting your immune system. Stress can make you sick by sapping your resistance, which puts your health at greater risk.

# Don't Be a Sourpuss

RECENTLY I WAS STRESSING about an obligation I had to complete by the end of the week and a friend called to tell me a joke she'd just heard. I listened sourly to her light-hearted tale and hardly harrumphed at the end. After her joke fell flat she asked, "So where are you right now—in the past or the future?" Her question stopped me short. She knows that when I lose my sense of humor, it's often because I'm re-living something painful in my past or obsessing over the future.

We often take life far too seriously and miss out on the joys of living in the present moment. If you find yourself being a sourpuss, try this simple technique: Take a deep breath and exhale. Scrunch your face into frown, imagining you've just tasted a sour lemon. Tense every muscle and hold for a count of five. Then relax your face, letting the tension drain away. Smile, not just with your mouth, but with your entire face. Hold for a count of five. Take one more deep breath. You'll know you've returned to the present moment when there is a chance you'll laugh at a joke.

# DAY 18

## WAKE-UP AFFIRMATION

*"Make no little plans. There is nothing in little plans to stir your blood. Make big plans. Once a big idea is recorded, it can never die."*

—*Daniel Burnham, architect*

## WAKE-UP WORKOUT

**1.** Let body slowly wake up
**2.** Take several deep breaths
**3.** Full-body tighten and release
**4.** Pelvic tilts
**5.** Pillow sit-ups
**6.** Hamstring stretch
**7.** Hands and knees yoga stretch

## CORE FOUR

**1.** Push-up
**2.** Sit-up
**3.** Sit and stand
**4.** Posture squeeze/biceps curl

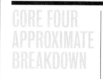

## PORTION CONTROL TIP

Never say "just a taste" unless you really mean it. Sometimes it's that "taste" that can lure you away from your healthy eating habits.

## ENERGY BALANCE BREAKFAST

*Pancake Morning*

> 2 5-inch whole-grain pancakes (made fresh or frozen)
> 1/2 cup blueberries
> 2 tablespoons trans-fat-free margarine
> Sprinkle of powdered sugar
> 1 egg and 4 egg whites

**1.** Serve the pancakes topped with blueberries, margarine, and sugar.
**2.** Scramble the eggs and egg whites and serve them on the side.

➤ If you want a larger meal: Add 1 chicken or turkey sausage link.

Drink water with lemon or 4 ounces of juice and 6 ounces of water, plus decaffeinated tea or coffee, if desired. Add low-fat creamer to taste.

| CORE FOUR APPROXIMATE BREAKDOWN | | |
|---|---|---|
| **PROTEIN**<br>➤ egg and egg whites: 20 grams<br>**CARBOHYDRATE**<br>➤ pancakes and blueberries: 25 to 30 grams | **FAT**<br>➤ egg yolk: 5 grams<br>➤ margarine: 5 grams<br>**FIBER**<br>➤ pancakes: 2 to 3 grams<br>➤ blueberries: 4 to 5 grams | |

# TAKE 10
## Seated biceps reverse curl

Strengthening your forearm muscles is particularly important for preventing carpal tunnel syndrome and remedying tennis and golf elbow as well as tendinitis.

1. Sit in a chair, lift your chest, contract your abdominals, press your shoulders back and down, align your head with your spine, and face forward.
2. Hold a 3- to 5-pound weight in each hand.
3. Straighten your arms by your sides with your elbows glued to your waist. Your elbows shouldn't move throughout this movement.
4. Turn your palms inward and keep your wrists in a straight line with your forearms.
5. Exhale as you bring the backs of your hands toward your shoulders.
6. Go as far as you can and then inhale as you lower your hands to the starting position.
7. Do as many as comfortable, rest a few seconds, and then do 2 more sets.

# SIT AND BE FIT
## Pulsing raise

This exercise will strengthen the fronts of your shoulders and the backs of your arms as well as some chest muscles.

1. Sit in a chair, lift your chest, contract your abdominals, press your shoulders back and down, align your head and spine, and face forward.
2. Hold a 3- to 5-pound weight in each hand with your palms facing each other and thumbs toward the ceiling. Your elbows should remain glued to your waist.
3. Exhale as you push your hands straight out in front of your body until fully extended, keeping a slight bend in your elbows.
4. Hold 1 second.

5. Lift up and down an inch or so with a pulsing motion, using very small movements, 10 times.
6. Return to the initial position and do 2 more sets.

# WATER BREAK

Operation Hydration. If you can't follow this program exactly, just remember this regime: 2 glasses of water in the morning, 2 more by noon, 2 prior to dinner, 1 with dinner, and 1 before bed.

# ENERGY BALANCE SNACK
## Three Cheese Quesadilla

　2 ounces cheese (mixture of 3 kinds)
　1 ounce shredded chicken
　1/2 flour tortilla
　1 teaspoon salsa

1. Grate the cheeses together.
2. Place the cheese and chicken on the tortilla.
3. Heat in a microwave for a few seconds or toast until the cheese is melted.
4. Top with the salsa and enjoy.

| CORE FOUR APPROXIMATE BREAKDOWN | PROTEIN ➤ chicken and cheese: 10 to 15 grams | FAT ➤ cheese: 5 to 10 grams |
|---|---|---|
| | CARBOHYDRATE ➤ tortilla: 10 grams | FIBER ➤ tortilla: 2 grams |

# WATER BREAK

If your skin is dry and flaky, it may be because you are dehydrated. Drink more water and keep your skin moisturized with a good topical lotion, too.

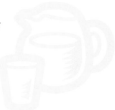

# ENERGY LIFT

## Raise and bend with a stretch

This exercise will raise your muscle temperature, allowing the muscles to become more pliant during the stretch.

1. Hold on to a chair for balance. Place your feet shoulder width apart, bend your knees slightly, contract your abdominals, place your shoulders down, lift your chest, and face forward.
2. Exhale as you rise up on your toes as high as you can. Do not roll your ankles inward or outward. Feel the contraction in your calf muscles.
3. Inhale and lower your heels to the floor. Make sure you don't bounce and use controlled movements to isolate your calf muscles.
4. Repeat 12 times.
5. Do 12 small squats. Make sure your knees are over your heels, not your toes.
6. Do this series, alternating exercises, for 3 sets.

### CALF STRETCH

1. Place one foot far enough behind the other to feel a slight stretch in your lower leg.
2. Keep your feet pointing forward and align your toes and heel in a straight line. The knee of your supporting leg should be slightly bent.
3. Hold the stretch at least 30 seconds.
4. Change legs and repeat on the other side.

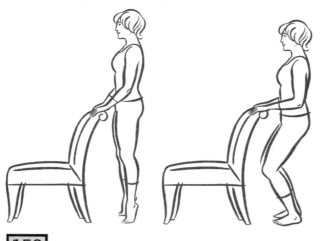

# ENERGY BALANCE LUNCH

## DINING IN

### Roast Beef Sandwich

1 baguette
Mustard and low-fat mayonnaise
Touch of creamed horseradish (optional)
4 ounces lean roast beef
Tomato and pickles

1. Hollow out the baguette: pull out most of the bread and leave a small amount near the crust.
2. Spread the mustard, mayonnaise, and horseradish (if using) on the baguette.
3. Pile on the roast beef, tomato, and pickles.
4. Serve with sliced vegetables and cole slaw made with low-fat mayonnaise.

## DINING OUT

Order a lean roast beef sandwich and ask for a hollowed out baguette or kaiser roll. Or eat only one 1/2 the bun. Add a side of cole slaw.

➤ If you want a larger meal: Add 1 to 2 ounces roast beef.

| CORE FOUR APPROXIMATE BREAKDOWN | PROTEIN ➤ roast beef: 20 to 25 grams CARBOHYDRATE ➤ hollowed-out baguette or 1/2 bun: 15 to 20 grams | FAT ➤ roast beef and mayonnaise: 10 to 15 grams FIBER ➤ cole slaw and vegetables: 5 to 10 grams |
| --- | --- | --- |

# SIT AND BE FIT

## Full spine roll-up

Besides being a good spine stretching exercise, this movement strengthens your lower back and relieves tension in your upper neck.

1. Sit on the edge of a chair or couch and place your hands behind your head at ear level.
2. Bend forward as far as you can, allowing your head to hang down with the weight of your arms, and gently stretch the back of your neck. If you are flexible, your chest will be resting on your thighs.
3. Contract your abdominals as you slowly roll up one vertebra at a time.
4. Hold at the top of the movement 10 to 20 seconds and repeat 2 times.
5. Breathing is reversed in this exercise, meaning your should exhale on the effort, because the rib cage is contracted. Exhale as you roll down and inhale as you roll up.

# WATER BREAK

Exposure to salt and minerals in high concentrations can eventually cause urinary tract infections as well as kidney stones. Water can prevent these occurrences. If you experience painful urination, drink more water and consult your doctor.

# ENERGY LIFT

## Hip stretch

This stretch, good for the sides of your hips and tops of your thighs, is especially beneficial to those who sit most of the day, which can make muscles tight and tired.

1. Lie on the floor with your hands interlaced behind your head. Keep your elbows wide, your knees bent, and your feet flat on the floor.
2. Bring your knees close together and cross your right leg over your left.
3. Allow your right leg to slowly and gently pull your left leg toward the floor until you feel an easy stretch.
4. Pull in your abdominals and keep your shoulders and elbows on the floor.
5. Breathing easily and deeply, hold a few seconds and release.
6. Repeat on the other side.

# WATER BREAK

If you are prone to muscle spasms, it could be because you are not drinking enough water. Consult your doctor if the spasms persist even when your water intake is increased.

# ENERGY BALANCE SNACK

## Nachos

4 tablespoons refried beans
4 whole-grain crackers
2 tablespoons grated cheddar cheese
2 tablespoons salsa

1. Spread the beans on the crackers.
2. Sprinkle with the cheese.
3. Toast or microwave until the cheese is bubbly.
4. Top with the salsa.

| CORE FOUR APPROXIMATE BREAKDOWN | PROTEIN ➤ beans: 3 grams ➤ cheese: 3 grams CARBOHYDRATE ➤ beans: 9 grams ➤ crackers: 11 grams | FAT ➤ cheese: 7 grams FIBER ➤ beans: 3 grams ➤ crackers: 2 to 3 grams |
|---|---|---|

# TAKE 10

## Hand and foot massage

This massage relaxes your hands and feet, which feels refreshing overall.

### HAND MASSAGE

1. Massage from the base of the hand out to the fingertips. Then massage your fingers from the base to the tips.
2. Massage the center, top, and bottom of your palm. Repeat on the other hand.
3. Clasp your hands together as if you were about to pray and squeeze tightly, release them, and shake them out.

## FOOT MASSAGE

1. With both hands massage from your heel to toes. At your toes take each toe and give it a good pressure massage. Then, go to the center of the foot and press and massage.
2. Place one hand on top of your foot and push your toes into a pointed position and hold a few seconds. Then pull your foot into a flexed position and hold for a seconds.
3. Release and repeat on the other foot.

# WATER BREAK

You can become dehydrated during cold weather without realizing it. Your body still perspires, and the moisture evaporates rapidly in cold, dry weather. So make sure to drink enough water regardless of the weather.

# ENERGY BALANCE DINNER

## DINING IN

Baked Chicken with Dijon and Lemon Juice

6- to 8-ounce chicken breast
1/2 cup lemon juice
2 tablespoons flavored mustard
1 teaspoon rosemary
1 teaspoon thyme

1. Coat a baking dish with olive oil spray.
2. Place the chicken breast in the dish and pour the lemon juice over it.
3. Brush with the flavored mustard and sprinkle with the herbs.
4. Bake in a preheated 350° oven 20 to 30 minutes or until the meat is no longer pink in the middle.
5. Serve with 1/2 cup rice or 1/2 baked yam and a large vegetable-laden salad with low-fat dressing.

## DINING OUT

Order a chicken dish you have never tried before. Ask for the sauce on the side and drizzle it over the chicken. Have a dinner salad to start and eat half the side dish that comes with the meal. If you are given a choice, ask for steamed broccoli with Parmesan cheese.

➤ If you want a larger meal: Add a chicken leg or thigh.

CORE FOUR APPROXIMATE BREAKDOWN

**PROTEIN**
➤ chicken: 20 to 25 grams
**CARBOHYDRATE**
➤ rice or potato: 25 grams
**FAT**
➤ entire meal: 10 to 15 grams
**FIBER**
➤ salad and vegetables: 10 grams

# ENERGY BALANCE SNACK

Cantaloupe and Prosciutto

1/2 cantaloupe
1 ounce prosciutto

1. Slice the cantaloupe lengthwise into small pieces.
2. Wrap the prosciutto around the cantaloupe slices and enjoy.

CORE FOUR APPROXIMATE BREAKDOWN

**PROTEIN**
➤ prosciutto: 7 grams
**CARBOHYDRATE**
➤ cantaloupe: 10 grams
**FAT**
➤ prosciutto: 7 grams
**FIBER**
➤ cantaloupe: 1 to 2 grams

# STRETCH, RELAX, AND SLEEP

1. Chest/posture stretch
2. Neck and upper spine stretch
3. Lower spine stretch

# STRESS RELIEF TIP

The next time you feel stressed, try listening to relaxing music. Sing along—it will calm your nerves and soothe your soul.

# Become a Massage Master

TO BECOME A certified massage therapist, you're required to take hours and hours of hands-on classes and pass a number of anatomy tests. But you can become an expert massage therapist for yourself simply by paying attention to the sore spots on your body, especially those tender places on the bottoms of your feet. All you need to do is sit in a comfortable chair and rest the ankle of one leg on the knee of the other. This position will allow you to use your thumbs to massage the bottoms of your feet. If this position is out of your range of motion, you can lean over and massage your feet with your fingertips. You'll get a bit more pressure and precision if you can use your thumbs, but either way will help release stored-up tension.

There's no need to learn about pressure points or memorize eastern foot-massage charts; simply feel around until you find a tender spot and massage it gently until the stress is released. Then move on to another spot. If you find a knot that is particularly stubborn, work on it for a while and come back to it another day. Not every point of tension in our bodies is ready to relax just because we will it to do so.

Be sure to massage gently. If you feel pain, the kind that causes you to hold your breath, you're pressing too hard and your muscles are resisting your efforts to make them relax. And certainly don't work so hard your thumbs or fingers start to ache. You'll be much more successful if you work within the "good sore" range, where you let out a big sigh of relief.

# DAY 19

## WAKE-UP AFFIRMATION

**"I finally figured out the only reason to be alive is to enjoy it."**

—*Rita Mae Brown, author*

## WAKE-UP WORKOUT

1. Let body slowly wake up
2. Take several deep breaths
3. Full-body tighten and release
4. Pelvic tilts
5. Pillow sit-ups
6. Hamstring stretch
7. Hands and knees yoga stretch

## CORE FOUR

1. Push-up
2. Sit-up
3. Sit and stand
4. Posture squeeze/biceps curl

## PORTION CONTROL TIP

You will often eat what is convenient. Keep Energy Balance foods, such as cut-up vegetables, low-fat dips mixed with cottage cheese, string cheese, and whole-grain crackers, handy.

## ENERGY BALANCE BREAKFAST

### Tunnel Bagel

> 1 large whole-grain bagel
> 2 tablespoons regular cream cheese
> 1 tablespoon jam or preserves
> 1 egg and 4 egg whites, scrambled

1. Slice the bagel and warm it 15 seconds in a microwave or a few minutes in a toaster. (Don't toast.) When the bread is soft, scoop out the inner part. You will have a bagel shell with a little bread left.
2. Fill with cream cheese and jam.
3. Enjoy with eggs on the side.

➤ If you want a larger meal: Increase amount of eggs to 2 eggs and 4 egg whites, scrambled.

Drink water with lemon or 4 ounces of juice and 6 ounces of water, plus decaffeinated tea or coffee, if desired. Add low-fat creamer to taste.

| CORE FOUR APPROXIMATE BREAKDOWN | PROTEIN ➤ egg and egg whites: 20 grams CARBOHYDRATE ➤ bagel: 15 to 20 grams ➤ jam: 10 grams | FAT ➤ egg yolk: 5 grams ➤ cream cheese: 5 grams FIBER ➤ bagel: 3 to 5 grams |
|---|---|---|

# TAKE 10
## Pelvic chair lifts

This exercise will lift and firm your buttocks and the backs of your thighs, as well as strengthening your abdominals and lower back.

1. Lie on your back with your knees bent at a 90-degree angle and your feet on a sturdy chair. Your toes should be pointing up, and the weight of your legs should be resting on your heels.
2. Exhale as you push your heels into the chair and lift your hips off the floor.
3. Inhale as you return to the starting position. Repeat 10 to 12 times.
4. Take a stretch break and place your arms behind your knees and hug them close to your chest. Hold 10 seconds and repeat 2 times.

# SIT AND BE FIT
## Front leg raise

This exercise will condition the fronts of your thighs, help stabilize your knees, and strengthen the fronts of your hips (hip flexors).

1. Sit in a chair, lift your chest, contract your abdominals, press your shoulders back and down, align your head and spine, and face forward.
2. Place either a book or rolled-up towel under your right thigh.
3. Slowly lift your right leg as high as possible, which may be as little as a few inches or all the way up. Keep your foot relaxed and your toes pointing up. At the top of the movement, tighten your knee and hold for a second.
4. Release your leg back to the floor.
5. Pause for a breath and repeat the exercise 6 to 8 times or as many as comfortable.
6. Rest for a second and do 2 more sets.
7. Repeat with your left leg.

# WATER BREAK

Fiber will cause constipation if there is not enough water to keep it moving through your system. If you are not used to a high-fiber diet, increase your fiber intake slowly to avoid abdominal distress.

# ENERGY BALANCE SNACK
## Strawberries and Cheese

1/2 cup ricotta cheese or low-fat cottage cheese
1 cup crushed fresh or frozen strawberries
1 tablespoon vanilla-flavored coffee creamer
1 tablespoon chopped toasted pecans

1. Put the cheese in a small bowl.
2. Combine the strawberries and creamer and place on top.
3. Sprinkle with the pecans.

| CORE FOUR APPROXIMATE BREAKDOWN | **PROTEIN** ➤ ricotta cheese or cottage cheese: 14 grams  **CARBOHYDRATE** ➤ strawberries and creamer: 10 grams | **FAT** ➤ pecans: 5 to 10 grams  **FIBER** ➤ strawberries: 3 to 5 grams |
|---|---|---|

# WATER BREAK

As we age, our intercellular reactions begin to slow down. This process is primarily caused by dehydration of the cells and the decreased ability of the cellular fluid to flow freely from one cell to another. Adequate water intake will slow this process.

# ENERGY LIFT
## Upper body chair stretch

This movement will stretch the large muscles of your back, elongate your spine, and open up your shoulder joint area.

1. Kneel at a comfortable distance from a chair.
2. Place both hands on the seat of the chair with your arms stretched out.
3. Put your head between your arms and sit back toward your heels.
4. Push down from the shoulders and feel the stretch along the sides of your waist and your back.
5. Hold 20 to 30 seconds and release.

# ENERGY BALANCE LUNCH

### DINING IN
## Smoked Turkey Club Wrap

    1 flour tortilla
    2 slices smoked turkey
    2 slices cooked turkey bacon
    1 tablespoon low-fat mayonnaise
    Chopped tomato and lettuce
    1 teaspoon cranberry sauce (optional)

1. Lightly toast the tortilla.
2. Place all the other ingredients on top and wrap it up.
3. Serve with a small dish of fresh fruit.

### DINING OUT

Ask for a turkey club with low-fat mayonnaise and only 2 slices whole-grain bread. Order a small amount of baked potato chips and iced tea.

➤ If you want a larger meal: Have more turkey on the sandwich.

| CORE FOUR APPROXIMATE BREAKDOWN | PROTEIN<br>➤ turkey and turkey bacon: 20 to 25 grams<br>CARBOHYDRATE<br>➤ bread: 15 to 20 grams | FAT<br>➤ mayonnaise: 10 to 15 grams<br>FIBER<br>➤ bread: 3 to 5 grams<br>➤ lettuce: 1 to 2 grams |
| --- | --- | --- |

# SIT AND BE FIT
## Countertop row

This exercise is good for your large back muscles in addition to strengthening the backs of your shoulders and the fronts of your arms.

1. Place a small pillow or soft towel over the edge of a countertop or the bathroom sink.
2. Hold a 3- to 5-pound weight in each hand.
3. Inhale as you bend over and place your forehead on the pillow. Your legs should be hip distance apart. Bend your knees, tighten your buttocks, and contract your abdominals.
4. Allow your hands to hang straight down with your palms facing each other.
5. Exhale as you bend your elbows and pull your arms all the way up to your sides until your elbows brush the sides of your waist. Squeeze your shoulder blades together.
6. Hold 1 second and release and then repeat 12 to 15 times. Rest and then do 2 more sets.

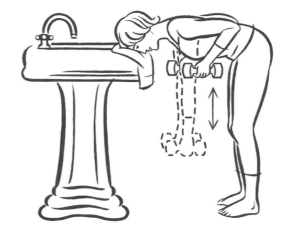

# WATER BREAK

About 40 percent of our fluids come from food—the balance comes from water, so drink up!

# ENERGY LIFT

Sitter's stress relief

This exercise will not only relieve your body after long hours of sitting; it will enhance the flexibility of your entire torso.

1. Find a private place where you can lie down.
2. Using a soft thick towel or a small exercise mat, lie on your side with your knees together and bent to form a right angle to your body.
3. Extend your arms in front of you, level with your shoulders, with your palms together.
4. Slowly lift your top arm up, out, and over to the side, twisting your back and turning your head to look at the ceiling.
5. Place your other hand on the outside of your top knee, to keep your knees down and in place.
6. If you are not flexible enough to do this torso stretch fully, go as far as comfortable. You will eventually be able to do the full stretch.
7. Hold this stretch 20 to 30 seconds and repeat on the other side.

# WATER BREAK

Drinking with your meals aids digestion and transports vital nutrients to your cells.

# ENERGY BALANCE SNACK

Repeat

Insert your favorite Energy Balance snack here. See the index for snack choices.

| CORE FOUR APPROXIMATE BREAKDOWN | PROTEIN<br>➤ 10 to 15 grams | FAT<br>➤ 5 to 10 grams |
|---|---|---|
| | CARBOHYDRATE<br>➤ 15 to 20 grams | FIBER<br>➤ 2 to 5 grams |

# TAKE 10

Contract and relax back stretch

This stretch will work your chest and back muscles while strengthening your abdominals.

1. Sit on the floor with your knees bent and your hands on the floor behind your back.
2. Lift your chest as you squeeze your shoulder blades back and together.
3. Hold 20 to 30 seconds and release.
4. Place your hands on your lower legs, contract your abdominals, and lean backward until you feel the stretch between your shoulder blades.

# WATER BREAK

Bad breath can be caused by a dry mouth and the buildup of bacteria, so drink water to keep your mouth fresh and clean.

# ENERGY BALANCE DINNER

## DINING IN

Angel Hair Pasta with Chicken

> 1 tablespoon olive oil
> 1/2 cup mixed broccoli, carrots, and any favorite vegetable (fresh or frozen)
> 1 clove garlic, minced
> 1 teaspoon dried basil

2/3 cup chicken broth

6 to 8 ounces grilled chicken breast, chopped

1 ounce whole wheat angel hair pasta (1/2 cup cooked)

1/4 cup parmesan cheese, grated

1. In a skillet, heat the olive oil over medium-high heat and add the vegetables; stir until lightly cooked.
2. Add the garlic, basil, and chicken broth; cook a few more minutes.
3. Add the chicken and stir. Remove from heat.
4. Cook the pasta according to package directions.
5. Drain it and place in a pasta bowl, add the skillet mixture, and sprinkle cheese on top.
6. Serve with a large green salad with a low-fat dressing.

### DINING OUT

Order angel hair pasta and chicken with a light cream sauce. Ask for the sauce on the side and half the pasta, and ask for more vegetables and chicken. Top with Parmesan cheese. Order a small Caesar salad with dressing on the side. Finish with a decaf cappuccino or latte.

➤ If you want a larger meal: Add more chicken and vegetables.

CORE FOUR APPROXIMATE BREAKDOWN

| PROTEIN | FAT |
|---|---|
| ➤ chicken: 20 to 25 grams | ➤ entire meal: 15 to 20 grams |
| **CARBOHYDRATE** | **FIBER** |
| ➤ pasta: 25 to 30 grams | ➤ salad, vegetables, and pasta: 5 to 10 grams |

# ENERGY BALANCE SNACK

Banana, Peanut Butter, and Low-Fat Cream Cheese

1 tablespoon low-fat cream cheese

1 tablespoon peanut butter

1 small piece whole-grain pita bread

1/2 banana, sliced

Spread the cream cheese and peanut butter on the warm pita bread and top the with banana slices.

CORE FOUR APPROXIMATE BREAKDOWN

| PROTEIN | FAT |
|---|---|
| ➤ cream cheese: 2 grams | ➤ peanut butter: 7 grams |
| ➤ peanut butter: 4 grams | ➤ cream cheese: 2 grams |
| **CARBOHYDRATE** | **FIBER** |
| ➤ banana: 5 grams | ➤ pita bread and banana: 1 to 2 grams |
| ➤ pita bread: 15 grams | |

# STRETCH, RELAX, AND SLEEP

1. Chest/posture stretch
2. Neck and upper spine stretch
3. Lower spine stretch

# HELPFUL HINT

What will cause our cells to age before their time? Answer: sugary, fatty foods laced with preservatives and additives. These foods tend to turn to acid in our bloodstream, upsetting our bodies' delicate pH balance. A steady diet of these foods causes our cells to age faster. This doesn't mean you can't have cakes and cookies from time to time; it means you should choose foods that feed your cells, not destroy them.

# Let's Talk Roughage

OKAY, NO WOMAN REALLY WANTS to talk in much detail about the state of her colon. But it's next to impossible to feel good if you're constipated or suffering from an irritated bowel. Healthy elimination can be achieved through a combination of three elements: fiber, fluids, and fun.

Fiber is found in edible plants, rather than animal foods, and aids in two ways. Insoluble fiber doesn't dissolve in water, and its bulkiness sweeps the sides of your intestines clean. Add insoluble fiber to your diet, with foods such as whole grains, broccoli, and nuts, if you're prone to constipation. Soluble fiber absorbs water and acts as a paste to hold your stool together. Increasing your intake of soluble fiber, with food such as bananas, oatmeal, and corn, will help if diarrhea is more of a problem. A balanced diet that includes both insoluble and soluble fiber will contribute to overall health and can help prevent diseases such as diverticulitis, irritable bowel syndrome, and even colon cancer.

But don't dive into those carrots, kidney beans, and bran flakes without also adding plenty of water to your diet. It's water that helps move insoluble fiber through your colon and turns soluble fiber into a pasty substance. Digestive problems are often aggravated by alcohol, coffee, and some soft drinks. . .so minimize your intake of these fluids and reach for a glass of purified water instead.

Lastly, have some fun! Mental attitude plays a major role in digestive health. Anxiety, anger and sadness can be primary sources of gastrointestinal distress. Rather than rely on medication to keep your digestive pipes clean and running smoothly, make sure you've ample opportunity to laugh and enjoy each day.

# DAY 20

## WAKE-UP AFFIRMATION

"It's easier to act your way into new ways of feeling than to feel yourself into new ways of acting."

—*Susan Glaser, musician*

## WAKE-UP WORKOUT

1. Let body slowly wake up
2. Take several deep breaths
3. Full-body tighten and release
4. Pelvic tilts
5. Pillow sit-ups
6. Hamstring stretch
7. Hands and knees yoga stretch

## CORE FOUR

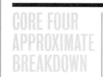

1. Push-up
2. Sit-up
3. Sit and stand
4. Posture squeeze/biceps curl

## PORTION CONTROL TIP

When a craving for high-fat, sugary foods strikes, try eating 1/2 sweet potato sprinkled with cinnamon and a slice of chicken. This snack will keep your blood sugar level for a few hours. If you still want the sweets, eat a small portion of whatever you want. After your Energy Balance snack, you won't overindulge.

## ENERGY BALANCE BREAKFAST

### Lox Baguette

1 baguette
2 tablespoons low-fat cream cheese
3 ounces lox
Red onion rings
1 slice green bell pepper
Sprinkle of capers.

1. Hollow out the baguette.
2. Spread with the cream cheese.
3. Top with the lox, red onion rings, and green bell pepper.
4. Sprinkle with the capers

➤ If you want a larger meal: Add more lox.

Drink water with lemon or 4 ounces of juice and 6 ounces of water, plus decaffeinated tea or coffee, if desired. Add low-fat creamer to taste.

| CORE FOUR APPROXIMATE BREAKDOWN | PROTEIN ➤ lox: 10 to 15 grams CARBOHYDRATE ➤ baguette: 15 to 20 grams | FAT ➤ cream cheese: 2 to 4 grams ➤ lox: 4 grams FIBER ➤ onion and bell pepper: 1 to 2 grams |
| --- | --- | --- |

## TAKE 10
### Walking improver

This exercise will wake up the muscles of your feet, ankles, and lower legs. Working this muscle group will encourage you to walk with your toes forward, which is better for your hips, knees, and feet.

1. Lie on your back with your left leg bent at a 90-degree angle, and your foot flat on the floor.
2. Clasp your hands behind your right knee and draw it toward your chest until your knee is directly over your hip.
3. Keep your left leg even with your right knee and your right shin parallel to the floor.
4. Circle your foot 20 times to the right, stop, and circle 20 times to the left.
5. Point and flex the foot 10 to 20 times.
6. Switch legs and repeat.

## SIT AND BE FIT
### Seated round over

Good for warming up the muscles of your back and shoulders, this exercise will also help increase the range of motion in your shoulder joints.

1. Sit in a chair, lift your chest, contract your abdominals, press your shoulders back and down, align your head and spine, and face forward.
2. Inhale as your raise both arms over your head with your elbows next to your ears, one hand on top of the other, and your palms facing forward.
3. Keeping your arms over your head, exhale as you round your back into a catlike arch and press your lower back into the chair. Keep your elbows close to your ears.
4. Repeat 4 times.

## WATER BREAK

Water helps flush out the lactic acid build-up in muscles that can lead to muscle cramps.

## ENERGY BALANCE SNACK
### Shrimp Cocktail

6 medium shrimp, deveined, cooked
2 tablespoons red cocktail sauce
4 whole-grain crackers

| CORE FOUR APPROXIMATE BREAKDOWN | PROTEIN ➤ shrimp: 14 grams | FAT ➤ shrimp and crackers: 5 to 10 grams |
|---|---|---|
| | CARBOHYDRATE ➤ crackers: 12 grams | FIBER ➤ crackers: 1 to 2 grams |

## WATER BREAK

Water has soothing and relaxing qualities, so take a water break whenever you feel stressed.

## ENERGY LIFT
### Stand, walk, and stretch

This energizing routine will increase circulation to all the muscles that support your back and torso all day long.

1. Stand up and walk around your chair 2 times.
2. Sit down and stand up 4 times.
3. Repeat this combination for at least 4 rounds.
4. Sit down with your knees together and lean your torso over your knees as far as you can. See if you can reach your ankles with your hands and allow your head and neck to hang down and relax.
5. Slowly roll up one vertebra at a time to an upright position. Take a few deep, full breaths.

# ENERGY BALANCE LUNCH

## DINING IN

### Bouillabaisse

1. Have 1 cup bouillabaisse, a fish soup made with seafood, tomatoes, and spices that can be found in most specialty grocery stores.
2. Add a large green salad with your favorite dressing and 1 small dinner roll.

## DINING OUT

Order bouillabaisse or a bowl of tomato soup and a side of grilled fish with vegetables. Finish with a decaf cappuccino or latte.

➤ If you want a larger meal: Add more fish to the soup.

| CORE FOUR APPROXIMATE BREAKDOWN | PROTEIN ➤ fish: 20 to 25 grams CARBOHYDRATE ➤ roll: 15 grams | FAT ➤ bouillabaisse broth: 7 grams ➤ fish: 10 grams FIBER ➤ entire meal: 5 to 10 grams |
| --- | --- | --- |

# SIT AND BE FIT

### Shoulder shrugs and rolls

This combination of shrugs and rolls will release tension in your upper neck and tone the muscles that support your head and shoulders.

1. Sit in a chair, lift your chest, contract your abdominals, press your shoulders back and down, align your head and spine, and face forward.
2. Shrug your shoulders up to your ears and rotate them backward, squeezing your shoulder blades together.
3. Hold the squeeze a few seconds. Breathe naturally.
4. Roll your shoulders in a circle forward 10 times and back 10 times.
5. Repeat the shoulder shrug.
6. Do the combination 2 more times.

# WATER BREAK

A hot bath at the end of the day can make for a relaxing evening. However, if the water is too hot, you can dehydrate your body due to perspiration. Drink a glass of water after a hot bath, steam, or sauna.

# ENERGY LIFT

### Curl and kickback

This combination will strengthen the fronts and backs of your arms and increase the strength of your upper back and abdominal muscles, which act as torso stabilizers.

## BICEPS CURL

1. Hold 3- to 5-pound weights, in your hands. Press your elbows against your waist and allow your arms to hang beside your thighs.
2. Exhale as you slowly bring your hands toward your shoulders.
3. Stop the movement before you actually touch your shoulders.
4. Hold 1 second and release to the starting position.
5. Repeat 12 to 15 times.

## TRICEPS KICKBACK

1. Return to the starting position.
2. Lean your upper body forward, bending from your hips, not your waist.
3. Keep your head and spine in a straight line without arching your lower back.
4. Bend your elbows slightly behind your waistline while pulling your shoulder blades together. Keep your shoulders pressed down; don't allow them to creep toward your ears. Your elbows do not move during this exercise.
5. Exhale as you slowly straighten your arms toward the ceiling, tighten the backs of your arms, and hold 1 second.
6. Return to the starting position but do not allow your elbows to move from their stabilized position.
7. Repeat 12 to 15 times.

## WATER BREAK

Some pipes hold lead residue. If you drink water from your household water source, let the water run for at least one minute before you fill your glass. This will help keep you and your family safe.

## ENERGY BALANCE SNACK

Poultry Dog

    1 turkey or chicken hot dog
    1 hollowed-out hot dog bun
    Mustard, onion, pickles, and relish to taste

1. Grill the hot dog.
2. Place it into the hollowed-out bun.
3. Add the mustard, onion, pickles, and relish.
4. Serve a variety of sliced vegetables with low-fat dip on the side.
5. Drink decaf iced tea.

| CORE FOUR APPROXIMATE BREAKDOWN | PROTEIN<br>➤ hot dog: 12 grams<br>CARBOHYDRATE<br>➤ bun: 15 grams | FAT<br>➤ hot dog: 5 grams<br>FIBER<br>➤ vegetables: 5 grams |
| --- | --- | --- |

## TAKE 10

Balance Ball wall squat

This exercise will strengthen the fronts of your thighs and your buttocks, helping protect your lower back from injury. Keep your knees over your heels to ensure less pressure on your knee joints, ligaments, and tendons.

1. Place the Balance Ball in the middle of your lower back and against a wall.
2. Place your feet hip distance apart. Move them out in front of you until you are a little off balance. (You will have to lean against the ball in order not to fall.)
3. Roll down the wall until your thighs are parallel to the floor.
4. Hold at the bottom of the movement 3 seconds.
5. Roll back up to the starting position. Don't lock your knees.
6. Repeat. Work up to 3 sets of 20 repetitions. Rest a few seconds between each set.

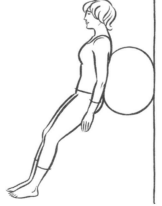
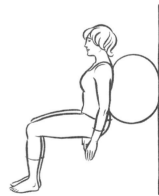

# WATER BREAK

If you are recovering from an illness in which you were vomiting or had diarrhea or a fever, make sure you replace that fluid with at least 8 glasses of water a day.

# ENERGY BALANCE DINNER

## DINING IN

### Apple Salad with Poppy Seed Dressing

- 1 small head iceberg lettuce
- 3 medium apples (Sprinkle cut-up apples with lemon juice to prevent them from turning brown.)
- 1/3 cup chopped walnuts
- 2 ounces raisins
- 2 tablespoons poppy seed dressing

1. Tear the lettuce into bite-size pieces and place in a large bowl.
2. Slice the cored, unpeeled apples thinly.
3. Toss with the lettuce, raisins, and dressing.
4. Add the walnuts just before serving.
5. Serve with 6 to 8 ounces lean meat or poultry.
6. Eat until you are full and save the rest for another meal.

## DINING OUT

Try any dish that resembles the above dinner. If there isn't anything that comes close, then be adventurous and order something you have never tasted before, keeping in mind the Energy Balance breakdown.

| CORE FOUR APPROXIMATE BREAKDOWN | PROTEIN | FAT |
|---|---|---|
| | ➤ meat or poultry: 25 to 30 grams | ➤ poppy seed dressing: 10–12 grams |
| | CARBOHYDRATE | FIBER |
| | ➤ apple salad: 20 to 30 grams | ➤ apple salad: 5 to 10 grams |

# ENERGY BALANCE SNACK
## Nutrition Bar

1 Balanced nutrition bar (see "Energy Balance Basics") and herbal tea.

| CORE FOUR APPROXIMATE BREAKDOWN | PROTEIN | FAT |
|---|---|---|
| | ➤ 10 to 15 grams | ➤ 5 to 10 grams |
| | CARBOHYDRATE | FIBER |
| | ➤ 15 to 22 grams | ➤ 1 to 2 grams |

# STRETCH, RELAX, AND SLEEP

1. Chest/posture stretch
2. Neck and upper spine stretch
3. Lower spine stretch

# STRESS RELIEF TIP

Writing in a journal will help you let off steam, and it may help you to look at what caused your stress in a different way. As an outlet for your feelings, a journal may provide insight and help to uncover a solution to a problem.

# Homemade Spa

THERE'S NO NEED to spend oodles of money at a spa to feel pampered. Indulge yourself with things you already have on hand. Invade your kitchen and try this simple spa treatment:

➤ Slice a piece of fruit (peach, orange, pineapple—whatever is in season) and place it on a plastic plate. Grab a box of oatmeal and head for the bathroom.

➤ Fill your tub with water and mix in a handful of oatmeal. Keep a little more nearby so that once you're in the tub, you can smooth it over your body. This natural cleanser gently removes dead skin cells and leaves your skin fresh and rejuvenated.

➤ Lean back and enjoy the warm water. To delight your taste buds, nibble on the fruit and let your mind drift to your favorite exotic location. Ahhhh . . .

# Internal Workout

**H**AVE YOU EVER COUGHED, sneezed, laughed, or began an exercise and felt a trickle of urine escape your bladder? Or have you experienced a total loss of bladder control without warning?

Urinary incontinence is a condition that affects more than half of all women at some time in their lives. Pregnant women are especially susceptible, but incontinence becomes more prevalent at menopause and occurs most frequently in senior years. The leakage associated with urinary incontinence is often caused by specific changes in your body functions such as infection, hormonal changes, disease, trauma, pregnancy, or the use of some medications. However, urinary incontinence is almost always treatable and, in most cases, can be well managed and even cured.

## TYPES OF INCONTINENCE

1. **STRESS INCONTINENCE** occurs when an activity, such as sneezing or laughing, increases the pressure in the abdomen (and therefore the bladder) and places an added stress on the bladder wall and the bladder sphincter (the tube that carries urine from the bladder to the urethra). This action causes urine to escape when coughing, sneezing, laughing, or exercising and is evident if you are paying frequent and urgent visits to the bathroom to prevent an accident or if you accidentally urinate upon waking in the morning or when getting up from a sitting position.
2. **URGE INCONTINENCE** happens when a stimulus, such as the sound of water running, triggers the urge to urinate and the bladder muscle suddenly spasms or contracts, often not allowing enough time to reach a restroom.

3. **OVERFLOW INCONTINENCE** occurs when the bladder fills beyond its capacity to hold urine. Symptoms can include the need to get up frequently in the night to urinate, taking a long time to urinate, when the urine stream doesn't have much force, and the need to urinate in small amounts without feeling completely empty afterward.
4. **TOTAL INCONTINENCE:** Occurs when the bladder sphincter completely fails and its symptom is a total inability to control the bladder.

Don't be discouraged! One way to treat incontinence is though exercise which strengthens the pelvic floor, a group of muscles that support the bladder, urethra, rectum, vagina, and uterus. However, before you begin any exercise program, speak with your doctor about your condition.

## EXERCISES TO IMPROVE INCONTINENCE

To isolate the large muscle groups used, try the following movements:
1. **BUTTOCKS:** Lie on your back and relax the buttock muscles. Tighten and hold them for five seconds, relax, then repeat five times.
2. **INNER THIGHS –** Contract the inner thigh muscles by squeezing a small pillow between your knees, holding a few seconds, relaxing, then repeating five times.
3. **ABDOMINALS –** Contract your abdominals, hold for five seconds, relax. Repeat five times.

After you have learned to contract one set of muscles at a time, move on to the Kegel muscle exercises that follow.

# KEGEL PELVIC FLOOR STRENGTHENERS

Dr. Kegel developed exercises in the 1930s to help women strengthen their pelvic floor muscles after giving birth. Many believe that Kegel's exercises not only help with urinary incontinence problems but they can help prevent them as well. To find and isolate your pelvic floor muscle group, try to stop the flow of urine as you go to the bathroom. These are the muscles you will want to squeeze and release during the day.

**WARNING:** Don't stop and start urine flow to strengthen your pelvic floor muscles—it can cause bacteria to lodge in your urinary tract. This should only be used to find and isolate the pelvic floor muscle group.

# KEGEL EXERCISE ROUTINE

1. Lie down in a comfortable bed with your legs relaxed; bend your knees with your feet flat on the bed. Relax all of your surrounding muscles and concentrate only on contracting the pelvic floor muscle group. Visualize your pelvic floor muscles, starting at the anus; squeeze the muscles around your anus tightly. Then relax, now focus on the muscles around the opening of your vagina. Squeeze them tightly and then relax. Imagine the muscles were on a drawstring and you could pull them together.

2. Now, contract these pelvic floor muscles and pull upward and tighten. Hold for five seconds and release. Repeat ten times.
3. After you have mastered the method while lying down, now try to do the same contract-and-hold exercise while standing and sitting.
4. When all of the positions are easy and comfortable, move onto the following rhythm method.

**SLOW SUSTAINED:** Contract and hold for 5 to 10 seconds, release and repeat five more times.

**QUICK AND FORCEFUL:** Pulse in quick rapid, forceful contractions twenty times.

Now combine the two contractions into one exercise. Breathe evenly and deeply as you perform five slow, ten fast, alternating for 4 sets.

One of the great things about this routine is that it can be worked in anywhere, anytime, such as when you are stopped at a red light or waiting in a line.

# DAY 21

## WAKE-UP AFFIRMATION

**"I can change the world around me by changing myself."**

—*Sanya Roman and Duane Packer, spiritual leaders and authors*

## WAKE-UP WORKOUT

**1.** Let body slowly wake up
**2.** Take several deep breaths
**3.** Full-body tighten and release
**4.** Pelvic tilts
**5.** Pillow sit-ups
**6.** Hamstring stretch
**7.** Hands and knees yoga stretch

## CORE FOUR

**1.** Push-up
**2.** Sit-up
**3.** Sit and stand
**4.** Posture squeeze/biceps curl

## PORTION CONTROL TIP

Low-sodium stocks, such as vegetable, chicken, and beef, can often be used to replace oil in cooking. For a flavor-intense meal, try using a stock instead of water when boiling a starch, such as rice, potatoes, or pasta.

## ENERGY BALANCE BREAKFAST

### Egg and Cheese Burrito

1 egg and 4 egg whites scrambled
1 corn tortilla
2 tablespoons black beans
1/2 cup grated low-fat cheddar cheese
Add salsa to taste

Place the hot eggs on the tortilla, top with beans, cheese, and salsa, and roll up.

➤ If you want a larger meal: Add 1 more egg.

Drink water with lemon or 4 ounces of juice and 6 ounces of water, plus decaffeinated tea or coffee, if desired. Add low-fat creamer to taste.

| CORE FOUR APPROXIMATE BREAKDOWN | PROTEIN ➤ egg, egg whites, and beans: 20 to 25 grams  CARBOHYDRATE ➤ tortilla and beans: 25 to 30 grams | FAT ➤ cheese: 5 grams ➤ egg yolk: 5 grams  FIBER ➤ tortilla and beans: 5 to 10 grams |
| --- | --- | --- |

## TAKE 10
### Wall squat

This exercise will not only strengthen the fronts of your thighs and buttocks, it will protect your lower back and keep your knees in the proper alignment to ensure less pressure on your knee joints, ligaments, and tendons.

1. Find a wall that has a slippery finish or place a bath towel behind your back to help you slide down the wall with more ease.  Place your feet hip distance apart and move them out in front of you until you are a little off balance. (You will have to lean against the wall in order not to fall.)
2. Keep your chest lifted, your abdominals contracted, your back pressed against the wall, your shoulders pressed back and down, your head and spine aligned, and face forward.
3. Slide down the wall until your thighs are parallel to the floor.
4. Keep your knees over your heels, not your toes.
5. Hold at the bottom of the movement 10 seconds or as long as comfortable.
6. Slide back up to the starting position. Don't lock your knees at the top of the position; keep them slightly bent.
7. Repeat 5 times. Work up to 3 sets of 10 repetitions, resting a few seconds between each set.

## SIT AND BE FIT
### Hips-stacked thigh stretch

This movement works the fronts of your thighs, your chest, and the fronts of your hips.

1. Lie on your left side with your head resting on your extended left arm, your knees bent together at a 90-degree angle, and your hips stacked on top of each other.
2. From behind, grab of the top of your right foot with your right hand. If you are not flexible enough to do this, use a small towel wrapped around your ankle.

3. Pull your foot toward your buttocks as you move your right hip slightly forward and contract your buttocks until you feel a gentle stretch in the top of your thigh. Hold an easy stretch at least 10 seconds and release.
4. Turn over and repeat on the other side.
Note: If you experience any pain in your knee joints with this or any other stretch, stop immediately, as you are overstretching the joint.

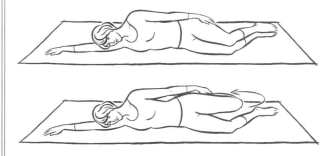

## WATER BREAK

A University of Washington study of dieters found that a glass of water quelled midnight hunger pangs as well as a snack.

## ENERGY BALANCE SNACK
### Sweet Potato Treat

    1/2 small sweet potato, baked
    2 ounces low-fat cheese
    2 tablespoons low-fat sour cream

Split open the potato and top with the cheese and sour cream.

| CORE FOUR APPROXIMATE BREAKDOWN | PROTEIN ➤ cheese: 7 grams ➤ sour cream: 2 grams CARBOHYDRATE ➤ sweet potato: 15 to 20 grams | FAT ➤ cheese: 5 grams ➤ sour cream: 2 grams FIBER ➤ sweet potato: 3 to 5 grams |
|---|---|---|

# WATER BREAK

A mere 2 percent drop in your level of body water can impair your short-term memory and cause difficulty focusing.

# ENERGY LIFT
## Sack ball

This game is not only good for raising your heart rate, it will improve your hand-eye coordination, balance, and timing.

1. Buy or make a beanbag filled with sand, beans, or pellets, large enough to kick off the side of your foot.
2. Throw the beanbag into the air and try to keep it in the air by kicking it off the side of each foot, back and forth.
3. By creating a circle, you can play this as a game with your kids, family, and friends.

# ENERGY BALANCE LUNCH

### DINING IN
## Tuna and White Bean Salad with Olives

### SALAD

6 ounces canned tuna in water, drained
1/2 cup canned white beans, rinsed, drained
1 small celery stalk, thinly sliced
4 Spanish olives, pitted, sliced
1 teaspoon chopped parsley

Combine all the ingredients in a small bowl.

### DRESSING

1 teaspoon red wine vinegar
1/4 teaspoon minced garlic
Dash salt and pepper
Dash paprika
1 tablespoon olive oil

Whisk the ingredients together and toss with the bean mixture. Serve at room temperature.

### DINING OUT

Order a grilled tuna steak with a small salad and small starch.

➤ If you want a larger meal: Add more tuna.

| CORE FOUR APPROXIMATE BREAKDOWN | PROTEIN ➤ tuna and beans: 15 grams | FAT ➤ olives and oil: 10 grams |
|---|---|---|
| | CARBOHYDRATE ➤ beans: 15 to 20 grams | FIBER ➤ beans: 5 to 10 grams |

# SIT AND BE FIT
## Lower back pillow stretch

This stretch relaxes your back and takes pressure off your spine for a few moments.

1. Sit on the edge of a chair or couch and place a pillow on your lap.
2. Lean over and rest your forehead on the pillow with your arms hanging down by your sides.
3. Hold 20 to 30 seconds and release. Do this whenever you need a quick back break.

# WATER BREAK

A recent study shows that 75 percent of Americans are dehydrated. Are you one of them? Take an 8-ounce water break now.

# ENERGY LIFT

Inner thigh squeeze with added stretch

This easy exercise tones your inner thighs and makes them more flexible. Strong, flexible inner thighs enable you to maintain better balance and aid in walking and climbing stairs.

**1.** Sit on the edge of a chair and hold a small pillow, rolled-up towel, or ball between your knees.
**2.** Squeeze and relax 15 to 20 times. Work up to 3 sets of 20 repetitions.
**3.** Place your hands on the insides of your knees.
**4.** Push your legs apart as far as comfortable.
**5.** Hold 10 seconds and release. Repeat both movements 2 times.

# WATER BREAK

A good way to get more fluids is by making your own popsicles. Buy a plastic popsicle mold, fill with low-carbohydrate fruit drinks, and freeze.

# ENERGY BALANCE SNACK

Lentil Soup with Chicken

1 cup lentil soup
2 ounces diced grilled chicken
1 ounce shredded cheese

Heat the soup, stir in the chicken, and top with the cheese.

| CORE FOUR APPROXIMATE BREAKDOWN | PROTEIN<br>➤ chicken: 15 grams<br>➤ lentil soup:<br>　3 to 5 grams<br>CARBOHYDRATE<br>➤ lentil soup:<br>　15 to 20 grams | FAT<br>➤ cheese: 7 grams<br>FIBER<br>➤ lentil soup:<br>　3 to 5 grams |
| --- | --- | --- |

# TAKE 10

Standing pelvic tilts

This subtle buttocks tilt and squeeze will not only firm your backside, it will help you isolate and contract your pelvic floor muscle group.

**1.** Stand with your feet a little more than shoulder width apart, your knees slightly bent, your chest lifted, your abdominals contracted, your shoulders pressed back and down, your head and spine aligned, and face forward.
**2.** Breathing deeply and evenly, squeeze your buttocks tightly as you push your pelvis forward, contracting your abdominal wall. As you hold a few seconds, contract and pull up your pelvic floor muscles (see "Internal Workout" to find them).
**3.** Release to a slightly arched back, and then pull your pelvis forward again and hold.
**4.** Repeat 10 to 15 times for 2 sets.

# WATER BREAK

Pure water is as important as enough water. From research results released in 1997, healthy water does not contain:

➤ excess sodium (added by water-softening systems)
➤ additives such as sugar
➤ chemicals and pesticides

Call your water company to find out the results of their most recent analysis.

## ENERGY BALANCE DINNER

### DINING IN

Stuffed Green Bell Peppers

4 large evenly shaped green bell peppers

1 pound extra-lean ground beef (less than 7 percent fat)

1/2 cup cooked rice

1 onion, chopped

1/2 cup chopped celery

1 egg

3 tablespoons low-fat half-and-half

3 tablespoons chopped parsley

1/2 cup tomato sauce

Salt and pepper to taste

1. Wash the peppers. Cut off the tops and remove the seeds and membrane. Reserve tops.
2. In a large mixing bowl, combine the ground beef, rice, onion, celery, and egg. Blend well.
3. Add the half-and-half, parsley, tomato sauce, salt and pepper and mix well.
4. Place the green peppers in an ovenproof dish that is large enough to hold the peppers upright.
5. Fill the peppers with the meat mixture, mounding a little on top of each. The filling will shrink while baking.
6. Bake at 400° for about 35 minutes, or until the filling is set and cooked through and the peppers are tender.
7. Have 2 peppers with a large vegetable salad with low-fat dressing. Add 1 small whole-grain dinner roll. Save the other two peppers for another day's snack.

### DINING OUT

Order either stuffed green bell peppers or a small portion of meat loaf and a large salad.

➤If you want a larger meal: Have a tall decaf latte with a taste of dessert.

| CORE FOUR APPROXIMATE BREAKDOWN | PROTEIN<br>➤ ground beef: 20 to 25 grams<br>CARBOHYDRATE<br>➤ rice: 10 grams<br>➤ roll: 20 grams | FAT<br>➤ entire meal: 10 to 15 grams<br>FIBER<br>➤ peppers: 3 grams<br>➤ salad and vegetables: 2 to 5 grams<br>➤ roll: 2 to 3 grams |
| --- | --- | --- |

## ENERGY BALANCE SNACK

Fresh Fruit with Low-Fat Vanilla Yogurt

1/2 small melon, chopped

8 pineapple chunks

1/2 cup low-fat vanilla yogurt

2 small graham crackers

Mix the fruit and yogurt and serve with the graham crackers.

| CORE FOUR APPROXIMATE BREAKDOWN | PROTEIN<br>➤ yogurt: 4 grams<br>CARBOHYDRATE<br>➤ yogurt: 11 grams<br>➤ graham crackers: 5 grams | FAT<br>➤ yogurt: 3 grams<br>FIBER<br>➤ fruit: 2 grams |
| --- | --- | --- |

## STRETCH, RELAX, AND SLEEP

1. Chest/posture stretch
2. Neck and upper spine stretch
3. Lower spine stretch

## STRESS RELIEF TIP

When you feel overwhelmed by a task, stop and take a breathing break. Slowly breathe in through your nose and out through your mouth 10 times. Then try to tackle the task in small steps.

# Yell "Enough Already!"

WOMEN ARE EXPECTED to be all things to all people! And we're as much to blame as those who expect so much from us because most of us try to make everyone happy. Rather than accept the roles of taxi driver, dinner fixer, bill payer, grocery shopper, energetic lover, ace employee, tub scrubber, elegant hostess, and super woman, stand in the middle of your living room and yell "Enough already!"

Other people will place unrealistic demands on you as long as you share in the fantasy that you really can do it all. Your body will be the loser as your stress level rises, the length and quality of your sleep declines, and you pick up bad habits such as grabbing a cup of coffee to get you through the afternoon. Eventually your health will suffer, and then you'll be of no benefit at all to yourself or anyone else.

# Core Four Lower Body

AS YOU BECOME STRONGER you may want to continue to expand your routine. Although some of the following lower body exercises can be found in other parts of this book and a few are new, this combination adds variety to your lower body conditioning program. For variety, I have designed three choices for each exercise and a bonus stretch for each body part exercised.

## BUTTOCKS, HIPS, AND THIGHS
Choose one of the following.

### Counter sit and hold

This knee bend will firm and shape the fronts of your thighs and your buttocks. You will also feel increased breathing and heart rates, indicating that you are conditioning your heart muscle and burning a small amount of fat.

1. Hold on to the counter with both hands for balance and sit back into a squat position.
2. Standing with your knees and toes pointing forward, sit back far enough so that your knees are directly over your heels. (If your knees are over your toes, there is too much pressure.)
3. Hold for 1 second and stand up. Repeat 10 times.

### Ballet knee bend

This exercise will improve your balance and strengthen the muscles involved in activities such as standing and walking. The stabilizing muscles being worked are your abdominals and lower back. The muscle groups being strengthened are the fronts of your thighs and your buttocks.

1. If possible, look in a mirror to ensure proper alignment of your spine and torso.

2. Hold on to a countertop, sink, or chair with one hand for balance.
3. Place your feet hip distance apart. Bend your knees slightly, lift your chest, contract your abdominals, press your shoulders back and down, align your head and spine, and face forward.
4. Inhale while bending your knees over your heels (make sure your knees do not go past your toes!) as you lower your buttocks toward the floor.
5. Hold a few seconds while slightly squeezing your buttocks.
6. Exhale as you return to the starting position. Repeat 10 times.

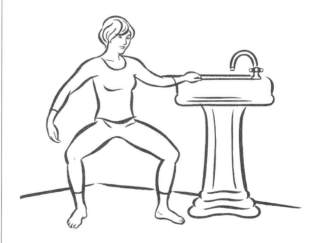

### Forward knee bend

This bend will work your hips and thighs and help protect your knees and lower back by strengthening your muscles.

1. Place a chair securely against a wall. Stand about 2 feet in front of the chair with your back

to it. Place your feet a little wider than hip distance apart, contract your abdominals, press your shoulders back and down, and align head and spine.

2. Slowly sit back. As your knees bend over your heels and your buttocks touch the chair, allow your torso to bend forward from your hips.

3. Extend your arms in front of your chest.

4. Touch the edge of the chair with your buttocks; exhale as you immediately stand back up without locking your knees. Once standing, tuck your pelvis under and squeeze your buttocks, release and sit back down.

5. If you have trouble balancing, hold on to a table or desk or the back of another chair.

6. Repeat 10 times for 3 sets, working up to 20 times for 3 sets.

### BONUS STRETCH

## Cross quadriceps stretch

1. Stand with your feet hip distance apart and bend your knees slightly.

2. Bend backward slightly, reach behind you, and grab your right ankle with your left hand. (You may also grab your sock or the heel of your shoe.) Slowly stand up to your full height as you bring your foot toward to your left buttock.

3. Keep your supporting leg (your left leg) bent slightly, and your foot pointing forward.

4. Hold for 10 to 20 seconds and then repeat with the other leg.

# HAMSTRINGS (BACKS OF THIGHS)

Choose one of the following.

## Lying hamstring lift

This lift will firm your buttocks and the backs of your thighs in addition to strengthening your abdominals and your lower back.

1. Lie on your back with your knees bent at a 90-degree angle and your feet resting on a sturdy chair. Turn your toes toward the ceiling and rest the weight of your legs on your heels.

2. Exhale as you push your heels into the chair and raise your hips off the floor. Hold a few seconds.

3. Inhale as you return to the starting position.

4. Repeat 10 to 12 times, rest a few seconds, and do 2 more sets.

5. Take a stretch break by placing your arms behind your knees and hugging them close to your chest. Hold for 10 seconds and do another set.

## Standing hamstring toner

This stretch will tighten the backs of your thighs and improve your balance.

1. Stand behind a chair, lift your chest, contract your abdominals, press your shoulders back and down, align your head and spine, and face forward.

2. Place your hands on the chair, bend your knees, and tighten your buttocks. Lift one leg behind you as far as possible without arching your lower back.

3. Bring your toes forward and flex your foot with your heel pointing up.

4. Exhale, bend your knee and slowly bring your heel toward your buttocks and hold for a second.

5. Release and repeat 4 times, working up to 12 repetitions per leg.

6. Switch legs and repeat.

**NOTE:** To add more resistance, wrap a 5-pound weight around your ankle or fill a large purse with a handle with a couple of cans of soup and hang it over your ankle.

## Standing buttocks lift

This exercise will tone the backs of your thighs and help to improve your balance.

1. Hold on to a chair or counter top. Stand up straight, place your feet hip distance apart. Lift your chest, contract your abdominals, press your shoulders back and down, align your head and spine, and face forward. Place both feet together, being careful not to lock your knees.

2. Squeeze the muscles in the back of your left thigh as you bend at the knee to bring your heel toward your buttocks.
3. Place a small water bottle or rolled up towel in the crook of your knee joint.
4. Hold this position for a count of 5 and release.
5. Change sides and repeat the lift 2 more times.
**Note**: if you feel a cramp in the back of your thigh, stop immediately and release your leg. Save this exercise for a later day when your hamstrings have become stronger.

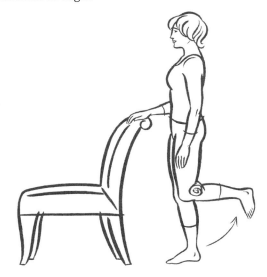

**BONUS STRETCH**

Standing hamstring stretch

This movement stretches the backs of your thighs and your lower back.
1. Stand up straight and place your feet hip distance apart. Bend your knees slightly, lift your chest, contract your abdominals, press your shoulders back and down, align your head and spine, and face forward.

2. Place your right leg on a low chair or couch, your toes pointing toward the ceiling and your knee unlocked.
3. Bend your left knee slightly to take pressure off your knee joint and lower back.
4. Place your hands together on your right thigh.
5. Contract your abdominals and slowly bend your upper body over your right leg.
6. Take the stretch to the point of comfort and hold 20 to 30 seconds.
7. Release and repeat with the left leg.
8. Repeat 3 times, alternating legs.

# CALVES AND SHINS

Choose one of the following.

These calf-raises help to prevent poor circulation in your lower extremities. They will also help improve your balance by strengthening the muscles of your calves and stabilizing your ankles.

Standing calf raise

1. Hold on to a chair for balance. Stand with your feet hip distance apart. Bend your knees slightly, lift your chest, contract your abdominals, press your shoulders back and down, align your head and spine, and face forward.
2. Take a deep breath and exhale as you rise up on your toes as high as you can without your ankles rolling inward or outward. Feel the contraction in your calf muscles.
3. Inhale and lower your heels to the floor. Make sure you don't bounce, and use controlled movements to isolate your calf muscles.
4. Do 2 sets of 12 times each.

**MORE CHALLENGING:** As you become stronger, and if you have access to stairs, you can get a more challenging lift and stretch by standing on the balls of your feet at the edge of a step and then lowering your heels to just a little below parallel. Don't press down too far at first; you could overstretch your Achilles tendon, which may not be ready for this much extension.

## One-leg heel raise

This is more of an advanced movement.

1. Hold on to a chair for support, lift your chest, contract your abdominals, press your shoulders back and down, and align your head and spine.
2. Wrap your left foot around your right ankle.
3. Slowly lift up your right heel and balance on your right toes.
4. Hold for a few seconds and return to the starting position.
5. Repeat 10 times on each leg, alternating legs for 2 sets.

## Shin strengthener

Walk on your heels 10 steps forward, stop, and walk 10 steps backward. Work up to 3 sets of 10 forward and ten backward. Take it easy; this is a subtle movement, and you can work your shins too hard, making them sore.

### BONUS STRETCH

## Two-part calf stretch

1. Stand a few feet from a wall, place your hands on the wall at shoulder height, bend your elbows and allow your forearms to rest gently on the wall, place your forehead on your forearms, allow your hips to drop forward, and tighten your buttocks.
2. Keep your knees straight but not locked and press your heels into the floor.
3. Keep your heels on the floor, holding the position for 10 to 20 seconds.
4. Bend both knees slightly, which will stretch your soler which lie under your calf muscles, an often ignored muscle in many people's workout routine.

# INNER THIGH

Choose one of the following.

Stretching and toning your inner thigh area will aid in preventing injury should you take a sudden step or stretch sideways.

## Inner thigh squeeze

1. Sit in a chair or on a couch, place a small pillow or rolled-up towel between your knees, and squeeze it with as much force as you can.
2. Breathing evenly and deeply, hold the squeeze for 5 seconds and release.
3. Do this 5 times, working up to 10 repetitions for 2 sets.

## Inner thigh toe touch

This easy toe touch will not only give you an energy rush and raise your heart rate; it will help tone and firm your inner thighs. Do this when there is no one else around, as it is a little funny-looking.

1. Stand up straight, and place your feet hip distance apart. Bend your knees slightly, lift your chest, contract your abdominals, press your shoulders back and down, align your head and spine, and face forward. Hold on to the back of a chair with your right hand for balance.
2. Lift your right foot toward your left hand.
3. Keep your left knee bent slightly to keep stress off your lower back.
4. Tap the inside of your right heel with your left hand.
5. Lower and tap again 10 times.
6. Repeat on the left side.

## Balance Ball inner thigh squeeze

If you relax your chest on top of the Ball during this exercise, you will stretch your entire spine in addition to firming and toning your inner thighs.

1. Sit on a chair or couch and hold the Balance Ball between your legs. Lift your chest, contract your abdominals, press your shoulders back and down, and face forward.
2. Place both hands on top of the ball for support, or, alternatively, lower the ball enough so that you can relax your torso on top of the ball.
3. Squeeze your thighs together, hold 1 second, and release.
4. Work up to 3 sets of 20 repetitions; rest 30 seconds between each set.

## Inner thigh tightener and release

This exercise will help tone, relax, and stretch your inner thighs, increasing flexibility to prevent injury should you lunge to either side quickly.

1. Sit on a carpeted floor with the soles of your feet together and your knees out to the sides. Lift your chest, contract your abdominals, press your shoulders back and down, align your head and spine, and face forward.
2. Place your right hand on the inside of your left knee and your left hand on the inside of your right knee.
3. Breathing evenly and deeply, push your knees against your hands and resist with your hands just enough to contract your inner thigh muscles. Hold 5 seconds.
4. Release and allow your knees to relax toward the floor.
5. Repeat both movements 3 times.

**BONUS STRETCH**

## Inner thigh stretch

1. Sit on a carpeted floor or mat and place a small pillow or rolled-up towel under your hips. Stretch your legs out in front of your body with your heels together, knees slightly bent, and your hands on your ankles. Keep your hips flat on the floor, lift your chest, contract your abdominals, press shoulders back, and align your head and spine.
2. Bend your knees and slowly pull your feet, heels first, toward your body; stop when you feel a gentle stretch in your inner thighs.
3. Hold 10 to 20 seconds and release.
4. Repeat 3 times.

# DAY 22

## WAKE-UP AFFIRMATION

"There is a fountain of youth; it's your mind, your talents, the creativity you bring to your life and the lives of the people you love. When you learn to tap this source, you will truly have defeated age."

—*Sophia Loren, actress*

## WAKE-UP WORKOUT

1. Let body slowly wake up
2. Take several deep breaths
3. Full-body tighten and release
4. Pelvic tilts
5. Pillow sit-ups
6. Hamstring stretch
7. Hands and knees yoga stretch

## CORE FOUR

1. Push-up
2. Sit-up
3. Sit and stand
4. Posture squeeze/biceps curl

## PORTION CONTROL TIP

Try to eat only when you are hungry. When you feel the impulse to binge, wait 10 minutes. During that time, take deep breaths, drink a large glass of water, go for a walk, call a friend, write a letter, or get involved in a fun project. Then, if you are still hungry, eat an Energy Balance snack.

## ENERGY BALANCE BREAKFAST

*Omelette Surprise*

1/2 cup egg substitute
1/2 cup spinach
2 tablespoons goat cheese or low-fat feta cheese
1 tablespoon diced onion
1 ounce Canadian bacon, diced
1 tablespoon olive oil
1 small whole wheat tortilla

1. Mix all the ingredients except the oil and tortilla in a medium bowl.
2. Heat the oil in a nonstick skillet over medium-high heat.
3. Pour the egg mixture into the skillet and shake the pan back and forth while stirring the eggs with your other hand, using a fork held flat just above the pan's bottom.
4. Once the eggs begin to set, stop stirring and let them cook all the way through.
5. Serve immediately with the warm, lightly buttered tortilla.

➤If you want a larger meal: Add another 1/2 cup egg substitute and 1 ounce Canadian bacon.

Drink water with lemon or 4 ounces of juice and 6 ounces of water, plus decaffeinated tea or coffee, if desired. Add low-fat creamer to taste.

| CORE FOUR APPROXIMATE BREAKDOWN | PROTEIN | FAT |
|---|---|---|
| | ➤ egg substitute: 18 to 24 grams | ➤ Canadian bacon: 2 to 3 grams |
| | ➤ Canadian bacon: 8 grams | ➤ goat cheese: 2 to 3 grams |
| | ➤ goat cheese: 5 grams | ➤ butter: 5 grams |
| | **CARBOHYDRATE** | **FIBER** |
| | ➤ tortilla: 15 to 20 grams | ➤ tortilla: 2 to 3 grams |

# TAKE 10
## Body balance

This exercise will not only improve your balance; it will help strengthen your core muscle groups, which include your abdominals and back muscles.

1. Kneel on a mat or carpeted area with your knees under your hips and hip distance apart, your hands directly under your shoulders and shoulder distance apart, and your abdominals contracted.
2. Carefully extend your right arm forward and your left leg back, keeping your balance with your left arm and right leg. Your extended leg and arm should be in a straight line with your spine, and your lower back should be tabletop flat.
3. Breathing evenly, hold for a count of 5 and release, change sides and repeat. Repeat 2 times on each side, alternating sides.

# SIT AND BE FIT
## Balance Ball reverse curl

This exercise will improve your balance and strengthen your lower back and abdominals at the same time.

1. Find a flat surface such as a wall, a securely closed door, or the side of your desk. Sit on the Balance Ball and roll forward until the small of your back rests on the ball and your knees touch the wall at a 90-degree angle, a little wider than hip distance apart. (This will prevent you from rolling too far forward, and if you have a balance concern, it will allow you to feel more secure.)
2. Cross your arms over your chest or, if you need to support your head, interlace your fingers behind your upper neck at ear level. Don't pull on your head; allow it to relax into your hands and rest there.
3. Tuck your pelvis forward and maintain this tilt.

4. Roll back slowly, keeping your torso in a straight line. Contract your abdominals and hold 1 second, then roll up to the starting position. Hold and repeat.
5. Do 5 to 10 repetitions, eventually working up to 3 sets of 20 repetitions.

# WATER BREAK

Be careful how much caffeine you drink, because it is readily absorbed from your intestinal system. Within an hour after you drink a cup of coffee, it reaches its peak concentration in your blood, penetrating your body's membranes and entering all your tissues. In pregnant women, it traverses the placenta. Caffeine metabolizes so slowly that half the amount ingested is still circulating three to six hours later.

# ENERGY BALANCE SNACK
## Con Queso Dip

>  2 ounces light processed cheese, cubed
>  1 tablespoon salsa
>  Dash chili powder

1. Microwave all the ingredients together on high for one minute, stirring at 30 seconds.
2. Serve with 3 ounces baked tortilla chips.

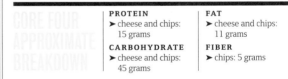

| CORE FOUR APPROXIMATE BREAKDOWN | PROTEIN ➤ cheese and chips: 15 grams | FAT ➤ cheese and chips: 11 grams |
|---|---|---|
| | CARBOHYDRATE ➤ cheese and chips: 45 grams | FIBER ➤ chips: 5 grams |

# WATER BREAK

To wean yourself off your morning coffee or tea, drink a large glass of water with lemon first. Wait 10 minutes and then have a half a cup of your regular beverage of choice. Then have another glass of water.

## ENERGY LIFT
### Take a hike

This series of movements will rejuvenate your whole body.

1. Take a brisk walk for at least 10 minutes.
2. Find a flight of stairs and walk up and down twice.
3. Stand a few feet from a wall, place your hands on the wall at shoulder height, bend your elbows and allow your forearms to rest gently on the wall, place your forehead on your forearms, allow your hips to drop forward, and tighten your buttocks.
4. Keep your knees straight but not locked and press your heels into the floor.
5. Keep your heels on the floor, holding the position for 10 to 20 seconds.
6. Bend both knees slightly, which will stretch your soler.

## ENERGY BALANCE LUNCH

### DINING IN
### Chicken Vegetable Stew

2 skinless, boneless chicken breasts, cut up
1 cup fat-free chicken broth
1/2 teaspoon Italian seasoning blend
1 teaspoon paprika
White pepper to taste
1 clove garlic, chopped
2 tablespoons chopped celery leaves
1 medium carrot, cubed
1 cup broccoli
2 medium celery stalks, cut into small pieces
1 small red potato, cut into small pieces
1/2 small yam, cut into small pieces
1 ounce grated cheddar cheese for garnish
2 tablespoons chopped parsley for garnish

1. Place the chicken, 1/2 cup broth, seasonings, and garlic in large saucepan. Bring to a boil, cover, reduce heat, and simmer over medium heat 10 minutes.
2. Add the vegetables and remaining 1/2 cup broth. Replace the cover and cook on low heat until the chicken and vegetables are done, 45 to 50 minutes.
3. Serve in bowls. Garnish with the cheese and chopped parsley. This stew makes about 4 servings and the remainder can be used as a snack, main course, or starter/appetizer.

### DINING OUT

Try a bowl of vegetable-based soup and a large green salad with low-fat dressing on the side.

| CORE FOUR APPROXIMATE BREAKDOWN | PROTEIN ➤ chicken: 10 grams CARBOHYDRATE ➤ vegetables: 15 to 20 grams | FAT ➤ stew: 3 grams ➤ cheese: 7 to 9 grams FIBER ➤ stew: 4 to 5 grams |
|---|---|---|

## SIT AND BE FIT
### Arm circles

This exercise will tone the sides of your shoulders with an isometric stabilizing contraction. It will also warm up your shoulder joints and help keep them flexible.

1. Sit on the edge of a chair or couch, lift your chest, contract your abdominals, press your shoulders back and down, align your head and spine, and face forward.
2. Hold your arms out to the sides, a little below shoulder height, keeping them parallel to the floor. Your hands should be flexed with your bent fingers pointing toward the ceiling. Keep your elbows bent slightly.
3. Breathing evenly and deeply, make large circles (of a size that is comfortable for you) with both arms in a slow and controlled manner.
4. Circle forward 10 times and then backward 10 times.
5. Lower your arms, shake them out, and give yourself a big hug. This will stretch your back and the sides of your shoulders.

# ENERGY LIFT

Seated row with resistance band

This exercise is not only good for your large back muscles (lats) it is also good for the fronts of your arms (biceps).

1. Sit on the floor with your back straight, your legs out in front of you, and your knees slightly bent.
2. Place an exercise band around the arches of your feet (wear shoes).
3. Hold an end in each hand, palms facing each other.
4. Keep your arms relaxed and the band taut but not pulled tight.
5. Exhale and squeeze your shoulder blades together as you pull your hands back until they are just below your shoulders and the sides of your chest.
6. Your elbows should be close to your body and pointing backward.
7. Hold, inhale, and return to the starting position.
8. Repeat 10 to 15 times, working up to 3 sets.
9. Stretch your back by clasping your hands and pushing your arms out in front of your chest as far as comfortable. Hold 20 seconds and release.

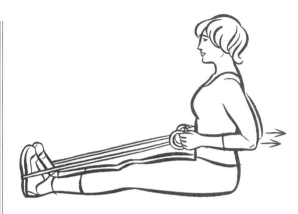

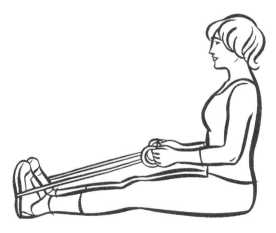

# WATER BREAK

Water helps metabolize fat, so running low on water can actually cause your body to store fat.

# ENERGY BALANCE SNACK

Tomato Soup

 1 cup tomato soup
 1/2 cup low-fat cottage cheese
 1 tablespoon croutons

1. Heat the tomato soup.
2. Add the cottage cheese and stir.
3. Serve in a bowl and top with the croutons.

| CORE FOUR APPROXIMATE BREAKDOWN | PROTEIN ➤ cottage cheese: 14 grams | FAT ➤ soup, cottage cheese, and croutons: 10 to 15 grams |
| --- | --- | --- |
| | CARBOHYDRATE ➤ soup and croutons: 15 to 20 grams | FIBER ➤ soup: 1 gram |

# TAKE 10

Toe point and flex

This exercise will relax and stretch your ankles and feet and strengthen your shins.

1. Lie face down on your bed with your head resting on a pillow and turned to the side.
2. Move your body to the foot of the bed and allow your feet to hang over the edge.

3. To stretch the tops of your feet, point your toes as much as possible.
4. Pull your toes back toward the edge of the bed, hook your toes on the edge of the mattress and pull. Your heels will be flexed and pointing toward the ceiling.
5. Feel the contraction in the fronts of your legs. Hold 10 seconds and release. Point your toes again and hold 5 seconds.
6. Repeat 5 times.

# WATER BREAK

To drink or not to drink . . . alcohol, that is. According to a four-state study of 15,000 women, just one alcoholic drink a day increases a woman's chance of breast cancer by 30 to 40 percent.

# ENERGY BALANCE DINNER

## DINING IN

### Curried Indian-Style Turkey

1 15-ounce can fat-free vegetable broth
1 tablespoon mild curry powder
1/2 teaspoon onion powder
1/2 teaspoon garlic powder
1/2 pound skinless, boneless turkey breast, cooked, sliced
2 teaspoons honey
1/2 cup frozen mixed vegetables
2 ounces raisins

1. Combine the broth with the curry, onion, and garlic powders.
2. Place the mixture in a large saucepan and bring to a boil.
3. Add the turkey and simmer 5 minutes.
4. Add the honey, vegetables, and raisins and cook 5 minutes.
5. Serve over 1/2 cup cooked whole-grain rice.

## DINING OUT

Order chicken or turkey curry with rice.

➤ If you want a larger meal: Add a salad with cucumber-yogurt dressing (found in supermarkets and specialty stores).

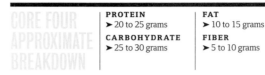

| CORE FOUR APPROXIMATE BREAKDOWN | PROTEIN ➤ 20 to 25 grams | FAT ➤ 10 to 15 grams |
|---|---|---|
| | CARBOHYDRATE ➤ 25 to 30 grams | FIBER ➤ 5 to 10 grams |

# ENERGY BALANCE SNACK

### Pastrami Wrapped Celery

2 slices low-fat pastrami
2 large celery stalks

1. Wrap the pastrami around the celery.
2. Serve with 5 whole-grain crackers.

| CORE FOUR APPROXIMATE BREAKDOWN | PROTEIN ➤ pastrami: 10 to 15 grams | FAT ➤ pastrami: 3 to 4 grams ➤ crackers: 3 grams |
|---|---|---|
| | CARBOHYDRATE ➤ celery and crackers: 10 to 15 grams | FIBER ➤ celery and crackers: 2 to 4 grams |

# STRETCH, RELAX, AND SLEEP

1. Chest/posture stretch
2. Neck and upper spine stretch
3. Bent-over lower spine stretch

# STRESS RELIEF TIP

In times of stress, you can do your health a favor by eating lots of antioxidant-rich foods, such as carrots, broccoli, and dark leafy vegetables, as well as taking antioxidant supplements. Stress increases the production of free radicals, destructive elements that damage healthy tissue and weaken your immune system. Antioxidants neutralize free radicals before they damage the body.

# Celebrate Yourself

YOUR HEALTH AND LONGEVITY are priorities for you, or you wouldn't be reading this right now. It takes a lot of commitment to make it into the fourth week of this program, so congratulations to you! As you may know, it takes about three weeks to form a new habit, and you've just passed the three-week mark.

I encourage you to celebrate yourself. Call a girlfriend and invite her over to toast your success, but don't break out the champagne. Instead, get out your blender and start with 8 ounces of fat free or soy milk. Add fresh fruit such as strawberries, cantaloupe, peaches, and bananas. Toss in a couple of ice cubes and blend away. Serve with a sprig of mint or a slice of lemon.

Ask your friend to make a toast in your honor, recognizing your many wonderful qualities such as endurance, commitment, stamina, and beauty (you might have to help her come up with these). Take some time to talk about how much better you feel and what you've learned and the habits you've established by following this program. It's so easy for us to work hard but fail to be congratulated for our efforts. You deserve to be celebrated.

# DAY 23

## WAKE-UP AFFIRMATION

*"We are free up to the point of choice, then the choice controls the chooser."*

—*Mary C. Crowley, writer*

## WAKE-UP WORKOUT

1. Let body slowly wake up
2. Take several deep breaths
3. Full-body tighten and release
4. Pelvic tilts
5. Pillow sit-ups
6. Hamstring stretch
7. Hands and knees yoga stretch

## CORE FOUR

1. Push-up
2. Sit-up
3. Sit and stand
4. Posture squeeze/biceps curl

## PORTION CONTROL TIP

Carry a small notebook or index cards in your purse, and each time you eat or drink something when you are not really hungry, make a note of what it is and how you feel. Include information about where you are and who, if anyone, is with you. This journal will help you get in touch with your feelings about food and what triggers an eating binge.

## ENERGY BALANCE BREAKFAST

The Liquid Breakfast

4 ounces nonfat milk

4 ounces vanilla soy milk

Small handful blueberries

1/2 banana

2 tablespoons soy protein powder (containing less than 2 grams of carbohydrate)

1 tablespoon flaxseed oil (found in health food stores)

2 ice cubes

Blend all the ingredients until smooth and serve with 2 to 4 vegetarian sausage patties.

➤If you want a larger meal: Add 1/2 cup scrambled egg substitute.

Drink water with lemon or 4 ounces of juice and 6 ounces of water, plus decaffeinated tea or coffee, if desired. Add low-fat creamers to taste.

| CORE FOUR APPROXIMATE BREAKDOWN | PROTEIN ➤ soy protein powder: 20 grams ➤ vegetarian sausage: 6 grams CARBOHYDRATE ➤ blueberries and banana: 10 to 15 grams ➤ milk: 10 grams | FAT ➤ flaxseed oil: 9 grams (heart-healthy omega-3 oil) ➤ vegetarian sausage: 5 grams FIBER ➤ blueberries: 3 to 5 grams |
|---|---|---|

# TAKE 10
Slouch stopper

This exercise will not only rejuvenate the muscles between your shoulder blades; it will wake up your shoulder "hinges" for better functioning.

1. Stand or sit with your chest lifted, your abdominals contracted, your shoulders pressed back and down, and your head straight in alignment with your spine. If you're standing, keep your buttocks tight, your knees unlocked, and your feet pointing forwards.
2. Inhale as you place you hands behind your head with your fingertips behind your ears, your thumbs resting on your jawline, your elbows pressed back, and your shoulder blades contracted.
3. Exhale as you bring your elbows together in front of your face and gently touch them together. Hold 1 second and release to the starting position.
4. Do 2 sets of 8 to 10 repetitions.

# SIT AND BE FIT
Say good-bye to painful wrists

This hand and wrist exercise helps restore circulation, improve the range of motion in your hands and wrists, and relieve pressure on the nerves in your hands, easing wrist and hand pain.

1. Sit in a chair, lift your chest, contract your abdominals, press your shoulders back and down, align your head and spine, and face forward. Extend your arms in front of your chest and bend your elbows slightly.
2. Gently flex your wrists up and down and then circle your hands for 1 to 3 minutes.

# WATER BREAK

Don't take your multi-vitamin with coffee, as caffeine impedes the absorption of iron and calcium. Take it with an Energy Balance meal or snack and a big glass of water, because food helps your body digest and assimilate vitamins.

# ENERGY BALANCE SNACK

6 hard-boiled eggs
2 tablespoons low-fat mayonnaise
2 teaspoons mustard
1 tablespoon sweet-relish
1 small celery stalk, finely chopped

1. Cut the eggs in half and spoon out the yolks.
2. Discard 3 yolks and put the other 3 in a bowl for the filling.
3. Mix the yolks with the mayonnaise, mustard, relish, and celery until fluffy and light. If you need salt and pepper, add sparingly. The sodium from the mustard, mayonnaise, and relish should be enough seasoning.
4. Fill the egg whites with the mixture and refrigerate.
5. Eat eggs with 5 whole-grain crackers. This recipe makes enough to last for at least 3 snacks.

| PROTEIN | FAT |
|---|---|
| ➤ egg whites with filling: 5 grams | ➤ egg filling: 8 to 10 grams |
| **CARBOHYDRATE** | **FIBER** |
| ➤ crackers: 10 grams | ➤ crackers and celery: 3 to 5 grams |

# ENERGY LIFT

This exercise, used by many physical therapists, stretches the rotator cuffs and shoulder joints, increasing flexibility. When your shoulder joints and the surrounding muscles are flexible and strong, you will be less likely to damage this area.

1. Stand or sit with your chest lifted, contract your abdominals, press your shoulders back and down, align your head and spine, and face forward. If you are standing, your buttocks should be tight, your knees unlocked, and your feet facing forward.
2. Place your right hand in the center of your back as high as possible.

3. Holding a towel in your left hand throw it over your left shoulder, retaining your grip on the end of the towel.
4. Grab the other end with your right hand and hold on.
5. Pull gently on the towel with your left hand, until you feel an easy stretch in your right shoulder. If you pull and feel pain in your right shoulder area, back up and take it easy.
6. Hold 10 seconds, release, and repeat on the other side.
7. Work up to holding 20 to 30 seconds.

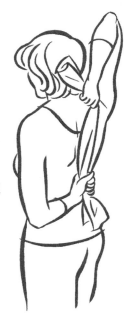

# ENERGY BALANCE LUNCH

## DINING IN

### Italian Meatballs

1 pound ground turkey
1/3 cup chopped onion
1/2 cup finely chopped celery
2 cloves garlic, chopped
1/2 teaspoon crushed dried oregano
1/2 teaspoon crushed dried basil
1/2 cup fat-free crackers, crushed to fine crumbs
1/2 cup cooked brown rice
2 egg whites

1. Combine all the ingredients and shape into small balls.
2. Place in simmering pasta sauce.
3. Cover partially and simmer gently 15 to 20 minutes, stirring often, until meat is no longer pink inside and evenly browned.

4. You may want to serve these meatballs over 1/2 cup cooked pasta, or try putting them on a hollowed-out French roll or stuffed into a piece of pita bread. Add a small green salad with olive-oil-and-vinegar dressing.

## DINING OUT

Order a side of meatballs and a French roll. Hollow out the roll and place the meatballs inside for a meatball sandwich. Add a small green salad.

➤ If you want a larger meal: Eat as many meatballs as you need to feel full.

| CORE FOUR APPROXIMATE BREAKDOWN | | |
|---|---|---|
| **PROTEIN**<br>➤ 4 to 6 meatballs:<br>20 to 25 grams<br>**CARBOHYDRATE**<br>➤ 4 to 6 meatballs:<br>4 to 6 grams<br>➤ hollowed-out<br>French roll:<br>15 to 20 grams | **FAT**<br>➤ 4 to 6 meatballs:<br>5 to 8 grams<br>➤ salad dressing:<br>9 grams<br>**FIBER**<br>➤ 4 to 6 meatballs:<br>2 to 3 grams<br>➤ salad: 1 gram | |

# SIT AND BE FIT

## Upper thigh and knee conditioner combo

These exercises will not only strengthen the fronts of your thighs; they will help strengthen your knee joint muscles as well. Start with the weight of your legs as resistance, and then as you get stronger add 5-pound ankle weights or place a few cans of soup in a purse with handles and hang it over your ankles.

### BENT LEG RAISES

1. Sit with your chest lifted, your abdominals contracted, your shoulders pressed back and down, your head in alignment with your spine, and your feet flat on the floor.
2. Exhale as you straighten one leg and hold for as long as comfortable, working up to 1 minute, breathing easily and deeply.
3. Inhale, bend your knee, and lower your leg halfway to the floor, to a 45-degree angle. Hold a few seconds and then straighten the leg again and hold. Work up to 4 times. Repeat on the other side.

### STRAIGHT-LEG RAISES

1. Assume the same seated position as for the bent-leg raises.
2. Lift your foot and leg as a unit, keeping your leg as straight as you can without hyperextending your knee.
3. Lift your leg off the chair as high as the strength of your thigh will allow.
4. Hold for as long as comfortable and release.
5. Return to the starting position and rest 10 seconds. Work up to 4 repetitions. Repeat on the other leg.

## WATER BREAK

Drink green or black tea. Tea contains enough fluoride to help protect against tooth decay and is also rich in polyphenols, which act as antioxidants that have been shown to protect against diseases such as cancer.

## ENERGY LIFT
### Posture lift and fly

This exercise strengthens your back and shoulders.

1. Sitting in a chair, place a pillow on your lap, bend forward from your waist, and place your chest on the pillow. Keep your head in alignment with your spine and your arms hanging to the floor.
2. Squeeze your shoulder blades together and lift your arms straight out to the sides, level with your shoulders.
3. Slowly lift your arms toward the ceiling as far as comfortable.
4. Lift and lower as if your were flapping your wings, keeping your neck muscles relaxed.
5. Do this flapping motion 10 times and relax your arms back to the floor.
6. Repeat 2 times.
7. Roll up to a seated position and give yourself a big hug to stretch your midback.

## WATER BREAK

Drink 8 glasses of water a day to flush excess sodium from your tissues. Excess sodium from a high-sodium diet can interfere with calcium absorption and increase the amount of calcium that is excreted from your system.

## ENERGY BALANCE SNACK
### Hawaiian Chicken

1/2 cup pineapple chunks
3 ounces grilled chicken, cubed
5 large lettuce leaves
1 tablespoon poppy seed dressing
1 teaspoon chopped walnuts

1. Mix together the pineapple chunks and chicken and place on a bed of lettuce.
2. Top with the poppy seed dressing and sprinkle with walnuts.

| CORE FOUR APPROXIMATE BREAKDOWN | **PROTEIN**<br>➤ chicken: 15 grams<br>**CARBOHYDRATE**<br>➤ pineapple:<br>  10 to 15 grams | **FAT**<br>➤ poppy seed<br>  dressing and<br>  walnuts: 10 grams<br>**FIBER**<br>➤ pineapple: 1 gram |
|---|---|---|

## TAKE 10
### Back pressure relief

This simple relaxation position will relieve lower back pressure and relax all your torso muscles.

1. Lie on your back on the floor with your legs at right angles and your lower legs resting on a chair or couch or the end of a bed and your knees over your hips.
2. Place your hands on your abdominals just below your rib cage and concentrate on breathing with your diaphragm. When you inhale the abdomen expands, and when you exhale it sinks.
3. Breathe and relax, letting both hips and your lower back sink into the floor.
4. Stay in this position, breathing evenly, until your feel your stress subside.

## WATER BREAK

Water evaporating from your skin cools your body, so when you take a drink, mist your face at the same time to refresh your body both inside and out.

## ENERGY BALANCE DINNER

### DINING IN

Sugar and Spice Barbecue Salmon

1 tablespoon sugar

1/4 teaspoon dry mustard

Dash cinnamon

1/2 teaspoon paprika

1/4 teaspoon cocoa

Dash chili powder (more if you like more of a kick)

1 teaspoon ground cumin

1/2 teaspoon freshly ground pepper

1/2 teaspoon coarse salt

6-to 8-ounce salmon fillet

3 tablespoons olive oil

1. Mix the first 9 ingredients together.
2. Dip the salmon in the oil and drag it through the spice mixture and coat on all sides.
3. Place the salmon on a barbecue grill or vegetable-sprayed broiler pan and cook until opaque in the center, about 5 minutes on each side.
4. Serve with a small baked red potato, mixed vegetables, and a green salad with low-fat dressing.

### DINING OUT

Order salmon prepared any way you like; if they have one, try the house specialty. Add lots of fresh vegetables and a starter salad.

➤If you want a larger meal: Eat a larger piece of salmon.

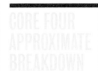

| CORE FOUR APPROXIMATE BREAKDOWN | PROTEIN<br>➤ salmon:<br>25 to 30 grams<br>CARBOHYDRATE<br>➤ potato: 20 grams<br>➤ vegetables and salad:<br>10 grams | FAT<br>➤ salmon and salad<br>dressing:<br>15 to 20 grams<br>FIBER<br>➤ salad and vegetables:<br>3 to 5 grams |
|---|---|---|

## ENERGY BALANCE SNACK

Granola and Cottage Cheese

1/2 cup low-fat cottage cheese or ricotta cheese

1/2 cup low-fat granola cereal

| CORE FOUR APPROXIMATE BREAKDOWN | PROTEIN<br>➤ cottage cheese:<br>14 grams<br>CARBOHYDRATE<br>➤ granola<br>20 grams | FAT<br>➤ cottage cheese:<br>4 grams<br>FIBER<br>➤ granola:<br>2 to 3 grams |
|---|---|---|

## STRETCH, RELAX, AND SLEEP

1. Chest/posture stretch
2. Neck and upper spine stretch
3. Lower spine stretch

## HELPFUL HINTS

Researchers at Georgia State University found that people tend to eat more in the presence of others. In the study, eating with one person increased food consumption by 28 percent, with two 41 percent, and with six or more 76 percent. The conclusion: Having company for meals allows you to linger over your meal longer and consume more food. The solution: Eat your meal slowly and have a cappuccino or decaf latte while you are lingering. When you're finished, drink a large glass of water with lemon.

# Make Time to Dine

**D**O YOU EAT THE SAME WAY you get gas for your car? Speed to the pump, fill up, and drive off in a cloud of dust? Your car may not need much ceremony when the gas gauge is on empty, but your body's needs are much more complex.

Rather than "eat" dinner, take time to "dine." It doesn't take a lot to turn a meal into an occasion to dine. Try these three easy steps:

➤ **SET THE MOOD.** Ambience for dining doesn't take much effort. Light a candle, turn on a soothing CD, and turn off the TV.

➤ **SET THE TABLE.** Rather than use the everyday dishes, set the table with the good dishes. Snip a few flowers from the garden and arrange them on the table. Without saying a word, you'll let your friends and family know this is a special occasion.

➤ **EAT SLOWLY.** Dining is a leisurely process, a chance to chew and savor and reflect. Conversation is enhanced when we slow down and actually listen to each other. Savoring each bite will increase our enjoyment of the moment, as well as aid in healthy digestion.

# DAY 24

## WAKE-UP AFFIRMATION

**"The future belongs to those who believe in the beauty of their dreams."**

—*Eleanor Roosevelt, former first lady and social activist*

## WAKE-UP WORKOUT

**1.** Let body slowly wake up
**2.** Take several deep breaths
**3.** Full-body tighten and release
**4.** Pelvic tilts
**5.** Pillow sit-ups
**6.** Hamstring stretch
**7.** Hands and knees yoga stretch

## CORE FOUR

**1.** Push-up
**2.** Sit-up
**3.** Sit and stand
**4.** Posture squeeze/biceps curl

## PORTION CONTROL TIP

If you eat on the go and have a hard time sticking to a healthful eating plan, you should try to plan ahead. Take a few hours one afternoon and make multiple portions of your favorite Energy Balance meals and snacks. Freeze or refrigerate the food in single servings so eating on the go will be quick and nutritious.

## ENERGY BALANCE BREAKFAST

### Takin' It Easy Italian Frittata

Make sure you have plenty of time to enjoy the fun of making this special breakfast.

    1/2 cup chopped onion
    2 cloves garlic, minced
    1/2 cup chopped zucchini
    1/2 cup chopped tomato
    2 to 4 tablespoons fat-free chicken broth
    4 ounces firm tofu, drained
    5 egg whites
    1/2 teaspoon honey
    1/2 teaspoon crushed dried basil
    1/2 teaspoon crushed dried oregano
    1/2 cup cooked brown rice
    1 ounce low-fat mozzarella cheese
    Dollop low-fat sour cream
    Dash paprika

**1.** In a 9- to 10-inch non-stick frying pan, sauté the onion, garlic, zucchini, and tomato in the broth 10 to 15 minutes, or until the vegetables are soft.
**2.** Puree the tofu with the egg whites, honey, basil, and oregano in a blender.
**3.** Spread the vegetables evenly in the skillet and pour the tofu mixture uniformly over them.
**4.** Cover and cook over low heat 1 to 2 minutes until partially set.

5. Stir in the brown rice, cover, and cook until the mixture is completely firm and nicely puffed, about 12 minutes.
6. Cut into 3 servings and freeze or refrigerate the other 2.
7. Top with the cheese, paprika, and sour cream.

➤If you want a larger meal: Eat until you are full.

Drink water with lemon or 4 ounces of juice and 6 ounces of water, plus decaffeinated tea or coffee, if desired. Add low-fat creamer to taste.

| CORE FOUR APPROXIMATE BREAKDOWN | PROTEIN ➤ tofu and egg whites: 15 to 20 grams CARBOHYDRATE ➤ frittata: 10 grams | FAT ➤ frittata: 2 grams ➤ sour cream: 3 grams ➤ cheese: 7 grams FIBER ➤ frittata: 3 grams |
|---|---|---|

# TAKE 10

Take a 20- to 30-minute walk and finish up with the following stretch.

## Standing hamstring stretch

**(BACKS OF THIGHS)**

1. Standing with your feet together, take a very large step forward with your right foot. Keep your right foot pointing forward and turn your left leg slightly so that your foot points a bit to the left.
2. Place your hands on your hips and bend your left leg while leaning your torso forward over your right leg as far as comfortable. Your back, neck, and head should be in a straight line, and your right knee should be unlocked.
3. Lift the toes of your right foot off the floor while maintaining pressure on your front heel. You should feel a comfortable stretch in the back of your right leg.
4. Breathing deeply and evenly, hold 20 to 30 seconds and repeat on the other side.

# SIT AND BE FIT

## Seated torso stretch

By stretching your entire torso, you will help your back become more flexible. This movement will also stretch the sides of your hips and help release tension in your lower back.

1. Sit on the floor with your left leg in front of you with your knee slightly bent.
2. Cross your right leg over your left knee or thigh and place your right foot flat on the floor.
3. With your arm straight and relaxed, press your left elbow against the outside of your right knee.
4. Keeping your hips on the floor, twist your torso to the right and look over your right shoulder.
5. Breathing deeply and evenly, hold 20 to 30 seconds and repeat on the other side.

# WATER BREAK

A new study has found that drinking just 2 to 3 cups of coffee a day not only raises blood pressure; it reduces aortic elasticity, which is essential for healthy heart function and coronary blood flow.

# ENERGY BALANCE SNACK

## Cheesy Barbecue Dip

2 tablespoons barbecue sauce
1/2 cup low-fat cottage cheese
1 cup cut-up vegetables
5 whole-grain crackers
1 1-ounce stick string cheese

1. Place the barbecue sauce in a small bowl.
2. Add the cottage cheese and mix thoroughly.
3. Serve with vegetables, crackers, and string cheese.

| CORE FOUR APPROXIMATE BREAKDOWN | PROTEIN ➤ cottage cheese: 14 grams ➤ string cheese: 6 grams CARBOHYDRATE ➤ crackers and vegetables: 10 to 15 grams | FAT ➤ string cheese: 7 grams FIBER ➤ vegetables and crackers: 2 to 5 grams |
|---|---|---|

# WATER BREAK

When your stomach is full, it stops grumbling for food. Try fooling it by drinking a big glass of water.

# ENERGY LIFT

Shoulder stabilizer

This exercise will strengthen and stabilize your shoulders and shoulder blades, your abdominals, and your lower back.

1. Get down on the floor on your hands and knees.
2. Lift your rib cage, contract your abdominals, and tighten your shoulder blades slightly so your upper back is flat. (The natural tendency is to let your back sag into a swayback.)
3. Exhale as you raise your right arm directly in front of you and hold a few seconds while balancing on your knees and left arm.
4. Inhale as you lower. Repeat 5 times, working up to 10 repetitions.
5. If you want to make this a little more effective, hold a 2- to 3-pound weight. Don't use anything heavier, as it would be too much for your shoulder at that angle.
6. Repeat on your left side.

# ENERGY BALANCE LUNCH

## DINING IN

Sloppy Joes

1/2 pound ground turkey breast, cooked
1/2 cup chopped onion
1 15-ounce can fat-free chili
1/2 cup chopped celery
1/2 cup chopped green bell pepper
1/2 cup fresh or frozen corn kernels
1/2 cup tomato sauce
1 teaspoon paprika
1/2 teaspoon dry mustard

1. In a medium saucepan coated in vegetable spray, heat the turkey and onion over medium heat 2 to 3 minutes.
2. Add the chili, celery, bell pepper, corn, tomato sauce, and seasonings.
3. Cover and simmer 30 minutes, stirring occasionally.
4. Serve over 1 piece hollowed-out French bread, 1 English muffin, or 1 small whole-grain hamburger bun with a green salad and low-fat dressing.

This recipe makes 4 servings so save the balance for other meals and snacks.

## DINING OUT

Order a turkey burger with vegetables on the side and a green salad.

➤If you want a larger meal: Eat another serving.

| CORE FOUR APPROXIMATE BREAKDOWN | PROTEIN ➤ sloppy joes: 15 to 20 grams | FAT ➤ sloppy joes: 2 to 5 grams |
|---|---|---|
| | CARBOHYDRATE ➤ bread: 25 to 30 grams | FIBER ➤ sloppy joes: 10 grams |

# SIT AND BE FIT

Foot and ankle stretch

This stretch for the lower legs is not only a good way to prevent injuries, it will help prevent leg cramps by increasing circulation.

1. Sit in a chair with your feet flat on the floor and your hands resting on your thighs. Lift your chest, contract your abdominals, press your shoulders back and down, align your head and spine, press your buttocks against the back of the chair, and face forward.
2. Extend your legs slightly so that your heels are 1 to 2 inches off the floor.
3. Point your toes toward the floor as far as you can; hold this stretch 20 to 30 seconds.
4. Point your toes to the ceiling, stretching your calves. Hold for 20 seconds.
5. Repeat both stretches 4 more times.

# WATER BREAK

Research has found that people who drink more than 2 glasses of wine or 4 ounces of hard liquor every day have less bone mass than people who don't drink. Alcohol not only has a direct toxic effect on bone cells; it also seems to take the place of calcium-rich foods in the diet.

# ENERGY LIFT

Prone buttocks lift

This exercise firms and tones your buttocks and helps strengthen your lower back.

1. Lie face down on a cushioned flat surface with your right leg extended straight behind you and your left leg bent at the knee, perpendicular to the floor, with your foot pointed toward the ceiling.
2. Your head should be aligned with your spine, with your forehead resting on your forearm. Your other arm should be extended above your head, flat on the floor.
3. Keeping your pelvis anchored to the floor and your knee bent, lift your left thigh a few inches off the floor. (This is not a large movement.) You will feel the contraction in your buttocks.
4. Hold 1 second and return to the starting position. Do 5 to 10 and repeat on the other side.

If you feel any strain in your lower back, stop and adjust your position and check your form. You may want to put a small pillow under your hips to take pressure off your lower back.

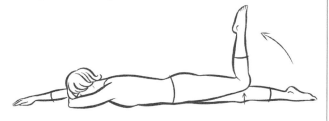

# WATER BREAK

A cup of low-sodium clear soup counts as fluid replacement and can also give you an extra hour of hunger abatement.

# ENERGY BALANCE SNACK

Turkey Dog

> 1 turkey dog
> 1 hollowed-out hot dog bun
> Mustard, relish, onions, and low-fat mayonnaise to taste

1. Place the hot dog on the bun.
2. Flavor with the mustard, relish, onions, and mayonnaise.
3. Serve with cut-up vegetables.

| CORE FOUR APPROXIMATE BREAKDOWN | | |
|---|---|---|
| **PROTEIN**<br>➤ turkey dog: 10 grams | | **FAT**<br>➤ turkey dog: 5 grams |
| **CARBOHYDRATE**<br>➤ bun: 10 to 15 grams | | **FIBER**<br>➤ vegetables: 5 grams |

# TAKE 10

Rib cage circles

This torso tension reliever wakes up stagnant muscles by allowing your abdominal and lower back muscles to work together to increase circulation.

1. Sit in a chair with your feet flat on the floor and your hands resting on your thighs. Lift your chest, contract your abdominals, press your shoulders back and down, align your head and spine, and face forward.
2. Slowly roll your upper torso from your rib cage in a small circle to the right 4 times. Stop and roll to the left 4 times.
3. Take 4 deep breaths and go back to your activities.

# WATER BREAK

Alcohol and PMS do not mix. Alcohol is a depressant, and when you drink your mood can be altered for the worse. If you are prone to angry outbursts, alcohol can accelerate impulsive emotions. Alcohol also dehydrates you and creates a roller coaster effect on your blood sugar.

# ENERGY BALANCE DINNER

## DINING IN

### Steak and Potatoes

6 ounces lean steak or ground beef

1. Grill the meat until cooked to your liking. A few minutes before you take the meat off the grill, brush with steak sauce and seasonings.
2. Serve with a small baked potato and a large green salad with low-fat dressing.

## DINING OUT

Start with a small Caesar salad; go easy on the dressing and croutons. Order a filet mignon or top sirloin steak, eat half, and save the rest for tomorrow. Add 1/2 baked potato with a small amount of sour cream and chives.

➤If you want a larger meal: Finish with a decaf cappuccino, latte, or herbal tea.

| CORE FOUR APPROXIMATE BREAKDOWN | PROTEIN ➤ steak: 25 to 30 grams CARBOHYDRATE ➤ potato, salad, and vegetables: 25 to 30 grams | FAT ➤ meal: 15 to 20 grams FIBER ➤ potato skin, salad, and vegetables: 5 to 10 grams |
|---|---|---|

# ENERGY BALANCE SNACK

Due to the large dinner, skip this snack. If you are even slightly hungry, have an 8-ounce glass of vanilla soy milk or nonfat milk.

| CORE FOUR APPROXIMATE BREAKDOWN | PROTEIN ➤ milk: 8 grams CARBOHYDRATE ➤ 10 grams | FAT ➤ soy milk: 5 grams FIBER ➤ 0 grams |
|---|---|---|

# STRETCH, RELAX, AND SLEEP

1. Chest/posture stretch
2. Neck and upper spine stretch
3. Lower spine stretch

# HELPFUL HINT

If you are sticking to this program, your body is probably feeling younger and more vital every day. Why not take this time to exercise your mind too? Once a week go somewhere you've never been or do something new—nothing radical, just slightly out of the norm. Walk a new way to work, try a dish you've never ordered, see a movie that's unfamiliar. By expanding beyond your normal parameters, you experience new and different ways of looking at the world.

# Rake for Health

MAINTAINING YOUR health can include taking up a hobby that gives you a mild workout—my favorite is gardening. The health benefits of gardening are threefold:

➤ **EXERCISE:** All that raking and weeding and mulching and hoeing provide excellent cardiovascular and strength training—rivaling any workout you could get in a gym.

➤ **STRESS RELEASE:** Gardening brings us into contact with nature in a way few traditional exercise programs can. Digging our fingers into the soil, smelling the fragrance of freshly cut grass, and enjoying the vibrant colors of flowers and vegetables can soothe away our cares.

➤ **NUTRITION:** Gardeners can reap an additional harvest from gardening—nutritious fruits and vegetables that go directly from the vines to their dinner tables. There's no need to worry about pesticides or other detrimental substances when you grow your own produce.

# DAY 25

## WAKE-UP AFFIRMATION

"Supposing you have tried and failed again and again, you may have a fresh start any moment you choose, for this thing that we call 'failure' is not the falling down, but the staying down."

—*Mary Pickford, actress*

## WAKE-UP WORKOUT

1. Let body slowly wake up
2. Take several deep breaths
3. Full-body tighten and release
4. Pelvic tilts
5. Pillow sit-ups
6. Hamstring stretch
7. Hands and knees yoga stretch

## CORE FOUR

1. Push-up
2. Sit-up
3. Sit and stand
4. Posture squeeze/biceps curl

## PORTION CONTROL TIP

Stave off hunger by having a stash of Energy Balance foods with you at all times, in your car, office, or purse. Keep a small insulated lunch box filled with string cheese, sliced apples, whole-grain crackers, and energy bars that are balanced with 10 grams of protein, no more than 23 to 25 grams of carbohydrates, and 3 to 6 grams of fat. If you plan for your blood sugar lows, you will always stay balanced.

## ENERGY BALANCE BREAKFAST

Hollow Banana Bagel

1 bagel
1/2 banana, sliced
1/2 cup low-fat cottage cheese
Sprinkle of cinnamon and sugar

1. Scoop out inside of the bagel.
2. Slice the banana and place on the bagel.
3. Fill with the cottage cheese.
4. Top with the cinnamon and sugar.

➤ If you want a larger meal: Add 1 scrambled egg and 3 egg whites.

Drink water with lemon or 4 ounces of juice and 6 ounces of water, plus decaffeinated tea or coffee, if desired. Add low-fat creamer to taste.

| CORE FOUR APPROXIMATE BREAKDOWN | PROTEIN ➤ cottage cheese: 14 grams CARBOHYDRATE ➤ bagel: 15 to 20 grams ➤ banana: 10 to 15 grams | FAT ➤ cottage cheese: 2 to 3 grams ➤ bagel: 1 gram FIBER ➤ 0 grams |
|---|---|---|

## TAKE 10

Tips for improving balance

Keep safety in mind when you practice balance training. Make sure walls, chairs, or other objects are nearby to use for support. Although no single factor is responsible for balance loss, some effects of aging, such as impaired vision, reduced reflex speed, and inner ear problems, can drastically reduce equilibrium. However, active older adults are better at maintaining balance and coordination than their inactive counterparts.

1. Practice standing on one leg whenever you are waiting in line.
2. If you are watching TV, stand up during commercials; see how long you can stand on one leg with your eyes closed. Change legs. (Note: Always have a chair nearby to catch your balance should you need it.)
3. Practice walking a straight line, placing one foot in front of the other. At the end of your outdoor walks, try doing a balance walk to finish.
4. Sit on a Balance Ball and lift one leg; see how long you can hold the position. Change sides. (See "Balance Ball Workout"). This exercise will aid in building greater pelvic mobility as well as strengthening your upper thighs, lower legs, and ankles, promoting increased stability.
5. Take large steps from side to side, using small squats to move from left to right. This movement also strengthens your heart muscle and burns fat, as it uses the large muscles of the body to raise your heart rate.

## SIT AND BE FIT

Tummy Toner

This exercise will not only tighten your abdominals, which will help your lower back, it will also improve your torso strength and overall posture. Do this movement any time you feel a slump. Many times just lifting your rib cage, tightening your abdominals, and breathing deeply with your diaphragm can make you look better and feel more energetic.

1. Sit in a chair with your feet together, flat on the floor. Lift your chest, press your shoulders back and down, align your head and spine, and face forward.
2. Inhale through your nose to a count of 5 as your belly expands.
3. Purse your lips and exhale forcefully for a count of 5 as you pull your navel in.
4. Repeat 10 times.

## WATER BREAK

Wake up and drink up. Start your day with a big drink, either herbal tea or a fresh glass of plain water, which will make up for the fluids you lost while you were sleeping.

## ENERGY BALANCE SNACK

Egg Salad Stuffed Celery

  2 hard-boiled eggs, finely chopped
  1 teaspoon sweet pickle relish
  1 tablespoon fat-free mayonnaise
  2 or 3 large celery stalks
  5 whole-grain crackers

1. Mix the eggs, relish, and mayonnaise.
2. Use it to fill the celery.
3. Serve with the crackers.

| CORE FOUR APPROXIMATE BREAKDOWN | PROTEIN<br>➤ eggs: 12 grams<br>CARBOHYDRATE<br>➤ crackers:<br>    10 to 15 grams | FAT<br>➤ egg yolks: 10 grams<br>FIBER<br>➤ celery: 1 to 2 grams<br>➤ crackers:<br>    1 to 2 grams |
|---|---|---|

## WATER BREAK

While it is recommended that you drink 64 ounces of water, many days you will need more: when you are sick, pregnant, or breast-feeding or if you spend a lot of time in overheated or air-conditioned environments. Drink a lot more if you are traveling via airplane, as recirculated air can leave you dehydrated at the end of your flight.

## ENERGY LIFT
### Inner thigh lift

This exercise will firm and shape your inner thighs as well as tone and lift your buttocks.

1. Lie on your back with your knees bent, your feet on the floor with your heels lifted, and your inner thighs squeezing a child's playground ball or small plush pillow between your knees.
2. Rest your head on a small pillow or rolled-up towel with your hands beside your hips, palms facing down.
3. Press your lower back to the floor and contract your abdominals.
4. Breathing easily and deeply, lift your buttocks slightly off the floor and squeeze gently while pressing your inner thighs against the ball.
5. Repeat 10 to 20 times. Rest and do 2 more sets. Work up to 2 sets of 30 times.

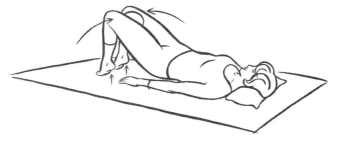

## ENERGY BALANCE LUNCH

### DINING IN
#### Special Taste Tuna

3 ounces water-packed tuna
1 dill pickle, finely chopped
2 radishes, finely chopped
1/2 teaspoon Dijon-style mustard
1/2 teaspoon lemon juice
1 tablespoon low-fat mayonnaise
1 to 2 cups shredded lettuce

1. Mix the tuna, pickle, radishes, mustard, lemon juice, and mayonnaise.
2. Place the lettuce on a plate and top with the tuna mixture.
3. Serve with whole-grain crackers or stuff a piece of pita bread to make a sandwich.

### DINING OUT

Order a tuna sandwich on bread or pita bread or tuna salad with pita bread on the side.

➤ If you want a larger meal: Add a decaf beverage and 1 cookie.

| CORE FOUR APPROXIMATE BREAKDOWN | PROTEIN ➤ tuna: 20 grams CARBOHYDRATE ➤ pita bread: 20 grams ➤ crackers: 15 to 20 grams | FAT ➤ mayonnaise: 3 to 5 grams FIBER ➤ lettuce, radishes, and pickle: 2 to 4 grams |
|---|---|---|

## SIT AND BE FIT
### Knee to shoulder

This exercise will help elongate the muscles of your hips and lower back, which will help prevent injuries, especially if you play golf or tennis.

1. Sit tall on a firm chair with armrests, lift your chest, contract your abdominals, press your shoulders back and down, align your head and spine, and face forward.
2. Place your right hand slightly behind you on the arm of the chair, fingers pointing out. Rest most of your weight on that hand.
3. Cross your right leg over your left at the knee and grasp your right knee with your left hand. Pull your right knee gently to the left. Press your right hip bone into the chair to maximize the stretch.
4. You should feel the stretch in your hip, buttocks, and lower back.
5. Hold the position for 20 to 30 seconds, breathing evenly and deeply.
6. Repeat on the other side.

# WATER BREAK

Read the labels of designer fitness waters because many are high in sugar and sodium. Often plain water is your best choice (and less expensive too!).

# ENERGY LIFT

## Kneeling ab crunch

This exercise will tighten your abdominals and strengthen your lower back, helping improve your balance and overall spinal flexibility. As an added plus, this crunch will really work your buttocks too. (This is a somewhat advanced movement, so take it slowly and don't get discouraged if it doesn't come easily the first few times.)

1. Get down on your hands and knees on a mat or carpeted area with your knees hip distance apart and your hands shoulder distance apart.
2. Inhale as your carefully extend your right arm and left leg straight out to the side and hold, keeping your lower back in a straight line.
3. Slowly exhale as you bring your right elbow and left knee together while tightening your abdominals and rounding your back toward the ceiling.
4. Repeat 5 times on that side and then change sides. Work up to 10 on each side.

# WATER BREAK AND ENERGY BALANCE SNACK

## Soup and Crackers

Combine this water break and Energy Balance snack with a bowl of clear soup such as low-sodium chicken or beef broth with 1/2 cup chopped chicken and vegetables. Add 5 low-salt, whole-grain crackers.

| CORE FOUR APPROXIMATE BREAKDOWN | | |
|---|---|---|
| **PROTEIN**<br>➤ chicken: 15 grams<br>**CARBOHYDRATE**<br>➤ crackers:<br>  10 to 15 grams | **FAT**<br>➤ broth: 3 to 5 grams<br>**FIBER**<br>➤ vegetables:<br>  3 to 4 grams | |

# TAKE 10

## Armchair dip

This exercise firms the backs of your arms, the large muscles of your back, your buttocks, and your abdominals, which are contracted to stabilize the torso during the movement.

1. Sit in a chair with your feet flat on floor, lift your chest, contract your abdominals, press your shoulders back and down, align your head and spine, and face forward.
2. Scoot forward to the edge of the chair and place your hands on the chair's armrests.
3. Exhale as you lift your body until your arms are fully extended, with your elbows slightly bent.
4. Keep your abdominals and buttocks contracted.
5. Repeat the movement 10 to 15 times or as many times as comfortable.
6. If you feel strain on your wrists, do only 2 or 3 until your wrists are flexible and strong enough to support your weight.

### TRICEPS STRETCH

1. Assume the prestretch position above.
2. Bring both arms overhead; place your right hand on the back of your right shoulder and hold your right elbow with your left hand.
3. Gently pull your elbow behind your head, creating a stretch.
4. Do this slowly and hold 15 to 20 seconds.
5. Repeat on the other side.

# WATER BREAK

Watch your alcohol consumption. Drink no more than a small glass per day, preferably with dinner. Alcohol appears to inhibit your body's ability to burn fat and encourages fat storage, in addition to increasing your appetite. Not a good combination for health or weight loss!

# ENERGY BALANCE DINNER

## DINING IN

Baked Salmon with Fruit Salsa

> 1/2 cup canned or fresh pineapple
>
> 1/8 each red, yellow, and green bell pepper, cored, seeded, cut into small pieces
>
> 1/2 small red onion, finely diced
>
> 1/2 cup chopped fresh mint or cilantro
>
> 2 tablespoons fresh lime juice
>
> Salt and pepper to taste
>
> 1/2 tablespoon brown sugar
>
> 1 6-ounce salmon steak, broiled or grilled

1. Combine the pineapple, bell pepper, and onion in a mixing bowl and gently toss.
2. Add the mint, lime juice, salt, pepper, and sugar to taste.
3. Place the salmon on a warm plate and top with the fruit salsa.
4. Serve with 1/2 cup brown rice or 1/2 baked yam with trans-fat-free margarine and a sprinkle of cinnamon and chopped walnuts.
5. Add a large green salad with low-fat dressing.

## DINING OUT

Order grilled salmon with fruit salsa. If fruit salsa is not available, order fruit on the side or top the salmon with regular salsa. Add a large green salad with vinegar-and-olive-oil dressing and 1/2 baked potato or a small side of rice.

➤If you want a larger meal: Start with a shrimp cocktail.

| CORE FOUR APPROXIMATE BREAKDOWN | PROTEIN<br>➤ salmon:<br>25 to 30 grams<br><br>CARBOHYDRATE<br>➤ fruit salsa: 15 grams<br>➤ rice or yam:<br>20 to 30 grams | FAT<br>➤ entire meal:<br>15 to 20 grams<br><br>FIBER<br>➤ entire meal:<br>10 grams |
| --- | --- | --- |

# ENERGY BALANCE SNACK

Carrot Raisin Salad

> 3/4 cup carrot raisin salad (Buy a premade salad or combine 1/2 cup shredded carrots with 2 ounces raisins.)
>
> 1/2 cup low-fat cottage cheese or 1/2 cup ricotta or farmers cheese

Mix the salad and cheese together and enjoy.

|  | PROTEIN<br>➤ cheese: 14 grams<br><br>CARBOHYDRATE<br>➤ carrot raisin salad:<br>15 to 20 grams | FAT<br>➤ cheese: 3 to 5 grams<br><br>FIBER<br>➤ carrot raisin salad:<br>3 to 5 grams |
| --- | --- | --- |

# STRETCH, RELAX, AND SLEEP

1. Chest/posture stretch
2. Neck and upper spine stretch
3. Lower spine stretch

# STRESS RELIEF TIP

Most people are healthier and happier when absorbed in something other than themselves. Volunteering or helping someone less fortunate than you can really put your problems in perspective.

# Exploit Your Wiggle Room

YES, WE ALL HAVE responsibilities, deadlines, and routines that direct, and sometimes limit, our choices. But no matter what our obligations may be, we all have a little wiggle room.

➤ Stuck in front of a computer all day? Make sure you take regular breaks, not to drink more caffeine but to refill your water container. Take off your shoes and lift your heels off the floor. This simple exercise will bring refreshing blood flow to your legs.

➤ Taking care of a houseful of kids? Don't plunk them in front of the television. Take advantage of their stamina and take them to the park. As they play on the equipment, you can enjoy nature while keeping an eye on them.

➤ Caught in rush hour traffic? Rather than rage at other motorists (and raise your blood pressure to dangerous levels), practice deep breathing exercises to destress before you get home. You'll arrive in much better shape, and everyone you live with will appreciate your relaxed mood.

# Shopping and Travel

WHENEVER YOU FIND your self waiting for service, whether its shopping or traveling, here are a few circulation, toning, and energy booster tips and exercises.

## SHOPPING SMARTS

These exercises will not only firm and tone your whole body, they will enable you to shop longer by supporting your spine and taking some of the tension off your lower back.

**PARKING:** Whenever it's safe, park your car as far away from the store as possible and walk briskly to store's entrance.

**REACHING:** When reaching up for a product that is on a high shelf, stand on your tip-toes and reach with your right arm as high as you can, stretching your waist line and opening up your shoulder joints. Hold for a second, take the product, and put it in your basket and move on. The next items that you need on a high shelf, perform the same movement with the left hand.

**LIFTING:** When reaching for an object below your waist, bend your knees, grasp the object, and use your thighs to stand back up. If you are lifting any object weighing more than 5 pounds, bend your legs so that one knee is on the ground and the other knee is bent perpendicular to your waist. Place the object on your bent knee and, holding the object with both arms, put both feet on the floor. Keeping both knees slightly bent, roll up, one vertebrae at a time, into a full standing position.

**LIFTING WEIGHT:** When you find yourself in the liquid detergent aisle, grasp in each hand a 3-5 pound handled bottle of liquid laundry detergent and lift in a bicep curl ten times and out for a side shoulder raise ten times (See "Core Four Upper Body" for form.)

**STANDING IN LINE:** Use this time to tone your buttocks, hips, thighs, and abdominals.
1. Stand with feet slightly apart, feet forward, chest lifted, shoulders pressed back and down, head in straight alignment with your spine.
2. Holding onto the shopping cart handle, lift your heels up, shifting your weight to your toes, and hold for 10 seconds. Return to starting position. Rock back on your heels; point your toes to the ceiling and hold for 10 seconds, then return to standing position.
3. Bend your knees over your toes and hold for 10 seconds. Release, repeat 5 times, and return to standing position.
4. Still holding on to the cart handle, place your feet so that your right heel supports most of your weight. Extend your left leg straight behind you, toes on the floor and heel lifted. Keep your right knee over your right heel—don't let it drift over your toes, which would place too much strain on your knee. Hold for 10 seconds. Now, take the left foot and put it on the cart's lower rail, bend your right knee and straighten the left leg until you feel a stretch in the back of your thigh. Hold for 10 seconds and repeat both movements with the right leg.
5. Return to standing position and bring one foot out in front of you until you have the space to tap your toe. Now, tap in a rapid rhythm, tap, tap, tap, tap fast. This will strengthen your shin

and release pent up frustration of waiting in line. Tap for a minute, then change sides.

**TAKING YOUR PURCHASES HOME:** Whenever you have purchases in plastic handled bags, use them as weights in exercises such as shoulder shrugs, side arm raises, biceps curls, triceps kickback, front arm raise, bent-over arm pulls, heel raises, or any of your favorite resistance exercises from this book. Just remember to always keep your knees bent, elbows bent, buttocks tight, shoulders back and down, and your head in straight alignment with your spine.

# TRAVEL SMARTS

**ON THE PLANE:** To make your flight more enjoyable, try the following.

➤ When stowing carry-on bags in the overhead bin, stand so that your hips are parallel to the bin and lift with your legs, biceps, chest, and front of your shoulders. Don't allow your lower back to arch, keep your knees bent, abdominals contracted, and buttocks tight.

➤ Before you buckle up, place a small airplane pillow or lumbar pillow behind your lower back for support. This will counteract the tendency to slump and decrease the risk of in-flight pain.

➤ If you are smaller than 5'4", rest your feet on a piece of luggage under the seat in front of you to bring your knees level with your hips and to take the strain off your lower back.

➤ Bring bottled water and drink 8 ounces an hour.

➤ To reduce the risk of deep vein thrombosis (DVT), a condition that can increase blood clots in your lower leg due to extended lengths of time in a stationary seated position, make sure you get up and walk around every two hours. One way to increase circulation in your legs is to point and flex your feet often during the flight, do twenty heel lifts in rapid succession, bounce your thighs, and squeeze your buttocks.

➤ To release lower back tension, try the following routine:

1. Place a small pillow on your lap, bend over and rest your chest on the pillow, allowing your head to hang down between your knees and your arms to hang beside your thighs. Hold for 10-20 seconds. Then, while contracting your abdominals, slowly roll up one vertebra at a time into an upright position.

2. Now tighten your abdominals, press your shoulders back and down, and align your head with your spine. Wrap your hands and arms around your shoulders and hug yourself, allowing your head to lower toward your chest. Hold for approximately 10-20 seconds.

3. Release and place the back of your hands behind you in the middle of your lower back, squeeze your shoulder blades together and hold for 10-20 seconds.

4. Reach up as high as you can and hold for 5 seconds and release.

5. Take 5 deep breaths. Inhale through your nose, pushing your abdominals out, and exhale through your mouth, pulling your abdominals in.

6. Press your lower back against your seat; hold for a count of 10 and release.

7. Bring your right leg up toward your chest. Place your right forearm behind your knee, and pull gently toward your chest. Hold for 10 seconds, release and do the left leg.

For the most energy when you get off the plane, stay away from alcohol and caffeine and try to eat in the Energy Balance:

➤ Call the airline before your flight to order a low-fat meal.

➤ If this isn't possible, eat all of the protein and half of the carbohydrate portions.

➤ Drink a large glass of water with lemon before and after your meal.

➤ If you are still hungry, eat a balanced energy bar (Fat: no more than 6 grams, Carbohydrate: no more than 23 grams, and Protein: at least 10 grams.)

# DAY 26

## WAKE-UP AFFIRMATION

*"I am learning from the past, I am planning for the future, and I am living for today."*

—*Stanley Black, real estate developer*

## WAKE-UP WORKOUT

**1.** Let body slowly wake up
**2.** Take several deep breaths
**3.** Full-body tighten and release
**4.** Pelvic tilts
**5.** Pillow sit-ups
**6.** Hamstring stretch
**7.** Hands and knees yoga stretch

## CORE FOUR

**1.** Push-up
**2.** Sit-up
**3.** Sit and stand
**4.** Posture squeeze/biceps curl

## PORTION CONTROL TIP

If you want to splurge on French fries, potato chips, or any other high-fat, high-sugar food, follow the dozen rule: Eat only 12 pieces or bites of the must-have food. With this rule in mind, you can eat whatever you want, in moderation.

## ENERGY BALANCE BREAKFAST

Waffle, Sausage, and Melon

1 small fresh or frozen whole-grain waffle
2 teaspoons trans-fat-free margarine
2 or 3 pieces vegetarian sausage, cooked
1/2 cantaloupe or honeydew melon

➤ If you want a larger meal: Add 1/2 cup egg substitute.

Drink water with lemon or 4 ounces of juice and 6 ounces of water, plus decaffeinated tea or coffee, if desired. Add low-fat creamer to taste.

| CORE FOUR APPROXIMATE BREAKDOWN | PROTEIN ➤ vegetarian sausage: 6 to 10 grams CARBOHYDRATE ➤ waffle: 10 grams ➤ melon: 5 grams | FAT ➤ vegetarian sausage: 3 to 4 grams ➤ margarine: 3 to 4 grams FIBER ➤ melon: 2 to 3 grams ➤ waffle: 2 to 4 grams |
| --- | --- | --- |

## WATER BREAK

Older people are five times more likely to be constipated than younger people are. Chronic constipation can lead to painful conditions such as hemorrhoids and diverticulitis. Water and fiber can relieve constipation, so drink up!

# TAKE 10

Tips for the computer-bound worker

1. Remember to fidget and keep your body moving when sitting for long periods.
2. Lift your rib cage and practice deep breathing, inhaling through your nose into your diaphragm. (Make your stomach push out.) Exhale through your mouth and contract your abdominals. Do this when you are feeling stiff and tired.
3. To exercise your hands and prevent carpal tunnel syndrome, keep a seed-filled balloon or a small soft ball nearby and take squeeze breaks.
4. Prevent eyestrain by looking up or off into the distance at a faraway object every 15 minutes. Roll your eyes in a slow circle to the left and then to the right. Squeeze your eyelids tightly, hold 1 second, and release. This will loosen up your eye muscles and help lubricate dry eyes. Repeat 2 times and go back to work.
5. Remember to change the side on which you hold the phone. If you hold the phone up to your right ear most of the time, change to the left. This will help release the strain in your neck muscles and keep them more balanced.

# SIT AND BE FIT

Inner thigh tightener

This exercise will help tone, relax, and stretch your inner thighs, increasing flexibility to prevent injury should you lunge to either side quickly.

1. Sit on a carpeted floor with the soles of your feet together and your knees out to the sides. Lift your chest, contract your abdominals, press your shoulders back and down, align your head and spine, and face forward.
2. Place your right hand on the inside of your left knee and your left hand on the inside of your right knee.
3. Breathing evenly and deeply, push your knees against your hands and resist with your hands

just enough to contract your inner thigh muscles. Hold 5 seconds.
4. Release and allow your knees to relax toward the floor.
5. Repeat this tense and relax 3 times.

# WATER BREAK

For a refreshing treat, freeze your favorite juice in an ice cube tray and then drop a few cubes into seltzer or club soda with a lime.

# ENERGY BALANCE SNACK

Chocolate Orange Shake

1 ounce chocolate-flavored protein powder
8 ounces orange juice
2 ice cubes

Blend all the ingredients in a blender until smooth.

| CORE FOUR APPROXIMATE BREAKDOWN | PROTEIN | FAT |
|---|---|---|
| | ➤ protein powder: at least 10 grams | ➤ protein powder: no more than 6 to 10 grams |
| | CARBOHYDRATE | FIBER |
| | ➤ protein powder: no more than 20 grams | ➤ protein powder: at least 5 grams |

# ENERGY LIFT

Standing buttocks lift

This exercise will tone the backs of your thighs and help improve your balance.

1. Hold on to a chair, wall, or countertop. Stand up straight and place your feet hip distance apart. Lift your chest, contract your abdominals, press your shoulders back and down, align your head and spine, and face forward. Place your feet together, pointing forward, being careful not to lock your knees.
2. Squeeze the muscles in the back of your right thigh as you bend your right knee to bring your heel toward your buttocks.
3. Place a small water bottle or rolled-up towel in

the crook of your knee and squeeze.

4. Hold this position for a count of 5 and release.
5. Change sides and then repeat the lift 2 times, alternating legs.

**NOTE:** If you feel a cramp in the back of your thigh, stop immediately and release your leg. Save this exercise for a later day when your hamstrings have become stronger.

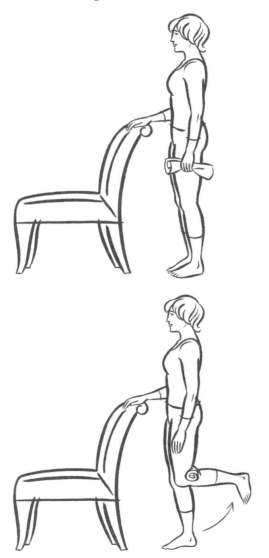

# ENERGY BALANCE LUNCH

### DINING IN

Reuben Sandwich

2 slices rye bread
3 or 4 slices lean corned beef
2 slices low-fat Swiss cheese
1/2 cup sauerkraut
Mustard to taste

1. Coat a large nonstick pan with vegetable spray and place over medium heat until warm.
2. Place the bread in the pan and let it brown.
3. Add the corned beef and cheese on top of the bread; allow the cheese to melt.
4. Add the sauerkraut and mustard and close the sandwich. Cook until the melted cheese holds the bread together.
5. Serve with cut-up vegetables and a decaf drink.

### DINING OUT

Order a Reuben sandwich with only 1 slice of cheese and lean corned beef. Ask to have it grilled in as little butter as possible. Enjoy with a decaf beverage.

➤If you want a larger meal: You shouldn't be hungry with this large sandwich. In fact, you may have to eat half and save the rest for later. If you are still hungry, try a large glass of water with lemon.

CORE FOUR
APPROXIMATE
BREAKDOWN

| **PROTEIN** | **FAT** |
|---|---|
| ➤ corned beef: 15 to 20 grams | ➤ corned beef: 10 to 15 grams |
| **CARBOHYDRATE** | **FIBER** |
| ➤ bread: 25 to 30 grams | ➤ bread: 1 gram |
| | ➤ vegetables: 3 to 4 grams |

## SIT AND BE FIT
Resistance band biceps curl

This biceps curl will strengthen the fronts of your arms, and using a resistance band is an easy way to increase the effectiveness of this exercise without the bulk of free weights.

1. Sit on the edge of a sturdy chair, lift your chest, contract your abdominals, press your shoulders back and down, and align head and spine.
2. Place a resistance band under your feet (wear non-skid shoes), which should be hip distance apart.
3. Grasp the ends of the band and press your elbows to your waist, holding your arms against your sides.
4. Exhale and slowly lift your hands toward your shoulders. Stop as soon as you feel the fronts of your arms tighten. Hold 1 second and release to a full arm extension, but don't lock your elbow.
5. Repeat 10 to 15 times for 2 sets.

## WATER BREAK

Prevent muscle soreness with more water. When you're physically active, your body taps the water that's stored in your muscles. That can decrease your strength and increase your risk of microscopic muscle damage, which is manifested as muscle soreness.

## ENERGY LIFT
Isometric chest booster

This chest toner will firm your entire chest while also strengthening your buttocks and abdominals, which stabilize your entire body during this exercise.

1. Lie face down on the floor with your legs straight, your feet together, and your toes tucked under.
2. Place your forearms on the floor, pull your elbows under your shoulders and close to your chest, and clasp your hands.
3. Slowly raise your body from the floor by straightening from head to toes. You will place your upper body weight on your elbows and forearms, and the balance of the weight on your toes.
4. Squeeze your buttocks tightly and contract your abdominals. Hold 2 to 5 seconds and lower.
5. Breathe evenly and deeply.
6. Repeat 3 to 5 times, working up to 10.

**Note**: This is not a beginner's movement; you need a certain amount of abdominal, lower back, and buttocks strength to complete it.

## WATER BREAK

Staying hydrated is especially important for women because we store less water than men do, since we generally have less muscle. If you are exercising with a male partner, realize that you will need a lot more water than he does to stay hydrated.

# ENERGY BALANCE SNACK

Three Bean Salad with Cottage Cheese

2/3 cup fresh or frozen green beans, cut in 1/2-inch pieces, cooked until tender

1 cup cooked or canned garbanzo beans

1 cup cooked or canned kidney beans

1/2 red onion, sliced

2 tablespoons chopped walnuts

1/2 cup apple cider vinegar

2 tablespoons honey

1/2 cup water

2 tablespoons frozen apple juice concentrate

1. If using canned beans, rinse well.
2. Combine all the beans, the onion, and the walnuts in a bowl.
3. Prepare the dressing by whisking the vinegar, honey, water, and juice concentrate with a fork until well blended.
4. Pour the dressing over the beans and mix well. Cover and chill at least 30 minutes.
5. Toss again before serving. Use a slotted spoon to strain the mixture when serving.
6. Serve with 1/2 cup low-fat cottage cheese on a bed of crisp green lettuce.

This salad will keep in the refrigerator at least a week. Have 2 or 3 large spoonfuls on 1/2 cup cottage cheese with a few chopped walnuts anytime you want a quick snack.

| CORE FOUR APPROXIMATE BREAKDOWN | PROTEIN ➤ beans and cottage cheese: 20 grams CARBOHYDRATE ➤ beans, honey, and juice concentrate: 20 to 25 grams | FAT ➤ walnuts: 5 to 10 grams FIBER ➤ beans: 10 grams |
|---|---|---|

# TAKE 10

Neck and chest stretch

This neck stretch, one of my favorites, will make your upper body more flexible as well as helping release tension from sitting too long in one position.

1. Sit on the edge of a sturdy chair, lift your chest, contract your abdominals, press your shoulders back and down, align your head and spine, and face forward.
2. Interlace your fingers and place them behind your head just above your ears.
3. Breathing evenly and deeply, allow your elbows to come forward and the weight of your hands and arms to gently pull your head toward your chest. Keep your spine straight.
4. Hold this position for 20 to 30 seconds and release to the starting position.
5. Press your elbows out to the sides and back far enough to feel a tightening in your midback and a stretch in your shoulders and chest.
6. Release and repeat the head drop and chest stretch 2 times.

# WATER BREAK

If you are going through menopause and its accompanying night sweats and hot flashes, you are perspiring and need more water.

# ENERGY BALANCE DINNER

## DINING IN

Chicken Breast Diabalise

4 large skinless boneless chicken breasts

1/2 teaspoon salt

1/2 teaspoon pepper

1 tablespoon olive oil

1 tablespoon butter or trans-fat-free margarine

3 tablespoons chopped fresh chives or green onions

Juice of 1/2 lemon or lime

3 tablespoons chopped parsley

2 teaspoons Dijon-style mustard

1/2 cup chicken broth

1. Place the chicken breasts between sheets of waxed paper or plastic wrap. Pound them slightly with a mallet, or buy them already thinly sliced or pounded. Sprinkle them with the salt and pepper.
2. Heat oil and butter in a large skillet over high heat.
3. Cook the chicken 4 minutes on each side, until no longer pink in the middle. Do not cook longer, or it will be dry. Transfer to a warm platter.
4. Add the chives, lemon juice, parsley, and mustard to pan. Cook 15 seconds while you whisk constantly.
5. Whisk in the broth. Stir until sauce is smooth.
6. Pour the sauce over the chicken.
7. Serve with lots of steamed vegetables and a large green salad with low-fat dressing.

This recipe makes 4 servings, so save some for tomorrow's lunch and possible snacks.

## DINING OUT

Try Chicken Piccata; ask for the sauce on the side and drizzle it yourself. Add lots of vegetables and a large green salad with vinegar-and-oil dressing. Finish with a decaf beverage and no more than 3 medium-size bites of dessert.

➤If you want a larger meal: Eat a little more chicken and drink a large glass of water.

| CORE FOUR APPROXIMATE BREAKDOWN | PROTEIN ➤ chicken: 20 to 25 grams CARBOHYDRATE ➤ salad and vegetables: 15 to 20 grams | FAT ➤ butter, oil, and salad dressing: 15 to 20 grams FIBER ➤ salad and vegetables: 5 to 10 grams |
|---|---|---|

# ENERGY BALANCE SNACK

Shrimp Cocktail

6 medium shrimp, deveined, cooked

2 tablespoons red cocktail sauce

4 whole-grain crackers

| CORE FOUR APPROXIMATE BREAKDOWN | PROTEIN ➤ shrimp: 14 grams CARBOHYDRATE ➤ crackers: 12 grams | FAT ➤ shrimp and crackers: 5 to 10 grams FIBER ➤ crackers: 1 to 2 grams |
|---|---|---|

# STRETCH, RELAX, AND SLEEP

1. Chest/posture stretch
2. Neck and upper spine stretch
3. Lower spine stretch

# STRESS RELIEF TIP

Some people find solace in religion. In many studies, faith, religion, and spirituality have been shown to help ease stress-related illnesses and medical problems such as depression and substance abuse. In many cases faith provides a sense of being cared for, loved, and valued—all feelings that enhance your well-being.

# Do Nothing

MY FAVORITE SPANISH proverb is "How beautiful it is to do nothing and then rest afterward." Doing nothing is a goal most of us have difficulty achieving, having been taught to overachieve, multitask, and generally run ourselves ragged. It is often in those "nothing" moments, however, that authentic living and spontaneous love are enjoyed. Here are a few of my favorites:

➤ Sip a cup of tea on the patio while watching the wisteria grow.

➤ Fill in a crossword puzzle, a really easy one that doesn't strain your brain.

➤ Get a piece of yarn and play with your kitties or play catch with your dog.

➤ Meditate for 15 minutes on the benefits of opposable thumbs.

➤ Call your mate just to say "I love you."

And then take a nap. After all this exertion, you deserve one.

# DAY 27

## WAKE-UP AFFIRMATION

"You have to accept whatever comes and the only important thing is that you meet it with the best you have to give."

—*Eleanor Roosevelt, former first lady and social activist*

## WAKE-UP WORKOUT

1. Let body slowly wake up
2. Take several deep breaths
3. Full-body tighten and release
4. Pelvic tilts
5. Pillow sit-ups
6. Hamstring stretch
7. Hands and knees yoga stretch

## CORE FOUR

1. Push-up
2. Sit-up
3. Sit and stand
4. Posture squeeze/biceps curl

## PORTION CONTROL TIP

Buy snacks in individual-size packages—this way you will not be tempted to eat more than 1 serving. Eat a protein source with any high-sugar snack to control insulin's fat-storing reaction.

## ENERGY BALANCE BREAKFAST

Baked Omelette

1 tablespoon butter or trans-fat-free margarine
2 eggs and 3 egg whites, or 1/2 cup egg substitute
1 ounce low-fat cheddar cheese
1/2 tomato, cut into bite-size pieces
2 tablespoons chopped green onion
1 teaspoon chopped coriander or parsley
Salt and pepper to taste

1. Heat the butter in a shallow ovenproof dish.
2. Beat the eggs and egg whites. Add the cheese, tomato, onion, coriander, salt, and pepper.
3. Pour the mixture into the dish.
4. Bake at 350° 10 minutes or until the eggs are fully set.
5. Serve with 1/2 whole-grain bagel, 1 whole-grain English muffin, or 2 slices whole-grain toast.

➤If you want a larger meal: Add more egg whites to make a larger omelette.

Drink water with lemon or 4 ounces of juice and 6 ounces of water, plus decaffeinated tea or coffee, if desired. Add low-fat creamer to taste.

| CORE FOUR APPROXIMATE BREAKDOWN | PROTEIN ➤ eggs and egg whites: 20 grams | FAT ➤ butter and cheese: 10 to 15 grams |
|---|---|---|
| | CARBOHYDRATE ➤ bread source: 30 grams | FIBER ➤ bread source: 3 to 5 grams |

213

# TAKE 10
## No pain in the neck

This stretch will help relieve tense, tight muscles in your upper neck. Due to the nature of the stretch position, it will also tighten your abdominals.

1. Lie on your back with your knees bent and your feet flat on the floor. With your fingers pointing toward your neck, place your hands behind your head. Allow your elbows to come forward in front of your face as far as comfortable.
2. With your hands, slowly lift your head until you feel a slight stretch in the back of your neck. Breathing evenly and deeply, press your lower back into the floor and tighten your abdominals.
3. Firmly press your head against your hands, resisting so your head does not move backward.
4. Hold for a count of 4. Release and repeat 2 times.

# SIT AND BE FIT
## Front of shoulder raise

This exercise will tone the fronts of your shoulders and strengthen your chest muscles.

1. Use a resistance band, a 3- to 5-pound weight, a large canned good, or a 3-pound bag of kitty litter.
2. Sit on the edge of a chair, lift your chest, contract your abdominals, press your shoulders back and down, align your head and spine, and face forward. With your feet flat on the floor, place your feet on the resistance band, hip distance apart.
3. Take hold of the band or weight, palm facing the floor, and keep a slight bend in your elbow. Exhale as you lift your right arm straight in front of you to shoulder height.
4. Hold 1 second and return to the starting position, inhale, and repeat 12 to 15 times.
5. Switch arms and repeat 2 more times, alternating arms, for a total of 3 sets of 12 to 15 on each arm.

# WATER BREAK

Reach for water the next time you crave a caffeinated beverage. Studies show that caffeine can leach valuable calcium from the body, increasing the possibility of osteoporosis.

# ENERGY BALANCE SNACK
## Tortilla with Brie

1 teaspoon honey mustard
1 ounce Brie cheese
2 thin slices chicken or turkey
1 small whole wheat tortilla

1. Place the honey mustard, cheese, and chicken on the tortilla.
2. Heat 10 seconds in a microwave or on medium in a toaster.
3. Serve with decaf vanilla tea.

| CORE FOUR APPROXIMATE BREAKDOWN | PROTEIN<br>➤ chicken or turkey: 15 grams<br>CARBOHYDRATE<br>➤ tortilla: 25 grams | FAT<br>➤ cheese: 4 grams<br>FIBER<br>➤ tortilla: 2 to 3 grams |
| --- | --- | --- |

# WATER BREAK

When drinking a lot of water, you may need to plan your restroom breaks. Your bladder will need relief about every hour to hour and a half after you drink 8 to 12 ounces of water, so make sure you plan accordingly.

# ENERGY LIFT

This exercise will firm and tone the fronts of your thighs and strengthen your buttocks and legs.

1. Stand up tall, lift your chest, contract your abdominals, press your shoulders back and down, and align your head and spine. Hold on to a countertop, sink, or doorway frame with your arms extended as far as comfortable and your elbows slightly bent.
2. Lift your left leg and wrap your left foot around your right ankle.
3. Hold on to the countertop, inhale, and slowly bend right knee. Sit back as far as you can Make sure your right knee is over your heel, not your toes.
4. Hold a few seconds, exhale, and stand back up to the starting position.
5. Repeat 12 to 15 times and change legs.

**BONUS STRETCH** Using the same position as above, bend your knee without sitting back. Allow your knee to bend over your toes while keeping your heel on the floor. This should create a stretch in your Achilles tendon.

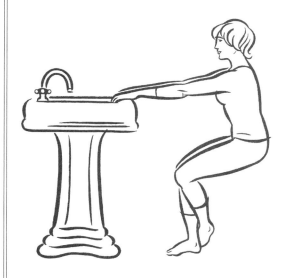

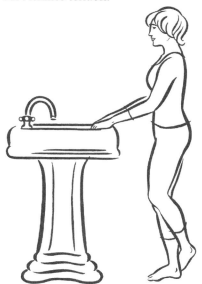

# ENERGY BALANCE LUNCH

### DINING IN

3 cups romaine lettuce

1/2 cup each corn, beets, asparagus, broccoli, and any other vegetable

2 tablespoons small croutons

2 tablespoons Parmesan cheese

2 tablespoons low-fat dressing

6 ounces extra-lean ground beef or ground turkey

1. Mix the lettuce and vegetables.
2. Add the croutons and sprinkle with the cheese.
3. Toss with the dressing.
4. Grill the meat until cooked to your preference and top with salad mixture.
5. Serve with a decaf beverage.

### DINING OUT

Order your favorite salad and a side of lean meat. Finish with a decaf beverage.

➤If you want a larger meal: Add more lettuce.

| CORE FOUR APPROXIMATE BREAKDOWN | PROTEIN<br>➤ beef: 20 to 25 grams<br>CARBOHYDRATE<br>➤ salad:<br>15 to 20 grams | FAT<br>➤ dressing:<br>12 to 15 grams<br>FIBER<br>➤ salad: 10 grams |
|---|---|---|

## SIT AND BE FIT
### Resistance band rotator cuff strengthener

This exercise will strengthen your shoulder rotator cuff and stabilizer muscle group, which is a difficult group to isolate. This movement has proved to be extremely beneficial with my clients who play golf or tennis or feel the wear and tear on their shoulder joint muscles in everyday activities.

1. Sit in a chair, lift your chest, contract your abdominals, press your shoulders back and down, align your head and spine, and face forward.
2. Place a resistance band securely under your feet, which are hip distance apart (wear nonskid shoes) with the left end of the band in your right hand and right end in your left hand.
3. Keep your knees apart with the band resting between your legs; your wrists and hands are crossed.
4. Pull the ends of the band up and glue your elbows against the sides of your waist. Your hands and forearms should form right angles.
5. Exhale as you slowly push your hands out to the sides and away from each other as you point your thumbs to the walls.
6. Hold 1 second and release.
7. Repeat 5 times, working up to 12. Do 2 sets.
**Note**: Don't do too many of these too soon—more is definitely not better with this exercise. This movement is subtle, and at first you may not feel

like it is doing anything, except creating a slight warm feeling in your shoulder joints. But you are working the rotator cuff muscle group. If you overdo this exercise, you can hurt or strain yourself.

## WATER BREAK

Healthy skin is 10 to 20 percent water, so for a natural glow, drink as much as you can.

## ENERGY LIFT
### Resistance band triceps extension

This is an excellent way to work the backs of your arms quickly, safely, and effectively with resistance.

1. Stand with your feet together, your knees bent slightly, and your buttocks tucked under tightly.
2. Drape a rolled-up towel over the back of your neck and place a resistance band over the towel.
3. Grasp the ends of the band with your elbows at your sides, exhale, and slowly straighten your arms, pressing them back behind your hips, but don't lock your elbows.
4. Hold for a few seconds and release your hands to waist height.
5. Repeat 12 to 15 times for 2 sets.

## WATER BREAK

Starting around the age of 30, your oil and sweat glands slow their production and your skin is less able to retain moisture. Keep your system hydrated and eat some heart-healthy fat, which will help moisturize your skin from the inside out.

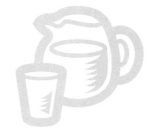

# ENERGY BALANCE SNACK

## Turkey Chili

Turkey chili (found in health food and specialty stores)

Serve 1 cup with 3 whole-grain crackers.

| CORE FOUR APPROXIMATE BREAKDOWN | PROTEIN ➤ turkey and beans: 15 grams | FAT ➤ turkey and crackers: 5 grams |
|---|---|---|
| | CARBOHYDRATE ➤ beans: 15 to 20 grams | FIBER ➤ beans and crackers: 3 grams |

# TAKE 10

## Pull-overs

This exercise will firm and tone your large back muscles, condition your triceps, and open up your rib cage, which will allow you to breathe more deeply. Due to the isometric stabilization, your chest muscles will also be slightly toned.

1. Lie on your back with your knees bent and your feet flat on the floor. Push your lower back into the floor as you contract your abdominals.
2. Clasp your hands and extend your arms straight out from your chest, keeping your elbows slightly bent.
3. Inhale deeply as you lower your arms over your head as far as they will go. At the top of the movement, bend your elbows and allow your hands to fall as far back as possible.
4. Hold, exhale, and return your arms to straight above your chest. Repeat 10 to 12 times.
5. Place your hands on the floor beside your hips with your palms up and relax completely with your eyes closed. Breathing deeply, think your whole body into a relaxed state for 2 minutes.

# WATER BREAK

Green or black decaf tea, steeped at least two minutes to make a strong brew, is a great replacement for coffee during the day. Tea is a strong antioxidant and may help neutralize some of the cancer-causing compounds in your body.

# ENERGY BALANCE DINNER

## DINING IN

### Real Meat Loaf

1 pound extra-lean ground meat
1/2 cup whole-grain cracker crumbs
1/2 cup cooked rice
1/2 cup chopped onion
1/2 cup grated carrot
1/2 cup finely chopped celery
1 1/2 teaspoons mustard (any kind)
1 teaspoon garlic
1/2 teaspoon each thyme and onion powder
1/2 cup tomato sauce
2 egg whites
6 tablespoons ketchup
2 tablespoons honey

1. Preheat oven to 350°.
2. Combine all the ingredients except the ketchup and honey.
3. Turn the mixture into an 8-inch loaf pan and bake at 350° for 40 minutes, until firm and brown on top.
4. After the meat loaf is done, combine the honey and ketchup and spread over the meat loaf. Cook an additional 5 minutes.
5. Eat a small (4- to 6-ounce) portion of meat loaf and save the rest for another meal.
6. Serve with a large green vegetable salad and 1 small roasted potato.
7. If you like gravy over your meat loaf, try one of the low-fat gravies found in your supermarket.

## DINING OUT

Order meat loaf and drizzle with gravy. Add lots of vegetables and a salad. Eat only 1/2 the potatoes. Finish with a decaf beverage.

➤If you want a larger meal: Eat additional, smaller piece of meat loaf.

| CORE FOUR APPROXIMATE BREAKDOWN | PROTEIN ➤ meat loaf: 20 to 25 grams | FAT ➤ meat loaf: 15 to 20 grams |
|---|---|---|
| | CARBOHYDRATE ➤ potato and salad: 20 to 25 grams | FIBER ➤ salad and potato: 5 to 10 grams |

## ENERGY BALANCE SNACK
### Pumpkin and Nonfat Plain Yogurt

1/2 cup canned pumpkin

1/2 cup nonfat plain yogurt

Sweetener to taste (noncaloric sweetener)

Sprinkle of cinnamon and/or nutmeg

Dollop of nonfat whipped topping

1 tablespoon chopped walnuts

1. Mix together the first 4 ingredients.
2. Top with nonfat whipped topping and walnuts.

| CORE FOUR APPROXIMATE BREAKDOWN | PROTEIN ➤ yogurt: 4 grams | FAT ➤ walnuts: 5 grams |
|---|---|---|
| | CARBOHYDRATE ➤ pumpkin: 9 grams ➤ yogurt: 8 grams | FIBER ➤ pumpkin: 5 grams |

## STRETCH, RELAX, AND SLEEP

1. Chest/posture stretch
2. Neck and upper spine stretch
3. Lower spine stretch

## 10 HELPFUL HINTS FOR OVERCOMING THE EFFECTS OF YOUR BODY'S CHANGES AS YOU AGE

1. Exercise with weights or resistance bands. There is nothing more youthful than muscle that is firm to the touch. No matter what your age, your muscles will respond to resistance exercise.
2. Do something that will get your heart pumping and your blood circulating every day.
3. Eat for your skin. Feed your skin the foods it needs to stay firm, moist, and healthy. Eat fresh fruits and vegetables and mix it up with lots of color. This will ensure a diet that is rich in antioxidants. Drink water and keep your protein intake in the balance.
4. Stay out of the sun. If you are in the sun, wear sunblock and a hat.
5. Cut out all the elements that destroy muscle and skin, including smoking, alcohol, caffeine, and high amounts of refined sugar.
6. Get plenty of rest. The only time you build, heal, and repair your immune system, muscle, and skin is when you sleep. Don't shortchange your body by not getting enough sleep—seven to eight hours is the average.
7. Consult your doctor to see if you need hormone replacement. For some women, this is the only answer to the uncomfortable side effects of menopause.
8. Give yourself permission to follow your interests and find the joy in living a life based on your wants and needs.
9. Laugh a lot. Nothing is going to stop you from aging. Only your attitude will ensure a happier transition.
10. Stay curious, keep learning, and find an activity that lights you up.

# Never Act Your Age

**W**E ARE CONFRONTED WITH two kinds of limitations as we age: genuine limitations inherent to being mortal and those we impose on ourselves through our attitudes. Past generations took for granted that getting older meant losing flexibility, facing more illnesses, and having to wear ugly shoes. But many of these misconceptions are being dispelled. Here are three attitudes that aren't based on reality:

➤ **OUR BODIES LOSE FLEXIBILITY AS WE AGE.** According to Lawrence Golding who conducted a study through the Adult Exercise Research Program at the University of Nevada at Las Vegas, "The stiffness many people associate with age actually comes from disuse." Not only do research findings support this assertion; so does Golding's personal experience—he is 72 and teaches fitness classes 5 days a week.

➤ **WE WILL ALL DIE OF SOMETHING.** My 93-year-old great-uncle went to work one morning as he had for decades and came home for lunch at his regular time. As was his habit, he took a nap after lunch before returning to work. But on this day, he never woke up. They found him with a peaceful expression on his face, having died in his sleep. Although it is true that we will all die, the cause of death does not have to be illness-related. At some point, our bodies will stop. According to a study of 1,731 University of Pennsylvania alumni published in the New England Journal of Medicine, people who were thin, refrained from smoking, and exercised at least two hours per week did not develop disabilities usually associated with age for up to seven years longer than their counterparts who were overweight, smoked, and remained sedentary.

➤ **WE SHOULD ACT OUR AGE.** Remember those big black shoes our grandmothers wore? And those shapeless house dresses? What about those hairnets? Gone are the days of ugly, sexless clothing for older women. Treat yourself to beautiful clothing, comfortable clothing, clothing that fits! Reject the notion that looking great is only for those who are younger or thinner. Wear whatever you want, bought from any department. Don't you dare act your age.

Both studies cited in Carol Krucoff's "High Blood Pressure? Walk It Off!" ivillage.com, 1998

# DAY 28

## WAKE-UP AFFIRMATION

"The principle goal [is] competing against yourself. It's about self-improvement, about being better than you were the day before."

*—Steve Young, NFL Quarterback*

## WAKE-UP WORKOUT

**1.** Let body slowly wake up
**2.** Take several deep breaths
**3.** Full-body tighten and release
**4.** Pelvic tilts
**5.** Pillow sit-ups
**6.** Hamstring stretch
**7.** Hands and knees yoga stretch

## CORE FOUR

**1.** Push-up
**2.** Sit-up
**3.** Sit and stand
**4.** Posture squeeze/biceps curl

## PORTION CONTROL TIP

When dining out, if a portion is obviously too large, before you begin eating, cut it in half and ask your waiter to wrap it to go.

## ENERGY BALANCE BREAKFAST

### Power Pancakes

1/2 cup low-fat cottage cheese
2 eggs
1 tablespoon soy protein powder
1 tablespoon trans-fat-free margarine
Salt to taste

**1.** Place all the ingredients in a blender and blend until smooth.
**2.** Heat a skillet coated with vegetable spray over medium-high heat.
**3.** Drop spoonfuls of the mixture onto the skillet.
**4.** Brown on both sides, flipping once.
**5.** Serve with low-sugar syrup and 1 whole-grain English muffin.

➤If you want a larger meal: Add 3 strips turkey bacon.

Drink water with lemon or 4 ounces of juice and 6 ounces of water, plus decaffeinated tea or coffee, if desired. Add low-fat flavored coffee creamers to taste.

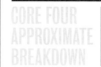

**CORE FOUR APPROXIMATE BREAKDOWN**

| PROTEIN | FAT |
|---|---|
| ➤ pancakes: 20 grams | ➤ cheese, margarine, and eggs: 10 to 15 grams |
| **CARBOHYDRATE** | |
| ➤ English muffin: 30 grams | **FIBER** |
| ➤ syrup: 5 grams | ➤ English muffin: 3 to 5 grams |

# TAKE 10
## Bicep and wrist stretch

This stretch is especially effective for anyone who does repetitive tasks such as data entry.

1. Sit on the edge of a chair, with your feet flat on the floor and your torso leaning slightly forward.
2. Place your hands on the sides of the edge of the chair with your fingers pointing backward.
3. Try to press the heels of your hands down flat on the chair seat. Take it easy; you may not be flexible enough to allow your palms to lie flat.
4. Hold 10 to 20 seconds, shake out your hands, and repeat 2 times.

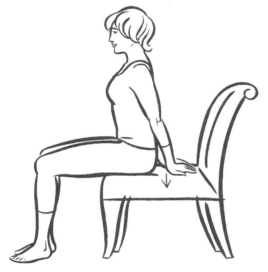

# SIT AND BE FIT
## Crossed legs with a long reach

This position will open up your hips and stretch your spine as well as your midback, chest, and shoulders. Try this stretch first thing in the morning and feel its invigorating results.

1. Sit on the floor with your legs crossed comfortably in front of your body, feet under your hips.

2. Lift your chest, tighten your abdominals, and align your head and spine.
3. Place one hand on top of the other on the floor right in front of you and straighten your arms with your elbows slightly bent.
4. Breathing evenly and deeply, lean forward from your hips as far as comfortable while sliding your hands along the floor as far as you can go.
5. As your back rounds over your legs, you will feel a stretch in your hips, back, and shoulders.
6. Hold 10 to 20 seconds and walk your hands back to the starting position.
7. Sit up straight, place your hands as far behind you as you can and pull your shoulder blades together. Hold 10 to 20 seconds.
8. Repeat both movements 2 times.

# WATER BREAK

If you feel a headache coming on, try drinking a large glass of water. One of the side effects of dehydration is a dull, pounding headache.

# ENERGY BALANCE SNACK
## Baked Apple with Goat Cheese

> 1 small apple
> Cinnamon to taste
> 1 tablespoon goat cheese
> 2 tablespoons low-fat cottage cheese

1. Cut up the apple and place it in a microwave-safe dish.
2. Heat on high until the apple is soft.
3. Sprinkle it with the cinnamon.
4. Top with the goat cheese and cottage cheese.

| CORE FOUR APPROXIMATE BREAKDOWN | PROTEIN<br>➤ goat cheese: 6 grams<br>➤ cottage cheese: 7 grams<br><br>CARBOHYDRATE<br>➤ apple: 20 grams | FAT<br>➤ goat cheese: 8 grams<br><br>FIBER<br>➤ apple: 3 grams |
|---|---|---|

## WATER BREAK

Drinking water will protect your kidneys against protein by-products. Anytime you eat protein, you need water to flush out your system to keep your kidneys healthy.

## ENERGY LIFT
### Leg extension toe tap

This exercise will tighten the fronts of your thighs and increase your heart rate.

1. Sit on the edge of a chair with your chest lifted, your abdominals contracted, your shoulders pressed back and down, your head and spine aligned, and your hands resting on the sides of the chair.
2. Breathing deeply and evenly, stretch your legs in front of your chair and tap your toes, alternating legs in rapid succession, while tightening the tops of your thighs. This motion will look similar to splashing your feet in a pool.
3. Keep tapping for 30 seconds.

## ENERGY BALANCE LUNCH

### DINING IN
### Tropical Chicken Salad

  1/2 small cantaloupe
  1/2 small honeydew melon
  1 skinless boneless chicken breast, cooked, chopped
  1/2 small orange, separated into segments
  1/2 cup green grapes
  1/2 cup fresh or frozen strawberries
  1/2 banana
  1/2 cup thinly sliced celery
  1 tablespoon finely minced green onion
  2 tablespoons poppy seed dressing

1. Cut the melons into small pieces or make melon balls.
2. Combine with the chicken, orange, grapes, strawberries, banana, celery, and onion. Toss to blend.
3. Add the dressing, toss again, and enjoy.

### DINING OUT

Order fruit salad and a broiled chicken breast.

➤If you want a larger meal: Add more chicken.

| CORE FOUR APPROXIMATE BREAKDOWN | PROTEIN ➤ chicken: 20 grams CARBOHYDRATE ➤ fruit salad: 20 to 30 grams | FAT ➤ dressing: 12 grams FIBER ➤ fruit: 5 to 8 grams |
|---|---|---|

## SIT AND BE FIT
### Chair slump leg extension

This combination exercise will tone your hip flexors and the tops of your thighs.

1. Scoot back into a chair until your buttocks are almost to the back edge of the seat, tighten your abdominals, and press your lower back into the back of the chair.
2. Lift your head and keep it aligned with your spine. Rest your hands on your thighs or the arms of your chair.
3. Breathing evenly and deeply, lift your right leg to a comfortable height with your knee bent and then slowly straighten your leg while pointing your toes. Hold 1 second, bend your knee, and return your foot to the floor.
4. Repeat 5 to 10 times and change legs.

# WATER BREAK

A study of more than 35,000 middle-aged women in Iowa found that those who drank at least 2 cups of black, green, or oolong tea a day significantly reduced their risk of getting digestive and urinary tract cancers.

# ENERGY LIFT
## Modified cobra pose

This yoga pose is excellent for stretching your abdominals and strengthening your lower back.

1. Lie on your stomach on a carpet or mat and raise your upper body by placing your elbows under your shoulders, keeping your hip bones touching the floor.
2. Push down on your elbows and forearms as you lift your torso off the floor, creating a gentle arch in your lower back.
3. Breathing evenly and deeply, hold for a count of 10 and release.
4. Repeat 2 times. Be careful not to overdo this pose; it can be too much, too soon for your lower back. With time, it will strengthen your lower back and you will be able to do more.

# WATER BREAK

If you are going through menopause, try to stay away from hot flash triggers, which can include caffeine, alcohol, and spicy foods. Drinking more water and staying hydrated will help make you feel better.

# ENERGY BALANCE SNACK
## Sardines and Crackers

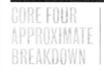

1 can boneless cleaned sardines packed in water or olive oil
1 tablespoon sweet pickle relish
1 tablespoon low-fat mayonnaise
5 whole-grain crackers

1. Drain the sardines and mash with a fork.
2. Add the relish and mayonnaise.
3. Place half the mixture on the crackers. Save the other for another snack.

| CORE FOUR APPROXIMATE BREAKDOWN | PROTEIN ➤ sardines: 14 grams CARBOHYDRATE ➤ crackers: 15 grams | FAT ➤ sardines: 6 grams FIBER ➤ crackers: 3 grams |
| --- | --- | --- |

# TAKE 10
## Family fun time

Take time to play with your family and show your kids how to engage in activities that will build health, burn fat, and create family fun time. (Plus, you may find something new that you enjoy!) Try the following activities and see which ones inspire participation, but don't insist anyone do something he or she doesn't like. Forced participation is the downfall of many fitness programs. Nothing inspires rebellion more than an activity that doesn't suit your abilities and at which your don't feel successful. As a fitness consultant, I have found the reason many people don't like to exercise stems from their early encounters with sports and movement.

1. Walking the dog for at least 30 minutes
2. Biking
3. Hiking and picnicking
4. Roller skating or blading (take lessons before you try this one)
5. Swimming
6. Boogie boarding at the beach
7. Going to a water park

223

8. Climbing jungle gyms, swinging on swings, and playing in the park. (You'll be surprised how much fun you can have working up a sweat!)
9. Playing ball games such as catch, basketball, handball, soccer, baseball, etc. An easy game that everyone can play is whiffleball, because the ball is easy to catch and hit.
10. Playing Ultimate frisbee or flag football.
    Note: If you don't have kids, plan the same activities with your friends.

## WATER BREAK

In the winter, central heating can dry out the air and subsequently your mucous membranes, which can increase your chances of catching a cold. Be sure to drink a lot of water and run a humidifier during winter.

## ENERGY BALANCE DINNER

### DINING IN

Broccoli Italian Style

1 bunch broccoli
2 tablespoons olive oil
1 tablespoon fresh lemon juice
Salt and pepper to taste

1. Trim the broccoli and cut into bite-size pieces.
2. Steam or microwave until tender.
3. In a bowl whisk together the oil, lemon juice, salt, and pepper.
4. Drizzle the mixture over the hot broccoli.
5. Serve with 6 to 8 ounces fish, lean meat, or chicken and 1/2 baked potato or 1/2 cup rice and a large green salad with low-fat dressing.

### DINING OUT

Order a large side of broccoli and drizzle it with olive-oil-and-vinegar dressing. Add lean meat, fish, or chicken and a large salad to start. Finish with a small dessert and decaf beverage. If you want a potato or rice, forgo the dessert.

➤ If you want a larger meal : Fill up on more broccoli and vegetables.

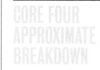

| CORE FOUR APPROXIMATE BREAKDOWN | PROTEIN ➤ fish, lean meat, or chicken: 20 to 25 grams CARBOHYDRATE ➤ potato or rice: 30 grams | FAT ➤ dressing: 10 to 15 grams FIBER ➤ broccoli and salad: 10 to 15 grams |
|---|---|---|

## ENERGY BALANCE SNACK

Soup or Juice

1 cup tomato soup or vegetable juice
Cut-up vegetables with 1/2 cup herbed low-fat sour cream dip

| CORE FOUR APPROXIMATE BREAKDOWN | PROTEIN ➤ dip: 7 grams CARBOHYDRATE ➤ soup or juice: 13 to 19 grams | FAT ➤ dip: 4 grams FIBER ➤ vegetables: 3 to 5 grams |
|---|---|---|

## STRETCH, RELAX, AND SLEEP

1. Chest/posture stretch
2. Neck and upper spine stretch
3. Lower spine stretch

## STRESS RELIEF TIP

Earlier in my career, I had the disease to please—I needed everyone to like me and think I was a good person. Over time I found I had set an impossible criterion. As I've matured, I've learned that RESPECT is the goal. Respect is standing up for yourself and others and living life on your own terms. This is a hard one for women, who often try to be the perfect wife, lover, mother, and caregiver. But being willing to be human, with all your foibles, is an amazing stress reliever.

# Don't Settle for Perfection

MANY WOMEN ARE ON A QUEST for a perfect body (whatever that means). As a result, they're never satisfied with themselves because of the simple fact that no one has a perfect body. No matter what you eat or don't eat, no matter how much you exercise or what parts of your body you exercise, and even if you have your entire body redone with plastic surgery—you'll still have a body someone could criticize. Pursuing perfection is living a life based on self-loathing. Don't settle for perfection; accept yourself as you are here and now.

I've heard women say "But if I accept myself, I won't lose the weight I need to lose" and "Why put effort into eating well if I already feel satisfied with myself?" Those are odd questions if you think about it. If you value yourself and enjoy your life then you'll take good care of yourself and do things that will prolong the length and quality of living. If you don't love yourself now, you won't love yourself when you're thinner or stronger or leaner because you still won't be perfect. Only a woman who genuinely loves herself as she is now can keep up healthy habits—day in and day out, year in and year out. So learn to love yourself first, and then focus on diet and exercise. You'll enjoy the entire process.

# Core Four Abdominals

WHEN YOU FEEL MOTIVATED to do more exercise, working your abdominals is a great place to start. The stronger your abdominals and lower back, the better you will be at all sports and activities. Your abdominal wall is a long band of vertical muscles attached to your rib cage and pubic bone. The small tummy bulge on most women is fat, not muscle. You can do abdominal exercises all day long and still have that tummy—decreasing your overall body fat is the only way to reduce it. For this you need fat-burning aerobic activity, like walking. However, strong abdominals will make you look thinner because they are your torso's natural girdle. A strong midsection will help your balance and posture as you mature.

## Tips for abdominal exercise safety

➤ Always move in a slow and controlled manner.
➤ When lifting from the floor, always come up to the midpoint of the movement. If you lift any higher, your strong hip flexor muscles will take over and pop you right up into a seated position.
➤ Never do straight leg sit-ups, which will eventually cause lower back pain by shortening the muscles that run from your lower back to the fronts of your hips and cause a slight compression in the disks of your lower back.
➤ Exhale as you lift and inhale as you lower.
➤ Support your head with a small pillow or place your hands on the round part of your skull, not the back of your neck. Do not interlace your fingers but allow your fingertips to cradle your head.
➤ When lifting, hold your head as if you have an orange or a baseball under your chin. This will help you keep your head steady throughout the exercise. Another way to keep your head stable

is to fix your eyes on a point in front of your knees. Don't look straight up at the ceiling, which may cause you to place too much pressure on the back of your neck.

## Basic Core Four sit-up (abdominals)

1. Lie on your back on the floor and place your feet on a chair, making sure your knees are directly over your hips.
2. Place a small pillow behind your head and keep your hands behind the pillow.
3. Look at a spot on the wall slightly above your knees and keep your gaze fixed on that spot.
4. Contract your abdominals, raise your head, and hold 1 second before returning to the starting position. Start with as many sit-ups as you feel comfortable doing, and gradually work up to 20. When 20 repetitions are easy, do another set. Eventually work up to 3 sets of 20 repetitions.

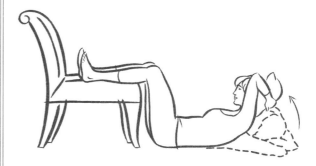

## Waist whittler (obliques)

1. Sit in a chair, lift your chest, contract your abdominals, press your shoulders back and down, align your head and spine, and face forward.
2. Allow your hands to hang by your sides. Gently bend over to the left as far as your torso will allow, keeping your hips glued to the seat of the chair. Hold 2 seconds and return to the starting position.
3. Repeat on the other side. Alternate sides for 5 sets.
**NOTE:** Because this stretch also works your lower back, discontinue if you feel any discomfort or strain.

## Twist again

1. Assume the same position used in the previous exercise, the waist whittler.
2. Raise your arms to shoulder level with your elbows bent, your palms facing down, and your hands in loose fists.
3. Very slowly twist to the right and hold, return to the center, and slowly twist to the left and hold.
4. Inhale in the center and exhale as you twist.
5. Repeat 5 to 10 times, alternating sides. If you feel any discomfort in your lower back, discontinue this series.

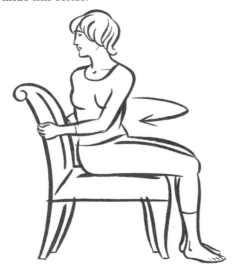

## Lower abdominal attachment crunch

1. Sit on the floor with your knees bent as close to your chest as possible and feet lowered so they are resting on the back of your thighs, ankles crossed.
2. Place your arms at your sides, palms down.
3. Exhale, contract your abdominals and push your lower back against the floor.
4. Start to slowly lift your hips up and off of the floor, so that your pelvis moves toward your rib cage.
5. Do not let your knees fall toward your chest as your spine curls up for your tailbone—let the abdominals do the work.
6. Return to starting position and work up to 12 to 15 repetitions.
**NOTE:** This is a very subtle movement, if you swing your legs you are not working these lower attachments but are working the hip flexors. This is also an advanced movement and you need strong abdominals in order to do it correctly.

## Seated reverse curl

This reverse curl is a little more challenging than the one in the Basic Core Four.

1. Sit on the floor, lift your chest, contract your abdominals, press your shoulders back and down, align your head and spine, and face forward. Bend your knees and place your feet flat on the floor, hip distance apart.
2. Stretch your arms in front of you with your hands clasped.
3. Maintain your lifted, abs-contracted posture, and exhale as you slowly round your spine into a catlike stretch. Your torso should resemble the letter C.
4. Note that it is the rounding of your spine and the contraction of your abdominals that allow you to lean back, not your hips or legs.
5. Repeat, working up to 12 to 15 repetitions.

## Abdominal stretch

This simple stretch is a great way to reduce stress.

1. Lie on your back and stretch your arms over your head.
2. Extend your legs in front of you as far as possible. Feel this stretch in your whole body.

## Lower back strengthener and stretch

This stretch will strengthen your lower back and help lift and firm your buttocks. Do this whenever you can lie down.

1. Lie face down, with a rolled-up towel under your hips and another under your forehead.
2. Extend both arms above your head, palms down.
3. Tighten your buttocks as you raise one extended arm and the opposite leg. Your arm should be straight with your fingers reaching for the wall.
4. Your toes should be reaching for the opposite wall.
5. Hold 5 to 10 seconds and release.
6. Repeat on the other side. Do 2 more sets, alternating sides.

## Lower back, spine, and buttocks stretch

This stretch is especially good for your buttocks and lower back.

1. Kneel on the floor with your buttocks resting on your heels. Your feet can be flexed underneath you or pointed with the tops of your feet on the floor, whichever is more comfortable.
2. Lean forward and slide your arms out in front of you and above your head with your palms down. Keep your buttocks on your heels.
3. Hold this pose 20 to 30 seconds.

# DAY 29

## WAKE-UP AFFIRMATION

"I don't ever look back—I look forward."

—*Steffi Graf, tennis player*

## WAKE-UP WORKOUT

**1.** Let body slowly wake up
**2.** Take several deep breaths
**3.** Full-body tighten and release
**4.** Pelvic tilts
**5.** Pillow sit-ups
**6.** Hamstring stretch
**7.** Hands and knees yoga stretch

## CORE FOUR

**1.** Push-up
**2.** Sit-up
**3.** Sit and stand
**4.** Posture squeeze/biceps curl

## PORTION CONTROL TIP

Change your unhealthy eating habits by changing your eating environment. Replace overeating trigger locations, like in front of the TV, with the kitchen table. Set your table with pretty dishes and utensils—make each meal a presentation, not an eat-on-the-run event.

## ENERGY BALANCE BREAKFAST

### Crepes and Poached Fruit

1/3 cup flour
1/2 teaspoon sugar
Pinch salt
1/3 cup milk
2 teaspoons water
1 egg
1 tablespoon unsalted butter, melted
1 cup water
Dash cinnamon
1/2 each fresh peach, pear, and apple

### FOR CREPES

**1.** Combine the flour, sugar, and salt in a mixer on high for 30 seconds.
**2.** With the mixer running, add the milk, water, egg, and butter.
**3.** Heat a nonstick skillet until very hot. Pour 3 tablespoons batter into the skillet and quickly tilt the pan to spread the batter evenly.
**4.** Cook until light brown, 30 to 40 seconds, flip, and cook an additional 15 seconds.
**5.** Repeat using all the remaining batter. As you finish, stack the crepes with waxed paper separating them to prevent them from sticking together while you prepare the fruit.
**6.** In a saucepan, bring the water and cinnamon to a boil.
**7.** Add the fruit, return to a boil, and cover. Reduce and simmer 5 to 6 minutes.
**8.** Lift the fruit out of the pan with a slotted spoon and place in a small bowl.
**9.** Place fruit on top of 2 crepes and roll them up.

**10.** Serve the two crepes with 2 eggs, 1/2 cup low-fat cottage cheese, or 2 slices Canadian bacon. Wrap the extra crepes in plastic wrap and re-frigerate. They will last 2 days.

➤ If you want a larger meal: Have either 1 additional crepe and more cottage cheese or 1 more slice Canadian bacon.

Drink water with lemon or 4 ounces of juice and 6 ounces of water, plus decaffeinated tea or coffee, if desired. Add low-fat creamer to taste.

| CORE FOUR APPROXIMATE BREAKDOWN | **PROTEIN** ➤ cottage cheese and Canadian bacon: 20 grams  **CARBOHYDRATE** ➤ fruit: 15 grams ➤ crepes: 15 to 20 grams | **FAT** ➤ egg and butter: 10 grams  **FIBER** ➤ fruit: 3 to 5 grams |
|---|---|---|

# TAKE 10
## Hip flexor stretch

This stretch is ideal for the muscles in the fronts of your hips and will help prevent an arched back, which can strain your lower back vertebrae and disks.
Your hip flexor muscles (where the fronts of your legs and your hips are attached) are some of the strongest muscles in your body while also some of the least flexible.

**1.** Kneel on a carpeted floor or mat. Move your right leg in front of you with your knee bent and your right foot flat on the floor.
**2.** Place both hands on your thigh; make sure your knee is directly over your heel, not your toes.
**3.** Breathing evenly and deeply, slowly slide your left leg behind your hip until you feel a gentle stretch in your left hip flexor.
**4.** Hold 10 seconds and release. Repeat on the other side.

# SIT AND BE FIT
## Upper body stretches

These stretches are excellent for your entire upper body since they will help increase the range of motion in your shoulder joints.

**1.** Stand and hold the ends of a medium towel in your hands. Make sure you have enough room to move through a full range of motion with your arms straight and your elbows slightly bent.
**2.** Hold the towel taut in front of your chest with your arms shoulder width apart. Pull it up and over your head and down behind your back as far as your shoulder joints will allow. Don't push, force, or strain yourself.
**3.** If you want to increase the stretch, move your hands closer together on the towel.
**4.** Breathing evenly and deeply, hold the stretch behind your back 5 to 10 seconds and release.
**5.** Hold the stretch at any point in the movement. (For example, if your shoulders are tight, hold the towel behind your head a little lower than your ears. If you need more chest flexibility, hold the towel behind your back a little lower.)
**6.** Repeat 2 to 3 times.

# WATER BREAK

A squeeze of lemon or lime juice in water is a refreshing way to boost your intake of vitamin C.

# ENERGY BALANCE SNACK
## Tea and Crumpet

1 pot decaffeinated green or flavored black tea
1 English crumpet or 1/2 whole-grain English muffin
2 tablespoons low-fat cream cheese
2 teaspoons low-sugar jam

**1.** Steep the tea.
**2.** Toast the crumpet or English muffin, spread it with the cream cheese, and top with the jam.

| CORE FOUR APPROXIMATE BREAKDOWN | PROTEIN ➤ cream cheese: 7 grams CARBOHYDRATE ➤ crumpet or English muffin: 15 grams ➤ jam: 5 grams | FAT ➤ crumpet: 3 grams FIBER ➤ crumpet or English muffin: 1 to 2 grams |
| --- | --- | --- |

## WATER BREAK

The average person loses approximately 2 cups of water a day simply by breathing.

## ENERGY LIFT

### Prone buttocks squeeze

This squeeze strengthens your buttocks and therefore increases the support for your back.

1. Lie on your stomach with your arms at your sides; place a small pillow under your hip bones for support and comfort.
2. Slowly tighten your buttock muscles.
3. Hold 5 to 10 seconds, breathing evenly and deeply. Slowly relax.
4. Repeat 2 times.

## ENERGY BALANCE LUNCH

### DINING IN

#### Taco Salad

   1 corn tortilla

   1/2 cup refried beans (if possible, without lard)

   1 small chicken breast, broiled, shredded

   1/2 cup low-fat cheddar cheese

   1/2 cup diced avocado

   1/2 cup combined: lettuce, cucumber, tomato, radishes, and green onion

   Taco sauce to taste

1. Place the tortilla in a microwave and heat for 15 seconds.
2. Spread the beans and chicken on the tortilla.
3. Top with the cheese and microwave until the cheese melts.

4. Form a taco and fill with the remaining ingredients.
5. Serve with low-calorie decaf beverage or a mixture of lemonade and iced tea.

### DINING OUT

Order a chicken soft taco with lemonade or iced tea.

➤If you want a larger meal: Make 2 tacos.

| CORE FOUR APPROXIMATE BREAKDOWN | PROTEIN ➤ chicken: 20 grams ➤ beans and cheese: 15 grams CARBOHYDRATE ➤ tortilla: 25 grams | FAT ➤ beans: 5 grams ➤ cheese: 4 grams FIBER ➤ beans: 1 grams ➤ vegetables: 3 grams ➤ tortilla: 1 gram |
| --- | --- | --- |

## SIT AND BE FIT

### Stand up and kick it

This stress-releasing activity will raise your heart rate and burn fat while helping tone and strengthen your buttocks, hips, and thighs.

1. Sit in a chair that won't slide, lift your chest, contract your abdominals, press your shoulders back and down, align your head and spine, and face forward.
2. Exhale as you stand up and kick your right foot in front of you. Sit back down.
3. Inhale as you sit and exhale as you stand and kick your left foot.
4. Sit, kick, sit, kick, back and forth until you have accelerated your breathing.
5. If you are unsure of your footing, place your chair close to a table for balance.
6. Walk in place until your heart rate has returned to normal.

## WATER BREAK

Caffeine is addictive. People who drink a lot of caffeinated beverages often develop a headache several hours after they have had their last beverage, or they may wake up with a headache that is relieved only with coffee, tea, or cola.

## ENERGY LIFT
### Wall hamstring stretch

This hamstring stretch will help relieve lower back strain by keeping the muscles in your lower back more flexible and relaxed.

1. Lie on your back in a doorway with your right leg through the doorway, your knee bent, and your foot flat on the floor.
2. Lift your left leg up until it is resting on the wall next to the doorway.
3. Slowly slide your heel up the wall, straightening your leg, until you feel a gentle stretch in the back of your thigh. Do not overstretch.
4. Breathing evenly and deeply, relax in this position for 20 to 30 seconds. Bend your knee to relieve the stretch, wait a few seconds then repeat stretch twice.
5. Switch legs and repeat on the other side.

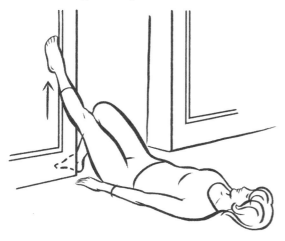

## ENERGY BALANCE SNACK
### Energy Bar

Favorite flavor energy bar that has at least 10 grams protein, no more that 23 grams carbohydrate, no more than 6 grams fat, and at least 2 to 4 grams fiber.

### CORE FOUR APPROXIMATE BREAKDOWN

| PROTEIN | FAT |
|---|---|
| ➤ 10 to 15 grams | ➤ 5 to 6 grams |
| **CARBOHYDRATE** | **FIBER** |
| ➤ 15 to 23 grams | ➤ 2 to 4 grams |

## TAKE 10
### Neck release and dorsal glide

This subtle neck exercise will help prevent stiffness and headaches by stretching the back of your neck. It will also release tension in your trapezius muscles (which run from the back of your head across the back of your shoulders).

1. Sit in a chair, lift your chest, contract your abdominals, press your shoulders back and down, align your head and spine, and face forward.
2. Slowly lower your chin as you glide your head backward over your shoulders.
3. Hold 5 seconds and release.
4. Repeat 5 to 10 times. If you feel pain, don't push your head so far back.

## WATER BREAK

Sip tranquilizing herbal teas made with chamomile, valerian, or passionflower. These ancient herbal remedies promote relaxation and sleep.

## ENERGY BALANCE DINNER
### DINING IN
### Raspberry-Glazed Cornish Game Hen

 1 small Cornish game hen
 1/3 cup raspberry preserves
 1 tablespoon lemon juice
 1 tablespoon grated orange peel

1. Remove skin and split game lengthwise in half.
2. Arrange the hen breast side up in a shallow baking dish.

3. In a small bowl, combine the preserves, lemon juice, and orange peel. Stir and blend well.
4. Brush the glaze over the hen.
5. Cover and bake at 350° 20 to 30 minutes.
6. Serve with vegetables, a large salad, and 1/2 baked potato or 1/2 cup rice.

### DINING OUT

Try a different game dish and add vegetables, 1/2 baked potato, and a large salad.

➤If you want a larger meal: Add 1 small dinner roll or double the recipe to make 2 hens.

| CORE FOUR APPROXIMATE BREAKDOWN | PROTEIN ➤ game hen: 20 to 30 grams CARBOHYDRATE ➤ potato: 15 to 20 grams ➤ rice: 30 to 40 grams | FAT ➤ game hen: 15 to 20 grams FIBER ➤ vegetables, salad, and potato with skin: 8 to 12 grams |
|---|---|---|

## ENERGY BALANCE SNACK
### Pita Pizza

1 small piece whole-grain pita bread

2 tablespoons tomato sauce

1/2 small chicken breast or any leftover meat

2 tablespoons grated mozzarella cheese

1. Place the pita bread in a microwave and heat 10 to 15 seconds, just enough to make it warm.
2. Spread with the tomato sauce, add the chicken, and sprinkle with the cheese.
3. Microwave 20 seconds or until the cheese melts.
4. Enjoy with a cup of relaxing herbal tea.

| CORE FOUR APPROXIMATE BREAKDOWN | PROTEIN ➤ chicken: 10 to 15 grams CARBOHYDRATE ➤ pita bread: 15 to 20 grams | FAT ➤ cheese: 5 to 6 grams FIBER ➤ pita bread: 2 to 3 grams |
|---|---|---|

## STRETCH, RELAX, AND SLEEP

1. Chest/posture stretch
2. Neck and upper spine stretch
3. Lower spine stretch

## EXTRA, EXTRA
### In bed inner thigh stretch

This stretch will release your inner thighs, stretch your hip joints, and help prevent groin pulls, a common injury in golfers and tennis players. If you sit for long periods, your hips become less flexible over time. Take time to release tension with this easy stretch.

1. Lie on your back in bed with your head resting on a pillow.
2. Bend your knees and bring the soles of your feet together with your knees out to the sides.
3. Slowly and gently lower your knees back toward the bed.
4. Let gravity do the stretching. Don't force this stretch and don't bounce or pulse.
5. If you are not flexible in this area and need extra support, place a pillow under each knee and allow your knees to rest on the pillows until you are more comfortable with this stretch.
6. Breathe deeply and steadily.
7. Hold 20 to 30 seconds and release. Work up to 3 repetitions.

## STRESS RELIEF TIP

Take a minute to lie on your bed and think *relax* to your whole body. Actually go from your head to your toes, muscle by muscle, commanding each one to relax.

# Live Luxuriously

**"I** NEVER GET MASSAGES," a girlfriend recently told me. "That seems like a luxury I can't afford. But," she admitted with a smile, "I get manicures every week. For me, manicures are necessities, not luxuries."

If you saw my nails, you'd know my values are the other way around. I'd spend my last dollar on a massage (to help me through the stress of financial ruin, of course), but I do my own nails to save money. Indulging in too much luxury, we're taught, is too much of a good thing. But in fact, one woman's luxury is another's necessity.

Here's a way to live luxuriously. Get a piece of paper and at the top write the word luxuries. Underneath, list at least ten ways to pamper yourself you rarely permit yourself to enjoy. My list would include pedicures, soaking in the tub amid rose petals, spending the day at the beach, and taking in a concert at the park. Once your list is complete, draw a line through the word luxuries and write above it, necessities. There! You no longer need to deprive yourself or feel guilty if you indulge in these nurturing pleasures. After all, they're not luxuries anymore; you *neeeeeeeed* them.

# DAY 30

## WAKE-UP AFFIRMATION

*"The most important factor for motivation is goal setting. You should always have a goal."*

—*Francie Larrieu Smith, long distance runner*

## WAKE-UP WORKOUT

**1.** Let body slowly wake up
**2.** Take several deep breaths
**3.** Full-body tighten and release
**4.** Pelvic tilts
**5.** Pillow sit-ups
**6.** Hamstring stretch
**7.** Hands and knees yoga stretch

## CORE FOUR

**1.** Push-up
**2.** Sit-up
**3.** Sit and stand
**4.** Posture squeeze/biceps curl

## PORTION CONTROL TIP

Stay away from value meal deals at fast food restaurants—they often contain an inordinate number of calories. Try to decide what you will order before you get to the counter so you are not tempted by a "bargain."

## ENERGY BALANCE BREAKFAST

### High-Protein Cereal

> 1/2 cup high protein, low-sugar cereal (8 to 10 grams of protein per serving)
> 1/2 cup vanilla soy milk or 1 percent milk
> Sugar substitute
> 1 tablespoon slivered almonds

Place cereal in a bowl, add the milk and sugar substitute, and top with the slivered almonds.

➤If you want a larger meal: Add 1/2 cup cottage cheese or 1/2 cup egg substitute, scrambled.

Drink water with lemon or 4 ounces of juice and 6 ounces of water, plus decaffeinated tea or coffee, if desired. Add low-fat creamers to taste.

| CORE FOUR APPROXIMATE BREAKDOWN | PROTEIN<br>➤ cereal: 8 to 10 grams<br>➤ cottage cheese: 7 grams<br>CARBOHYDRATE<br>➤ cereal: 20 to 25 grams | FAT<br>➤ milk: 5 grams<br>FIBER<br>➤ cereal: 4 to 6 grams |
|---|---|---|

## TAKE 10

### Exaggerated stair climb

**1.** Climb the stairs in your home, office, or local mall. Try tackling two steps at a time for two flights.
**2.** Work up to adding some arm pumps in front of your chest no higher than shoulder height as you climb.
**3.** Exaggerate your motions, taking each step slowly.
**4.** Cool off by descending the stairs slowly, taking full, deep breaths as you go.
**5.** Repeat 3 times, working up to 3 sets of 3 repetitions each.

## SIT AND BE FIT

Forward flexion

This is a good stretch for your lower back and hamstrings. It will protect you from overstretching your lower back. Reversing the flow of blood to your head is helpful for improving your complexion and increasing oxygen flow to your brain.

1. Begin by standing with your feet hip distance apart. Bend over and place your hands on a chair or couch, keep your knees bent, and your abdominals contracted.
2. Slowly straighten your knees to a comfortable position. Always keep a slight bend in your knees to keep strain off your lower back.
3. Drop your head and let it relax. This will increase circulation to your face and brain.
4. Hold this position for as long as comfortable.
5. Keep your knees bent as you return to the starting position.
6. Repeat 2 times.

## WATER BREAK

Some people get a rash where their thighs rub together during exercise, which may be caused by dehydration. Dehydration can cause sweat to dry as irritating salt crystals. Drink water, wear fabrics that keep sweat away from your skin, and if the area is very sensitive, apply petroleum jelly for lubrication.

## ENERGY BALANCE SNACK

Dijon Mustard Dog

2 turkey or chicken hot dogs
1 slice whole-grain bread
1 teaspoon Dijon-style mustard
2 teaspoons pickle relish

1. Toast turkey dogs until heated throughout.
2. Spread the bread with the mustard and relish.
3. Fold the bread around the hot dogs.
4. Enjoy with decaf herbal tea (hot or cold).

| CORE FOUR APPROXIMATE BREAKDOWN | **PROTEIN** ➤ turkey dogs: 10 grams **CARBOHYDRATE** ➤ bread: 13 grams | **FAT** ➤ turkey dogs: 5 grams **FIBER** ➤ bread: 3 to 5 grams |
|---|---|---|

## WATER BREAK

Different types of water

➤ Sparkling water: carbonated water (some are naturally carbonated; others are injected with carbon dioxide).
➤ Spring water: must reach the earth's surface naturally from a spring, but this is no guarantee that it is pure.

## ENERGY LIFT
### Push-ups with weights

This exercise will tone your chest muscles and the fronts of your shoulders as well as improving your upper body strength.

1. Lie on your back on the floor with your legs on a chair, couch, or bed. Contract your abdominals and press your lower back into the floor. Rest your head on a pillow, keeping your head and spine aligned.
2. Hold 5- to 8-pound weights with your hands facing each other. Keep your elbows close to your waist and your forearms at a 90-degree angle to the floor.
3. Exhale as you push the weights straight up, extending your arms but keeping your elbows slightly bent.
4. Hold when fully extended and tighten your chest muscles, and then release to the starting position.
5. Repeat 12 to 15 times, rest, and do 2 more sets.

## ENERGY BALANCE LUNCH

### DINING IN
### Tuna Casserole with Cashews

- 1/2 cup thinly sliced celery
- 2 tablespoons chopped onion
- 1 teaspoon butter or margarine
- 3 ounces water-packed tuna, drained
- 1/2 cup frozen peas
- 1/2 cup condensed fat-free cream of mushroom soup, undiluted
- 2 tablespoons chopped cashews

1. In a microwave-safe bowl, combine the celery, onion, and butter.
2. Cook in a microwave uncovered on high 3 to 4 minutes, or until the vegetables are tender.
3. Add the tuna, peas, soup, and cashews.
4. Cover and microwave 3 to 5 minutes, or until piping hot.
5. Serve over 1/2 small baked potato with a large green salad.

### DINING OUT

Order a tuna Niçoise salad and 1 small dinner roll.

➤If you are still hungry: Finish with a decaf cappuccino or latte.

| CORE FOUR APPROXIMATE BREAKDOWN | PROTEIN ➤ tuna: 20 grams CARBOHYDRATE ➤ peas and soup: 25 to 30 grams | FAT ➤ cashews and butter: 10 to 15 grams FIBER ➤ vegetables, salad, and potato with skin: 5 to 10 grams |
|---|---|---|

# SIT AND BE FIT
## Seated pull-over stretch

Your entire shoulder area will benefit from this stretch, which will also lift and expand your rib cage to allow for deeper breathing.

**1.** While sitting in a chair, lift your chest, contract your abdominals, press your shoulders back and down, and align your head and spine.

**2.** Clasp your hands, interlacing your fingers, with your arms straight in front of your chest.

**3.** Inhale as you bring your arms straight over your head and push them as far behind your head as comfortable. Do not allow your head to drop forward; keep your elbows close to your ears. Exhale at the top of the movement hold a few seconds, feeling the stretch and the opening of your rib cage. Breathe evenly and deeply.

**4.** Inhale deeply and exhale as you allow your hands to slowly return to the starting position.

**5.** At the end of the movement, tighten your chest muscles by pressing your arms together.

**6.** Relax and repeat 5 times.

This movement can also be done lying on the floor with your knees bent, your feet flat, and your abdominals contracted and pressed into the floor.

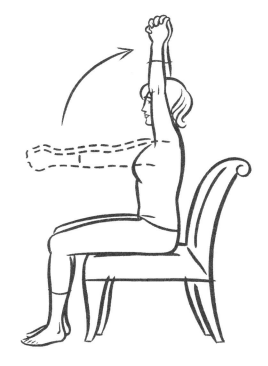

# WATER BREAK

If you question the purity of your water source, for a fee usually under $100, you can send a sample of your water to a laboratory and have it analyzed. To find a water-testing lab in your area, check with your local state health, water, or environmental resources department.

## ENERGY LIFT
### Side-to-side rock

This exercise is an excellent way to stretch and release your lower back muscles, especially toward the end of the day, when they are tired and need a break.

1. Lie on a carpeted floor or mat, bring your knees to your chest, and place your forearms behind your knees.
2. Hold your legs loosely and gently and rock from side to side. Don't overrock; just let the weight of your legs take you from one side to the other.
3. Let this rocking motion gently massage your back and spine.
4. Continue this motion for 20 to 30 seconds, breathing evenly and deeply.
5. When you are ready to get up, roll onto your right side and into a fetal position.
6. Place both hands on the floor, and gently push yourself onto your hands and knees. Stand up slowly by placing your right foot in front of you with your knee bent.
7. Using your thigh, a bed, or a chair for support, stand up with your knees bent and your upper body bending forward.
8. Slowly roll up to a straight standing position one vertebra at a time. By standing this way, you will take all strain off your lower back.

## WATER BREAK

Water that sits overnight in pipes tends to accumulate lead. To lessen the possibility of drinking contaminated water, allow your cold water to run at full force at least two minutes. Place a large pan in the sink to collect the water and use it for household chores. Avoid using the hot water, because it tends to absorb lead and other metals more readily.

## ENERGY BALANCE SNACK
### Chili con Queso Dip

14 1/2-ounce can diced tomatoes, undrained

10-ounce can diced tomatoes and green chilies, undrained

1 teaspoon olive oil

1/2 cup chopped onion

2 garlic cloves minced

8 ounces fat-free cheese

1 teaspoon chili powder

6 ounces light processed cheese (such as Velveeta light), cubed

Cilantro (optional)

1. Drain the tomatoes and tomatoes with chilies in a colander over a bowl, reserving 1/3 cup liquid; set the tomatoes and reserved liquid aside.
2. Heat the oil in a medium saucepan over medium heat. Add the onion and garlic and sauté for 4 minutes.
3. Add the cheese and cook until the cheese melts, stirring constantly.
4. Add the tomatoes, reserved liquid, and chili powder; bring to a boil.
5. Add the processed cheese; reduce heat and simmer 3 minutes or until the processed cheese melts, stirring constantly. Garnish with cilantro, if desired.
6. Serve 1/2 cup warm with 1 large piece whole-grain pita bread, cut into sections and baked into chips. Save the balance for a later snack.

| CORE FOUR APPROXIMATE BREAKDOWN | PROTEIN<br>➤ cheeses: 14 grams<br>CARBOHYDRATE<br>➤ pita bread and tomatoes: 15 grams | FAT<br>➤ oil and cheeses: 5 to 10 grams<br>FIBER<br>➤ tomatoes and pita bread: 3 to 5 grams |
|---|---|---|

# TAKE 10

One-leg stand

Good for your buttocks, hips, and thighs, this exercise will improve the strength of your ankles and your balance. Since this is an advanced movement, make sure you are strong enough in both legs before you try it.

1. Move a chair next to a sturdy table or desk for balance. Sit down, lift your chest, your abdominals, pull your shoulders back and down, align your head and spin, and face forward.
2. Place your feet flat on the floor, far enough from the chair so you can easily stand up. Place your left foot behind your right ankle and wrap your toes around your ankle and foot.
3. Hold on to the table and exhale as you stand up using your right leg.
4. When you reach the full standing position, tighten your right buttock. Keep your knee slightly bent.
5. Do 3 to 5 and work up to 12.
6. Take a break and repeat on the other leg.

# WATER BREAK

Every time you have an alcoholic beverage, chase it with a glass of water. Alcohol dehydrates your cells and suppresses your nervous system, causing poor attention and an inability to concentrate, leading to fatigue.

# ENERGY BALANCE DINNER

## DINING IN

Curried Chicken with Sweet Peppers

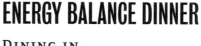

1/2 clove garlic, minced
1/2 teaspoon minced ginger
Dash cumin
1 teaspoon olive oil or canola oil
Dash ground coriander
1/8 teaspoon curry powder
Dash cayenne pepper (optional)
Dash salt
1/2 each red, yellow, and green bell pepper, cut into small strips
Diced onion to taste
1/2 tablespoon lemon juice
1/2 tomato, cut into bite-size pieces
6-to 8-ounce chicken breast, grilled, cubed

1. Place the garlic, ginger, cumin, and oil in a large microwave-safe bowl.
2. Microwave on high 2 minutes.
3. Stir in the coriander, curry powder, cayenne pepper, salt, bell peppers, onion, lemon juice, and tomato.
4. Microwave on high 3 minutes.
5. Stir in the chicken, cover, and microwave on high for another 1 to 2 minutes, or until all the ingredients are hot.
6. Serve over 1/2 cup brown rice with a large green salad.

## DINING OUT

Order curried chicken. Place 1/2 the rice on a plate and top it with the chicken. Start with a cucumber salad and 1 piece pita bread.

➤If you want a larger meal: Add more chicken.

| PROTEIN | FAT |
|---|---|
| ➤ chicken:<br>20 to 25 grams | ➤ entire meal:<br>15 to 20 grams |
| **CARBOHYDRATE** | **FIBER** |
| ➤ rice: 30 grams | ➤ entire meal:<br>10 grams |

## ENERGY BALANCE SNACK

### Nutty Nectarine Sundae

1 small ripe nectarine

2 ounces low-fat vanilla ice cream

2 tablespoons water

1 tablespoon sliced almonds

1. Slice the nectarine and place in a small bowl with water and microwave on high heat 2 minutes.
2. Put the ice cream in a dessert dish and top with the poached nectarine and almonds.

| PROTEIN | FAT |
|---|---|
| ➤ almonds:<br>2 to 4 grams | ➤ ice cream:<br>5 to 10 grams |
| **CARBOHYDRATE** | **FIBER** |
| ➤ ice cream:<br>20 to 25 grams | ➤ nectarine: 3 grams |

## EXTRA, EXTRA

### Buttocks and outer hip stretch

This stretch will increase flexibility in your outer hips and lower back while opening up your shoulders and chest.

1. Lie on your back or the floor and bend your knees, with your left leg over your right knee.
2. Interlace your fingers behind your head.
3. Use your left leg to pull your right leg toward the floor until you feel a mild stretch along side of your hip and your lower back.
4. Keep your upper back, shoulders, and elbows flat on the floor.

5. Stretch your knee toward floor.
6. Hold 20 to 30 seconds. Repeat on the other side.

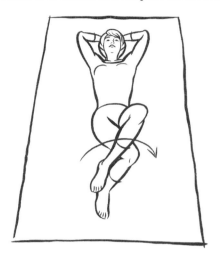

## STRETCH, RELAX, AND SLEEP

1. Chest/posture stretch
2. Neck and upper spine stretch
3. Lower spine stretch

## HELPFUL HINT

Exercise doesn't waste time—it creates time. After the first few weeks of an easy exercise program, many of my clients report having more energy and greater productivity.

# Toss Out Your Hammer

C AN YOU THINK OF A GOOD REASON to smash your thumb with a hammer? Me neither.

We are neurologically wired to withdraw from pain and make a beeline toward pleasure. Touching a hot stove taught us to wear oven mitts. Hiking in new shoes that rubbed blisters all over our feet motivated us to wear BandAids the next time out. Getting sunburned so badly on the backs of our legs we had trouble sitting for several days is the best advertisement for sunscreen. And yet so-called fitness experts still promote excessive exercise resulting in painfully sore muscles and fatigue. We're promised instant thinness through nutritionally bankrupt diet schemes. Why do any of us buy into the exercise myth of "No pain, no gain"?

Aiming for the perfect body is a recipe for failure, often resulting in poor nutrition, injurious exertion, and, ultimately, diminished health. The next time you contemplate starting the newest fad diet or buying a quick-fix get-in-shape-in-three-minutes exercise gadget, think of hitting your thumb with a hammer. It will hurt.

In contrast, the success of this program rests on the belief that fitness is a healthy, pleasurable, doable way of life, void of pain and deprivation. Congratulations for coming this far! Now that Jeanne's program has helped you establish healthy habits, I hope you continue them for the remainder of your long and healthy life.

# Your Day

HERE'S YOUR CHANCE to create a personalized routine incorporating your favorite exercises and food from the Fit Forever program.

## EXERCISES

For a well-rounded workout, try to pick exercises that work each of the following areas of your body:

➤ Abdominals
➤ Back of arms
➤ Calves and shins
➤ Chest
➤ Front of arms
➤ Hips, thighs, and buttocks
➤ Lower back
➤ Midback

Whenever possible, be sure to include aerobic activity in your routine, even if it is only a 10-minute walk.

## FOOD

Any meal or snack you choose from the program will be in the Energy Balance. If you want to create your own combinations, remember the Nutritional Core Four—protein, complex carbohydrates, a little fat, and fiber.

## WAKE UP WORKOUT

## CORE FOUR

## SIT AND BE FIT

## BREAKFAST

**PROTEIN:** 15 to 20 grams
**CARBOHYDRATE:** 25 to 30 grams
**FAT:** 10 to 15 grams
**FIBER:** 5 to 10 grams

## WATER BREAK

## TAKE TEN

## ENERGY LIFT

## SIT AND BE FIT

## WATER BREAK

## SNACK

**PROTEIN:** 10 to 15 grams
**CARBOHYDRATE:** 15 to 20 grams
**FAT:** 5 to 10 grams
**FIBER:** 3 to 5 grams

## WATER BREAK

## TAKE TEN

## SNACK

**PROTEIN:** 10 to 15 grams
**CARBOHYDRATE:** 15 to 20 grams
**FAT:** 5 to 10 grams
**FIBER:** 3 to 5 grams

## WATER BREAK

## WATER BREAK

## DINNER

**PROTEIN:** 15 to 20 grams
**CARBOHYDRATE:** 25 to 30 grams
**FAT:** 10 to 15 grams
**FIBER:** 5 to 10 grams

## ENERGY LIFT

## SNACK

**PROTEIN:** 10 to 15 grams
**CARBOHYDRATE:** 15 to 20 grams
**FAT:** 5 to 10 grams
**FIBER:** 3 to 5 grams

## LUNCH

**PROTEIN:** 15 to 20 grams
**CARBOHYDRATE:** 25 to 30 grams
**FAT:** 10 to 15 grams
**FIBER:** 5 to 10 grams

## STRETCH, RELAX, AND SLEEP

# Conclusion

IF THIS BOOK HAS INSPIRED YOU to take action, any action, toward a healthier, more balanced life, then I have done the job I set out to do. A few things to remember as you set out:

➤ *Fit Forever* is based in fact, not fiction. The movements have evolved from years of practical application, and the combinations of foods both satisfy and build health as you burn stored fat for energy.

➤ Eat the foods you love in moderation, combine the Core Four of protein, complex carbohydrates, fat, and fiber into a meal, and you will not be hungry.

➤ Start moving every day and you probably won't want to stop. Who knows? One "Sit and Be Fit" may lead to more challenges, making for a happier, healthier you.

➤ By the end of this book, the Core Four and Energy Balance should have become habit. So if you must have that hot fudge sundae, go ahead, but remember that you are always one meal and movement away from being Fit Forever.

➤ Be kind to yourself and try to make peace with your body. As you go through life, your body and mind will change and evolve with each passing year. Only a true familiarity with your strengths and desires will keep you prepared for what is to come.

Take care of yourself for a lifetime...

— Jeanne

# Index

## FOODS

### BREAKFAST
Almond French Toast...............136
Bagel with Cream Cheese ..........38
  and Lox
Baked Omelette ......................213
Baked Potato and ...................142
  Poached Eggs
Balanced Energy Drink .............80
Breakfast Hash .......................126
Breakfast of Champions ...........56
Cantaloupe Cooler ..................106
Cheddar Veggie Omelette .........44
Cinnamon French Toast ............86
Crepes and Poached Fruit........230
Egg and Cheese Burrito............168
Eggs Benedict Energy .............100
  Balance Style
Eggs, Toast and Lox..................32
High-Protein Cereal.................236
Hollow Banana Bagel...............198
Lox Baguette...........................160
Muffin Treat............................66
Oat Bran Breakfast ..................72
Omelette Surprise ...................180
Pancake Morning....................148
Parmesan Egg Bagel................112
  Sandwich
Power Pancakes......................220
Strawberry Omelette ..............118
Takin' It Easy Italian Frittata ...192
The Liquid Breakfast ..............186
Through the Garden .................92
  Omelette
Tunnel Bagel .........................154
Waffle and Eggs......................50
Waffle, Sausage, and Melon ....206

### LUNCH
Barbecue Chicken Pizza...........102
Bouillabaisse ..........................162
Chicken Caesar Salad ...............34
Chicken Tabbouleh Salad ..........94
Chicken Vegetable Stew...........182
Chicken Waldorf Salad..............74
Cranberry, Feta, and ................52
  Walnut Salad
Falafel with Cucumber Salad ...128
Hamburger and Salad .............215
Italian Meatballs.....................188
Low-Fat Ham Sandwich ..........120
  with Fruit Salad
Reuben Sandwich ...................208
Roast Beef Sandwich ..............150
Salmon Salad Sandwich ...........81
Salsa Pita..................................40
Shrimp Salad..........................144
Sloppy Joes............................194

Smoked Salmon and Goat..........58
  Cheese Sandwich
Smoked Turkey Club Wrap ......156
Smoked Turkey Salad................87
Special Taste Tuna ..................200
Taco Salad .............................232
Tropical Chicken Salad.............222
Tuna and Apple Salad ...............68
Tuna and White Bean .............170
  Salad with Olives
Tuna Burger ..........................138
Tuna Casserole with ...............238
  Cashews
Tuna Cheese Spread................108
Tuna Pasta Salad ......................46
Turkey and Smoked ...............114
  Gouda Sandwich

### SNACK
An Apple a Day .........................41
Baked Apple .............................73
Baked Apple with ...................221
  Goat Cheese
Banana Bites.............................83
Banana, Peanut Butter, and.....158
  Low-Fat Cream Cheese
Black Bean Soup .....................103
Cantaloupe and Beef Jerky........69
Cantaloupe and Proscuitto ......152
Carrot Raisin Salad .................202
Celery and Peanut Butter ..........75
Cheesy Barbecue Dip..............193
Cheesy Soup.............................60
Cheesy Veggies .........................84
Chili con Queso Dip................240
Chocolate Orange Shake ..........207
Con Queso Dip.......................181
Crackers and Cheese ................35
Crackers and Cheese ................42
Deviled Eggs ..........................187
Dijon Mustard Dog .................237
Edamame ................................87
Egg Salad Stuffed Celery .........199
Fresh Fruit with Low-Fat.........172
  Vanilla Yogurt
Frozen Fruit ...........................130
Fruit and Cheese .......................33
Fruit Cocktail Surprise ............146
Fruit Plus.................................76
Gelatin Sundae.......................122
Got Milk?.................................90
Graham Cracker Treat.............116
Granola and Cottage Cheese ....190
Grapefruit Compote ................139
Grapes.....................................52
Hawaiian Chicken ..................189
Healthy Trails.........................143
Hot Chocolate ..........................96
Hummus and Pita Bread...........81
Jicama Chips with Fruit Salsa ..113
Lentil Soup with Chicken........171

Mushroom Pita Pizza................59
Nachos ..................................151
Nuts ......................................47
Nutty Nectarine Sundae..........242
Oatmeal Delight .....................140
Pastrami Wrapped Celery ........184
Peanut Butter and Cheese ........95
Peanut Butter and ..................110
  Something
Peanut Butter from the Jar......145
Peanut Butter Pretzel .............137
Pear Sandwich .......................121
Pineapple Cottage Cheese .......129
Pita Pizza ..............................234
Ploughman's Snack .................107
Poultry Dog ...........................163
Pretzel Trail Mix ......................54
Pumpkin and Nonfat ..............218
  Plain Yogurt
Roast Turkey Wrap ...................67
Salmon Snack Balls...................93
Salty and Sweet ......................119
Sardines and Crackers.............223
Shrimp Cocktail...............161, 211
Soup and Crackers .................201
Soup or Juice .........................224
Strawberries and Cheese..........155
Strawberry Shake ...................104
Super Celery ............................57
Sweet Potato Treat..................169
Tall Decaf Latte ........................45
Tea and Crumpet....................231
Three Bean Salad with ............210
  Cottage Cheese
Three Cheese Quesadilla..........149
Tomato Soup ..........................183
Tortilla with Brie ....................214
Tuna Wrap ...............................53
Turkey Chili............................217
Turkey Dog ............................195
Veggies, Chips and Dip .............89
Vegetables and Dip.................115
Yogurt .....................................48
Yogurt Fruit Parfait...................70
Yogurt Parfait ..........................36

### DINNER
Almond-Crusted Turkey ............84
  Cutlets
Angel Hair Pasta ....................157
  with Chicken
Apple Salad with ....................164
  Poppy Seed Dressing
Baked Chicken with Dijon .......152
  and Lemon Juice
Baked Salmon with ..................202
  Fruit Salsa
Baked Turkey-Stuffed Tomato .121
Beef Fajitas .............................42
Broccoli Italian Style................224
Broccoli, Sausage, and ............140

Pesto Penne
Chicken Breast Dijonaisse........211
Chicken Stuffed with Spinach .110
  and Ricotta Cheese
Chicken Walnut Pita ...............104
Chicken, Lean Steak, or ............60
  Shrimp Waldorf Salad
Curried Chicken with ..............241
  Sweet Peppers
Curried Indian-Style Turkey ....184
Grilled Fish with Tropical Salsa ..96
Grilled Salmon with ..................90
  Parmesan Broccoli
Lamb Chops with Couscous .......54
Lemon Chicken Piccata.............70
Orange Shrimp ........................116
Out-of-the-Ordinary ................48
  Cheeseburger
Pasta Bowl ...............................76
Raspberry-Glazed Cornish........233
  Game Hen
Real Meat Loaf .......................217
Simply Stir-fry ..........................36
Spinach Filled Salmon.............130
Steak and Potatoes .................196
Stuffed Green Bell Peppers.....172
Sugar and Spice ......................190
  Barbecue Salmon
Turkey Meat Loaf ....................146

## EXERCISES

### BALANCE BALL WORKOUT.....132-135
Abdominal stretch ...................134
Basic sitting position ...............132
Bounce the stress and.............133
  day away
Desk sit .................................133
Inner thigh squeeze ................135
Lower back lift .......................134
One-foot balance ....................133
Relax the back ........................134
Reverse roll abdominal toner...134
Sides of the waist (obliques) ...134
Wall squat ..............................135

### CORE FOUR ABDOMINALS .....227-229
Abdominal stretch ...................229
Basic Core Four sit-up..............227
  (abdominals)
Lower abdominal ....................228
  attachment crunch
Lower back, spine, and ............229
  buttocks stretch
Lower back strengthener.........229
  and stretch
Seated reverse curl .................229
Twist again..............................228
Waist whittler (obliques).........228

**CORE FOUR LOWER BODY** .....175-179
Balance Ball inner ....................179
    thigh squeeze
Ballet knee bend .......................175
Counter sit and hold ................175
Cross quadriceps stretch ..........176
Forward knee bend....................175
Inner thigh squeeze ..................178
Inner thigh stretch ...................179
Inner thigh tightener ...............179
    and release
Inner thigh toe touch ...............179
Lying hamstring lift ..................176
One-leg heel raise ....................178
Shin strengthener .....................178
Standing buttocks lift ..............176
Standing calf raise ....................177
Standing hamstring stretch .....177
Standing hamstring toner .......176
Two-part calf stretch ...............178

**CORE FOUR ROUTINE, THE**.........9-11
Posture squeeze .........................11
Push-up ........................................9
Sit-up ..........................................10
Sit and stand .............................11

**CORE FOUR UPPER BODY** .....124-125
Chest stretch ............................125
Lying arm press with ...............124
    a wrist cross
Midback and shoulder .............125
    stretch
Rotator cuff raise .....................125
Rotator cuff stretch ................125
Side of the shoulder raise ........124
Sink pull....................................125
Standing biceps curl.................124
Triceps and biceps stretch ......125
Triceps kickback ......................124

**ENERGY LIFT**
15-minute walk .........................74
Arm circles.................................81
Back scratcher...........................187
Cat curl stretch.........................139
Chair straddle.............................69
Curl and kickback .....................162
Doorknob knee bend .................88
Doorway push and stretch .......145
Fidgets ........................................34
Front of thigh stretch ...............103
Get up and dance! .....................75
Hand shake .................................52
High and low march..................144
Hip stretch ................................151
Inner thigh lift .........................200
Inner thigh squeeze with .........171
    added stretch
Isometric chest booster.............209
Kick out the stress.....................82
Kneeling ab crunch...................201
Leg extension toe tap ...............222
Marching knee bend .................102
Modified cobra pose .................223
One-leg squat ...........................215
Overhead stretch.......................129
Overhead triceps stretch...........120
Pace it out..................................87
Pivot point knee bend .............138
Posture lift and fly ..................189

Prone buttocks lift....................195
Prone buttocks squeeze............232
Push-ups with weights .............238
Raise and bend with ...............150
    a stretch
Raise and squat..........................46
Resistance band triceps ...........216
    extension
Roll-down/roll-up ...................108
Sack ball ...................................170
Seated row with ......................183
    resistance band
Shake, shake, shake .................114
    your booty
Shake with stretch .....................95
Shoulder stabilizer ...................194
Side-to-side rock ......................240
Sitter's stress relief...................157
Side-to-side lunge ......................47
Squat and lift .............................40
Stairs to nowhere.......................59
Stand, walk, and stretch ..........161
Standing box step.....................107
Standing buttocks lift ..............207
Standing calf raise .....................39
Standing cat stretch....................68
Standing kickbacks....................114
Stationary lunge .........................58
Take a hike ...............................182
Toe touch ...................................53
Twist and shout .........................94
Up, down, and out ....................35
Upper back lat stretch ..............127
Upper body chair stretch..........156
Wall hamstring stretches .........233
Wall sit and hold ......................119

**EXTRA, EXTRA**
Buttocks and outer hip ...........242
    stretch
In bed inner thigh stretch........234
Sit and stretch............................90

**INTERNAL WORKOUT**.........166-167
Kegel pelvic floor ...................167
    strengtheners

**MORE FROM CHORES**.............62-63
Push-and-pull chores ...............63
Reaching outward chores .........62
Reaching upward chores ...........62
Shoveling chores .......................63
Standing chores .........................62

**SIT AND BE FIT**
Arm circles...............................182
Assisted chair stand..................143
Balance Ball reverse curl..........181
Bear hug....................................114
Biceps curl..................................58
Buttocks bounce and squeeze ...46
C is for crunch............................33
Car care ......................................51
Chair pull and push...................127
Chair slump leg extension........222
Chest stretch .............................119
Countertop row.........................156
Crossed legs with a long ..........221
    reach
Do the monkey ...........................74
Foot and ankle stretch..............194
Forearm rotation........................52

Forward flexion ........................237
Front leg raise ...........................155
Front of shoulder raise .............214
Full spine roll-up .....................150
Hamstring stretch.......................67
Hand squeeze and release .......113
Hips-stacked thigh stretch .......169
Inner thigh tightener ...............207
Isometric biceps curl .................88
Knee to shoulder ......................200
Lower back pillow stretch.........170
Lower back stretch .....................81
Leaning-over triceps ................120
    extension
Neck strengthener ......................87
Neck warm-up and stretch .......101
One leg at a time .......................144
Overhead extension....................57
Palm push ..................................94
Posture fix .................................128
Posture in line.............................73
Posture pull and stretch.............39
Pulsing raise .............................149
Reach for the stars....................107
Resistance band biceps curl.....209
Resistance band rotator............216
    cuff strengthener
Roll away fatigue .......................68
Say good-bye to .......................187
    painful wrists
Seated hamstring stretch .........137
Seated pull-over stretch ...........239
Seated round over ....................161
Seated torso stretch .................193
Shoulder shrugs .........................34
Shoulder shrugs and rolls ........162
Side stretches.............................82
Stand up and kick it .................232
Stress releasing neck ................138
    stretches
Tummy toner .............................199
Thumbs up..................................40
Toe taps.....................................108
Upper body stretches ...............231
Upper thigh and knee ..............188
    conditioner combo
Waist whittler ...........................102
Wrist workout ............................93

**STRETCH, RELAX, AND SLEEP**....12-13
Chest/posture stretch.................12
Lower spine stretch ...................13
Neck and upper spine stretch....12

**TAKE 10**
Armchair dip.............................201
    Triceps stretch ......................201
Armchair lifts.............................83
Away from the wall .................143
    torso stretch
Back pressure relief .................189
Balance Ball wall squat ...........163
Balance practice.........................73
Ballet bend .................................38
Bicep and wrist stretch ...........221
Body balance ............................181
Buttocks firmer ........................137
Buttocks lift ...............................80
Buttocks lift ..............................129
Chest and shoulder stretch .......59
Contract and relax back ..........157
    stretch

Cross-triceps extension .............69
Doorway chest stretch...............45
Exaggerated stair climb............236
Eyes wide open..........................66
Family fun time ........................223
Foot massage .............................53
Hand and foot massage ..........151
    Hand massage ......................151
    Foot massage.......................152
Hip and back balancer .............121
Hip flexor stretch......................231
Hip toner break.........................57
Inner thigh stretch ...................139
Just walk away .........................36
Knee lifts ....................................41
Mini-vacation deep breathing.109
Neck and chest stretch .............210
Neck massage .............................93
Neck release and dorsal glide ..233
No pain in the neck .................214
One-arm fly ..............................119
One-leg stand ...........................241
Pelvic chair lifts .......................155
Pull-overs .................................217
Reach for it...with a ................145
    side stretch
    Overhead arm punches .......145
    Side stretch ..........................145
Reach for the floor....................113
Reverse stationary lunge ..........106
Rib cage circles .........................195
Rotator cuff stretch....................89
Seated biceps reverse curl.........149
Seated hamstring stretch ..........103
Shoulder rotation......................75
Sink push-up .............................87
Sit and hold ...............................33
Slouch stopper.........................187
Standing hamstring stretch .....115
Standing hamstring stretch .....193
    (backs of thighs)
Standing stretch.........................47
Standing pelvic tilts.................171
Tips for the computer-.............207
    bound worker
Toe point and flex ....................183
Twist and stretch ......................51
Wall squat ................................169
Walk and stretch.......................127
Walking improver ....................161
Wrist and forearm stretch .......95

**WAKE UP WORKOUT** ...................7-8
#1 ................................................7
#2 ................................................7
#3 ................................................8
#4 ................................................8
#5 ................................................8
#6 ................................................8
#7 ................................................8